USMLE STEP 1 SECRETS

USMLE STEP 1 SECRETS

Thomas Brown
West Virginia University School of Medicine
Morgantown, West Virginia

Dave Brown
Arizona College of Osteopathic Medicine of Midwestern University
Glendale, Arizona

HANLEY & BELFUS, INC.
An Affiliate of Elsevier

HANLEY & BELFUS
An Affiliate of Elsevier

The Curtis Center
Independence Square West
Philadelphia, Pennsylvania 19106

Note *to the reader*: Although the techniques, ideas, and information in this book have been carefully reviewed for correctness, the authors, editor, and publisher cannot accept any legal responsibility for any errors or omissions that may be made. Neither the publisher nor the editor makes any guarantee, expressed or implied, with respect to the material contained herein.

Library of Congress Control Number: 2003110772

USMLE STEP 1 SECRETS   ISBN 1-56053-570-9

© 2004 by Hanley & Belfus, Inc. All rights reserved. No part of this book may be reproduced, reused, republished, or transmitted in any form, or stored in a database or retrieval system, without written permission of the publisher.

Printed in the United State

CONTENTS

v

CONTRIBUTORS

Dave Brown
Fourth-year medical student, Arizona College of Osteopathic Medicine of Midwestern University, Glendale, Arizona

Thomas Andrew Brown
Fourth-year medical student, West Virginia University School of Medicine, Morgantown, West Virginia

Bahair H. Ghazi
Fourth-year medical student, West Virginia University School of Medicine, Morgantown, West Virginia

Benjamin R. Lafferty
Fourth-year medical student, West Virginia University School of Medicine, Morgantown, West Virginia

Robin R. Parmley, Ph.D.
Assistant Professor, Department of Microbiology, Midwestern University, Glendale, Arizona

Y. Gloria Yueh, Ph.D.
Associate Professor, Department of Basic Science, Midwestern University, Glendale, Arizona

PREFACE

Step 1 of the USMLE now focuses predominantly on an *understanding* of basic science *concepts*. It does so primarily in a clinical vignette format, in which you are expected to understand and apply basic science concepts in a clinical context. The thought occurred to us to develop a review book that provides ample opportunity to do just that with high-yield test material. We believe that this approach will be a refreshing change from the numerous review books that contain endless series of laundry lists. Consequently, we developed a systems-based chapter organization, in which you can test your skills at diagnosis of frequently tested diseases of a given system and also answer predominantly conceptual questions that review the relevant anatomy, biochemistry, pathology, physiology, and pharmacology of the diseases. We used the questions in each case to provide a more integrated understanding by covering the various aspects of a given disease in one setting so that it is easier to see how everything connects.

The nature of the highly popular *Secrets Series*® lends itself perfectly to this style of review. Its question-and-brief answer format facilitates understanding and retention.

Inasmuch as the traditional heavy hitters on Step 1 have been pathology, physiology, and pharmacology, we have attempted to reflect that same emphasis in the cases. We have also included separate chapters on neuroscience, microbiology, immunology, and genetics/biochemistry, again covering high-yield material in a conceptual and case-based format.

In each chapter we lay the groundwork with high-yield basic concepts pertaining to a specific system. These concepts are important to review before digging into the cases. Doing so helps to create a mindset for reading about the diseases of that system and also facilitates an understanding of the various aspects of the diseases.

On several occasions, to create a clearer overall picture of heavily tested diseases, we have included some information that is not typically found in first- and second-year medical textbooks; it is usually found instead in clinical subspecialty texts. We have done so only when it appeared that a slight amount of additional information may make a topic substantially more comprehensible and therefore easier to master and remember. Along a similar vein, we have simplified some explanations for the sake of clarity and comprehensibility, doing so only if we anticipated that the simplification would enhance performance on the boards without compromising clinical competency. Finally, a select few of the explanations taken from the textbooks are considered "current theory"—not established concepts.

We have a few suggestions for getting the most out of the book. The first is to attempt to answer the questions yourself before reading the answers. You gain a much greater understanding if you think about the subject first than if you simply read the answer right away and say, "That makes sense." Also, once you have read and understood the questions and answers in the cases, reading back through the case vignette and understanding (immediately) why various manifestations are seen helps consolidate your knowledge; it is also highly satisfying.

We have also attempted to entertain in various places. Hopefully our sense of humor at least does not offend anyone and may make studying for boards a little more enjoyable. We had fun writing this book. We hope that you'll have fun reading it.

Dave Brown
Thomas Brown

ACKNOWLEDGMENTS

A project as enormous in scope as this necessarily depends on the expertise of a diverse group of people. We owe particular gratitude to Dr. Gloria Yueh, who was instrumental in helping us develop the style, nature, and consistency of the book from its early stages. Dr. Yueh also reviewed the biochemical, metabolic/endocrinologic, and genetic concepts throughout the book as well as wrote the chapter about genetic and metabolic diseases. We also express significant thanks to Anne Marie Chomat, the student reviewer at Hanley & Belfus, who scored in the 99th percentile on both Steps 1 and 2 of the USMLE, for her enthusiasm throughout the project and her helpful suggestions and comments on what constitutes high-yield material. Similarly, we thank Dr. Robin Parmley for joining us and writing the immunology chapter on short notice. We also acknowledge the other reviewers, especially Jame Abraham, MD (hematology-oncology) and Chris Martin, MD (epidemiology-biostatistics), as well as the physicians who reviewed individual chapters in their specialty area, either anonymously or as direct favors to the authors. Two student reviewers, Bahair Ghazi (MSIV) and Benjamin Lafferty (MSIV), deserve special recognition for their additional input as contributing authors for the infectious diseases and behavioral sciences chapters, respectively. Finally, we have to thank the demanding Stan Ward, our editor at Hanley & Belfus, for his incessant pressuring to get this project completed on time.

1. GASTROINTESTINAL SYSTEM

Dave Brown and Thomas Brown

BASIC CONCEPTS

1. What is the <u>major stimulus for gastrin secretion</u>? What are the physiologic actions of gastrin in the stomach?

<u>Protein</u> in the stomach is the primary stimulus for the secretion of gastrin by G cells. The secreted gastrin stimulates the secretion of hydrochloric acid and intrinsic factor by the gastric parietal cells and stimulates secretion of pepsinogen by the chief cells. Note that all of these secretions are important in protein/meat digestion, since the acidic environment helps hydrolyze proteins and also creates an optimal pH in which pepsin works (pH of about 2). Additionally, the secreted intrinsic factor binds and protects the vitamin B12 that is present in meat. A major inhibitor of gastrin secretion is decreased gastric pH, which is essentially a negative feedback mechanism to keep the stomach from becoming too acidic.

2. List the main pancreatic enzymes and their functions.

Pancreatic enzymes are involved in digestion (degradation) of food macromolecules. **Amylase** degrades starch/complex carbohydrate; **trypsin** and **chymotrypsin** degrade proteins; and **lipase** hydrolyzes triglycerides. **DNase** and **RNase** enzymes are also present in pancreatic secretions. In addition, the pancreas secretes **bicarbonate**, which neutralizes acidic chyme entering the duodenum and creates the pH necessary for pancreatic enzymes to work.

Note: The pancreatic acinar cells are rich in secretory granules full of enzymes, and the pancreatic ductal cells are principally responsible for bicarbonate and fluid secretion.

3. What are the primary hormonal stimuli for the pancreatic exocrine secretions? How do these secretions differ in content?

Cholecystokinin (CCK) primarily stimulates the secretion of enzymes (e.g., proteases such as trypsinogen) from the pancreatic acinar cells, whereas secretin primarily stimulates the secretion of a bicarbonate-rich fluid from pancreatic ductal cells.

4. What are the primary stimuli for the secretion of CCK and secretin? Where are these hormones secreted?

Cholecystokinin is secreted primarily in response to fatty acids entering the duodenum, whereas secretin is released primarily in response to acidification of the duodenum. Both are secreted from the duodenum.

5. What other digestive processes does CCK stimulate?

CCK also stimulates contraction of the gallbladder and relaxation of the sphincter of Oddi (where the common bile duct enters the duodenum). Together these actions release bile into the duodenum. By stimulating pancreatic secretion of lipolytic enzymes as well as the delivery of bile to the small intestine, CCK creates the appropriate milieu for the digestion of fats.

Note: CCK also delays gastric emptying. This explains why the sensation of fullness lasts longer after a fatty meal.

6. What is the function of the bile salts? How are they formed?

The bile salts solubilize fats in meals, creating a bigger surface area on which pancreatic lipase can work. They also form micelles that facilitate the delivery of fatty acids to the intestinal

1

enterocytes for absorption. Bile salts are formed from the degradation of cholesterol in the liver. Of interest, this is the body's primary method for eliminating cholesterol.

7. What is the enterohepatic circulation? Why is it important in the digestion of fats?

When substances are secreted by the liver into the intestinal tract, then reabsorbed by the intestine and returned to the liver, this pathway is known as enterohepatic recirculation. The majority of the bile salts delivered to the intestine during digestion are from intestinal reabsorption of secreted bile salts. Diseases that decrease bile salt reabsorption impair the enterohepatic circulation and cause fewer bile salts to be secreted by the liver; thus, fat digestion is impaired.

8. What is the chemical difference between conjugated and unconjugated bilirubin? How are these substances formed?

Bilirubin is a breakdown product of the heme moiety found in red blood cells, bone marrow, liver, and mitochondrial cytochrome enzymes. **Unconjugated** bilirubin is the breakdown product formed in the peripheral tissues, whereas **conjugated** bilirubin is formed in the liver by conjugating glucuronic acid to bilirubin to make it more water-soluble.

Note: Jaundice is a yellowish discoloration of the skin and sclera due to elevated levels of either conjugated (direct) or unconjugated (indirect) bilirubin.

9. Why is unconjugated bilirubin not normally excreted in the urine?

Unconjugated bilirubin is hydrophobic and circulates bound to albumin. Albumin, a negatively charged protein, cannot cross the glomerular basement membrane because the glycosaminoglycans that form this membrane are negatively charged and repel the albumin.

10. What defines the foregut, midgut, and hindgut anatomically? Which main arteries provide the blood supply to each segment?

The **foregut** comprises the upper GI tract down to a site just distal to the ampulla of Vater (where the common bile duct empties into the second part of the duodenum). Its main vascular supply comes from the celiac artery. The **midgut** extends from the second part of the duodenum down to the splenic flexure of the colon and is served by the superior mesenteric artery. The **hindgut** extends from the splenic flexure of the colon to the anus and is supplied by the inferior mesenteric artery.

Note: The pancreas and liver are embryologic outgrowths of the foregut and share its vascular supply (i.e., celiac artery).

11. Which veins feed into the portal vein?

All the veins of the foregut, midgut, and hindgut, which includes the gastric veins, splenic vein, and superior and inferior mesenteric veins. Consequently, portal hypertension can have manifestations in any and all of these vascular beds (e.g., congestive splenomegaly from splenic vein hypertension, esophageal varices from gastric vein hypertension).

12. What are the anatomic layers of the gut wall?

From the lumen outward, the layers of the gastrointestinal tract are as follows:
1. **Mucosa**, composed of the mucosal epithelium, lamina propria, and muscularis mucosae
2. **Submucosa**, which contains the submucosal (Meissner's) nerve plexus
3. **Muscularis propria**, composed of an inner circular smooth muscle layer, myenteric plexus, and outer longitudinal smooth muscle layer
4. **Serosa** (adventitia), which is the fibrous outer covering

Note: The teniae coli are band-like muscles comprising the outer longitudinal smooth muscle layer of the large intestine, except in the appendix and rectum.

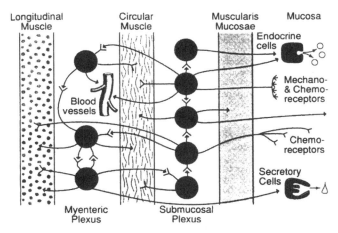

Layers of the gut wall. (From Johnson LR: Gastorintestinal Physiology, 4th ed. St. Louis, Mosby, 1991, with permission.)

CASE 1

A 52-year-old obese man complains of a long history of chest discomfort after heavy meals. He describes this discomfort as a substernal burning sensation that radiates to his neck and is often exacerbated by lying down. He also complains of difficulty with swallowing solid foods. When questioned, he recalls that exams done years ago showed some type of diaphragmatic disorder, but he does not know whether it is related to his current condition. A cardiac stress test is negative, and a 1-week therapeutic trial with omeprazole causes substantial relief of pain.

1. What is the likely diagnosis?
Gastroesophageal reflux disease (GERD), also called reflux esophagitis.

2. Discuss the pathophysiology of GERD.
GERD is caused by the reflux of acidic and/or bilious gastric contents into the esophagus, which irritate the esophageal mucosa and causes pain. Many factors can predispose to reflux. One of the most important factors is abnormal transient relaxation of the lower esophageal sphincter (LES) unrelated to swallowing. An atonic (continually relaxed) LES also allows reflux. Increased intra-abdominal pressure (e.g., obesity, pregnancy, Valsalva maneuver) may also cause reflux of gastric contents into the esophagus.

3. With what diaphragmatic disorder was the patient probably diagnosed?
Sliding hiatal hernia.

4. Explain why a rolling (paraesophageal) hiatal hernia is not likely to cause GERD, whereas a sliding hiatal hernia often does.
In a **sliding** hiatal hernia, the esophagogastric junction herniates upward through the esophageal hiatus in the diaphragm. The additional sphincteric pressure that is provided by the diaphragm is then lost and allows reflux of gastric contents to occur more easily. In contrast, in a **rolling** hiatal hernia, a portion of the gastric fundus "rolls into" and herniates through the diaphragm, but the esophagogastric junction remains in place. Although rolling hiatal hernias usually do not cause reflux, they are more serious because they can become incarcerated and ischemic.

5. What complication of GERD is most likely to lead to the following conditions?
Gastrointestinal bleeding: esophageal ulceration.
Esophageal adenocarcinoma: Barrett's esophagus, which is columnar metaplasia of strati-fied squamous esophageal epithelium.
Difficulty with swallowing: esophageal stricture.

6. Why would a patient with Sjögren's syndrome be more susceptible to esophageal pathology in GERD?

Sjögren's syndrome is an autoimmune disease due to lymphocytic infiltrations of the lacrimal and salivary glands, causing dry eyes and dry mouth due to deficient secretions. Because saliva is rich in bicarbonate, it functions to neutralize acid in the esophagus. The absence of this protective function predisposes patients with this condition to esophageal damage with even min-imal gastroesophageal reflux.

7. Cover the left-hand column and attempt to list the class of drug, mechanism of action, and primary side effect of the drugs used in the treatment of GERD.

DRUG	CLASS	MECHANISM OF ACTION	PRIMARY SIDE EFFECT
Cisapride	GI stimulant	Prokinetic drug; stimulates release of acetylcholine from myenteric plexus (increases gastric emptying and LES tone)	Cardiac arrhythmias
Cimetidine Ranitidine Nizatidine Famotidine	H_2 receptor antagonists	Inhibits histamine-stimulated release of hydrochloric acid by blocking H_2 receptors on parietal cells	Cimetidine inhibits hepatic cytochrome P450 enzymes.
Metoclopramide	Antiemetic/GI stimulant	Prokinetic drug (increases gastric emptying and LES tone) via cholinergic side effects	Parkinsonian symptoms
Omeprazole Lansoprazole Rabeprazole	Proton pump inhibitors	Irreversibly inhibits the parietal cell H^+-K^+-ATPase pump	Hypergastrinemia

H^+-K^+-ATPase = hydrogen-potassium-adenosine triphosphatase.

8. Which of the above drugs are contraindicated when bowel obstruction is suspected? Why?

Prokinetic drugs (cisapride, metoclopramide) should be avoided whenever bowel obstruction is suspected, because they can exacerbate the obstruction and potentially cause perforation.

9. Why may omeprazole cause hypergastrinemia?

Proton pump inhibitors such as omeprazole inhibit gastric secretion of hydrochloric acid by irreversibly inhibiting the H^+-K^+-ATPase pump on gastric parietal cells. This process raises gas-tric pH, but since it is low gastric pH that inhibits gastrin production by G cells, gastrin produc-tion continues uninhibited.

CASE 2

A 50-year-old woman complains of recent difficulty with swallowing (dysphagia) solids and liquids, chest pain with eating, a cough at night, and an unintentional loss of 15 pounds over the past 2 months. A few weeks ago she suffered from a bout of pneumonia. A barium swal-low reveals a dilated esophagus (megaesophagus) with a "bird's beak" narrowing at the lower esophageal sphincter (LES). Esophageal manometry shows an increased LES pressure with incomplete LES relaxation and a complete absence of peristalsis in the lower esophagus.

1. What is the diagnosis?
Achalasia.

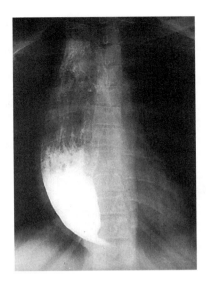

Radiographic appearance of achalasia. (From Katz DS, Math KR, Groskin SA (eds): Radiology Secrets. Philadelphia, Hanley & Belfus, 1998, p 93, with permission.)

2. Is the LES normally tonically constricted or tonically relaxed?
The LES is normally tonically constricted, generating an intraluminal pressure of approximately 30 mmHg. This pressure prevents reflux of gastric contents into the esophagus. During the esophageal phase of swallowing, the LES relaxes in response to a food bolus descending through the esophagus, a phenomenon called *receptive relaxation.*

3. What is the major histopathologic finding in the esophagus of patients with achalasia?
Destruction of the myenteric plexus.

4. How does this finding help explain the dilated esophagus and constricted esophageal sphincter?
The myenteric plexus mediates receptive relaxation of the LES in response to a food bolus coming down the esophagus. The myenteric plexus also mediates esophageal peristalsis (hence the aperistalsis). The failure of the LES to relax, together with the failure of the distal esophagus to undergo peristalsis, allows food to accumulate and dilate the lower esophagus, creating the bird's beak appearance.
Note: The myenteric plexus is located between the inner circular and outer longitudinal smooth muscle layers (muscularis propria) of the esophagus.

5. Describe the pathologic mechanism of achalasia in Chagas disease. What organism is the primary culprit?
Achalasia in Chagas disease is also due to destruction of the myenteric (Auerbach's) plexus in the esophagus. This disease is caused by the protozoan parasite *Trypanosoma cruzi.* In Chagas disease the myenteric plexus of the colon may also be destroyed, causing toxic megacolon.

6. What was the likely cause of this patient's previous episode of pneumonia?
Aspiration of esophageal contents, especially during sleep, due to the presence of undigested material in the esophagus.

7. Injection of botulinum toxin into the LES is a treatment option for this patient. What is the drug's mechanism of action in this context?
Much of the tonic constriction of the LES is due to vagal cholinergic innervation. Because botulinum toxin exerts its effects by inhibiting the release of acetylcholine from nerve endings, it reduces this input to LES tone.

CASE 3

A 33-year-old man complains of a burning epigastric pain that develops 1–3 hours after meals. The pain is particularly bothersome at night and often awakens him around 2:00 or 3:00 AM in the morning. For several months he has been taking antacids, which give some degree of relief from the pain. A barium swallow of the upper GI tract reveals a well-demarcated crater in the proximal duodenum, and a urea breath test is positive. His physician prescribes triple antibiotic therapy for 14 days and cimetidine for 6 weeks.

1. **What is the most likely diagnosis?**
Peptic ulcer disease of the proximal duodenum.
Note: Acute gastritis secondary to head trauma is called Cushing's ulcer, whereas acute gastritis with severe burns may be called Curling's ulcer.

2. **Describe the classic difference in timing of pain with gastric and duodenal ulcers.**
Gastric ulcers generally become painful during or immediaely after eating, whereas duodenal ulcers become painful a few hours after a meal. Gastric ulcers typically hurt when the stomach is most active (i.e., with meals), whereas duodenal ulcers hurt when the duodenum is most active (i.e., 1–3 hours after a meal). There can be significant variation among different patients, however.

3. **If this patient's ulcer caused bleeding, would he more likely present with melena or hematochezia?**
He would more likely present with melena, which is a dark, tarry stool typically caused by an upper GI bleed. Hematochezia is bright red blood per rectum that generally occurs in lower GI bleeds but may also occur in massive upper GI bleeds.

4. **What is gastric heterotopia? How can it cause peptic ulcer disease?**
The term *heterotopia* refers to the presence of normal tissue in an abnormal location. In gastric heterotopia, gastric mucosa located in the duodenum or even at more distal sites of the small intestine (e.g., Meckel's diverticulum) can lead to peptic ulcer disease by the inappropriate secretion of acid.
Note: When peptic ulcers are refractory to aggressive therapy, when multiple ulcers are present, or when ulcers are located in abnormal positions such as the jejunum, Zollinger-Ellison syndrome (due to a gastrin-secreting tumor, or gastrinoma) should be suspected. The increased gastrin secretion by these tumors causes excessive secretion of acid by the parietal cells.

5. **Why was this patient given triple antibiotic therapy?**
Helicobacter pylori and nonsteroidal anti-inflammatory drugs (NSAIDs) are the two predominant causes of peptic ulcers, both duodenal and gastric. This patient is not taking NSAIDs but does have a positive urea breath test, which is indicative of an *H. pylori* infection that needs to be eradicated. The principal benefits of eradicating *H. pylori* with triple antibiotic therapy are substantial reductions in rate of ulcer recurrence and risk of developing gastric adenocarcinoma.
Note: H. pylori produces the enzyme urease, which breaks down urea to liberate ammonia and carbon dioxide (CO_2). Consequently, *H. pylori* can be detected by having a patient ingest ^{13}C- or ^{14}C-labeled urea and then determining whether the patient's breath contains radiolabeled CO_2. Interestingly, the liberation of ammonia by *H. pylori* neutralizes gastric acid and facilitates the organim's survival in the stomach. Infection can also be detected by serum antibodies to *H. pylori*, but this test does not discriminate between current and previous infection.

6. **After a while on his treatment plan, the patient developed gynecomastia. What is the most likely cause?**
He was taking cimetidine. One of its distinctive side effects is gynecomastia.

Note: Cimetidine is the only H_2 antagonist that inhibits one of the hepatic cytochrome p450 enzymes. This effect can be particularly dangerous in combination with warfarin, which is metabolized through this pathway.

7. What pharmacologic treatment strategies for peptic ulcer disease are available for this patient?
- Proton pump inhibitors (omeprazole, lansoprazole, pantoprazole)
- H_2 antagonists (cimetidine, ranitidine)
- Anticholinergics (atropine)
- Mucosal protective agents (misoprostol, sucralfate)
- Antacids (calcium carbonate, magnesium hydroxide, aluminum hydroxide)

Note: Magnesium causes diarrhea, whereas aluminum causes constipation. The two compounds are often comined in antacid formulations to balance these effects.

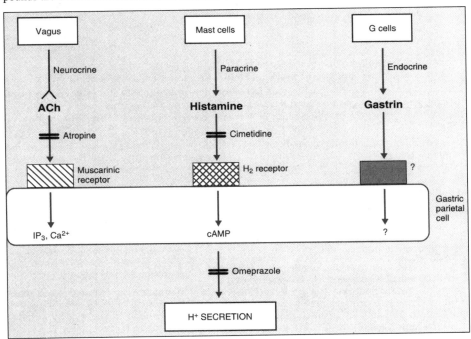

Regulation of H^+ secretion. (From Costanzo L: STARS Physiology. Philadelphia, W.B. Saunders, 1998, p 309, with permission.)

8. For gastric ulcers refractory to medical treatment, partial gastrectomy is an option. Why is the vagus nerve to the stomach often selectively severed during this procedure?

Selective vagotomy eliminates the cholinergic input to the parietal cells, which reduces parietal cell acid secretion.

9. How are NSAIDs thought to predispose to the formation of gastric ulcers?

NSAIDs inhibit the production of prostaglandins in the gastric mucosa. These prostaglandins normally function to protect the gastric mucosa by increasing mucus and bicarbonate secretion and by stimulating local vasodilation, which maintains a steady energy supply to the gastric mucosa and prevents ischemic injury.

10. Why may misoprostol be beneficial when given in combination with NSAIDS?

Misoprostol is a prostaglandin E_1 analogue, and its presence in the gastric mucosa negates some of the deleterious effects of NSAIDs.

Note: Because misoprostol is a prostaglandin that can induce smooth muscle contraction (e.g., of the uterus), it should be avoided in pregnant women.

11. If the patient desires to take a cyclooxygenase (COX) inhibitor for an arthritic condition, which class of COX inhibitor (NSAIDs or COX-2 inhibitors) is preferable? Explain.

The COX-2 inhibitors are preferred because COX exists as two primary forms in the body: a constitutive form (COX-1) and an inducible form (COX-2). COX-1 is present in multiple tissues, and in the stomach it is responsible for the production of protective prostaglandins. The inducible form, COX-2, is present primarily in inflammatory cells (e.g., neutrophils), and is responsible for the production of proinflammatory substances. COX-2 inhibitors such as **celecoxib** (Celebrex) and **rofecoxib** (Vioxx) have minimal inhibitory effects on COX-1 but are potent inhibitors of COX-2, thereby causing fewer gastrointestinal side effects.

CASE 4

A 40-year-old man complains of worsening anorexia and a weight loss of 20 lb over the past 2 months. He indicates that he has pain in his upper stomach that is exacerbated every time he eats, and he is often nauseated. He admits to drinking a 12-pack of beer every day for the past 3 months. On physical exam he has epigastric tenderness. A barium swallow reveals no apparent ulcerations of the gastric or duodenal mucosa. An endoscopy is performed, and tissue biopsy reveals inflammation of the gastric mucosa. There are no duodenal lesions.

1. What is the likely diagnosis, based on endoscopy?

Acute gastritis.

2. What are the two primary classifications of *acute* gastritis?

Acute gastritis can be classified as infectious and noninfectious types. Infectious acute gastritis is typically caused by *H. pylori*, whereas noninfectious acute gastritis is generally caused by exposure to toxins and drugs (e.g., ethanol, NSAIDs) or severe physical stress (e.g., head trauma, burns, surgery). The severe physical stress may cause ulcers because stress increases cortisol production, and cortisol inhibits prostaglandin synthesis (in addition to various other effects). In addition, gastric ischemia may develop because of mesenteric vasoconstriction during severe physical stress.

3. What are the two primary classifications of chronic gastritis?

Chronic gastritis is also subdivided into two types: type A (noninfectious) and type B (infectious). Type A chronic gastritis is caused by autoimmune destruction of parietal cells in the fundus and body of the stomach. Type A gastritis causes pernicious anemia and is also called fundal gastritis and/or autoimmune gastritis. Type B chronic gastritis is associated with *H. pylori* colonization of the gastric antrum. (See figure, top of next page.)

Note: Type B chronic gastritis is more common than type A, accounting for approximately 80% of cases of chronic gastritis.

4. Why may G-cell hyperplasia develop in type A chronic gastritis?

Reduced acid secretion (due to destruction of parietal cells) in type A chronic gastritis reduces the negative feedback on gastrin-producing cells, causing both G-cell hyperplasia and elevated levels of gastrin. This process is similar to the mechanism by which long-term use of proton pump inhibitors causes hypergastrinemia.

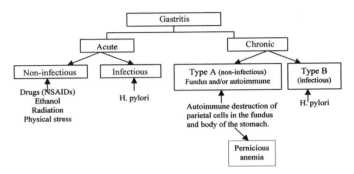

Acute vs. chronic gastritis. (Courtesy of Gloria Yueh, Ph.D., Midwestern University.)

5. How does destruction of the parietal cells in type A (autoimmune) chronic gastritis result in pernicious anemia?

The parietal cells produce intrinsic factor, which is needed for proper absorption of B12 in the small intestine. Vitamin B12, in turn, is required for DNA synthesis in rapidly proliferating erythrocyte progenitor cells. A deficiency of vitamin B12, therefore, may result in a macrocytic anemia.

6. Why are patients with type A chronic gastritis predisposed to gastric and enteric infections?

Destruction of the parietal cells can cause achlorhydria (absence of hydrochloric acid), which increases gastric pH and makes it more "friendly" to infecting bacteria, particularly *Salmonella* spp.

CASE 5

A 38-year-old alcoholic presents to the emergency department with severe epigastric abdominal pain that radiates to his back. He also complains of nausea and vomiting. Physical exam reveals fever (101° F), tachycardia, blood pressure of 98/60 mmHg, epigastric tenderness, and absent bowel sounds. Lab tests reveal significantly elevated serum amylase and lipase, hypocalcemia, and leukocytosis.

1. What is the diagnosis?

Acute pancreatitis.

2. What are the most common causes of acute pancreatitis?

Alcohol abuse and gallstones are the most common causes. Other less common but well-established causes of pancreatitis include hypertriglyceridemia and hypercalcemia.

3. How can gallstones cause pancreatitis?

Gallstones can pass into the lower common bile duct and obstruct the egress of bile into the intestine. The bile can then back up into the pancreatic duct, irritating and inflaming the pancreatic tissue. In addition, because the pancreatic duct cannot empty, pancreatic secretions may build up and contribute to the inflammatory process.

Note: Patients with cystic fibrosis often develop chronic pancreatitis because thick pancreatic secretions can block the pancreatic duct.

4. What is fat necrosis? How does pancreatitis cause its development?

Fat necrosis is simply focal areas of fat destruction, not a specific pattern of necrosis such as coagulative or liquefactive necrosis. Fat necrosis develops in pancreatitis because pancreatic lipases that are released liquefy fat cell membranes and destroy the cells.

5. How can chronic pancreatitis lead to persistent diarrhea?

Chronic pancreatitis can lead to deficiency of various pancreatic digestive enzymes, which leads to profound malabsorption of many nutrients. These would-be nutrients are subsequently catabolized/fermented by bacterial flora in the large intestine. The final products of this catabolism are typically osmotically active and draw water into the lumen of the intestine, leading to an osmotic diarrhea.

6. Why might insulin-dependent diabetes develop in patients with chronic pancreatitis?

The chronic inflammation can eventually destroy the beta cells of the islets of Langerhans.

CASE 6

A 2-week-old boy is brought to the emergency department with nonbilious projectile vomiting that began earlier in the day. Physical exam reveals a firm, palpable abdominal mass in the epigastric region, and ultrasound reveals a thickened and elongated pylorus muscle. The parents are assured that the condition is easily treated by surgery, although the boy may have to be fed small meals after surgery to avoid symptoms associated with dumping syndrome.

1. What is the diagnosis?

Congenital hypertrophic pyloric stenosis.

2. What condition may predispose to hypertrophic pyloric stenosis in adults?

Peptic ulcer disease, when the ulcer is located in close juxtaposition to the pylorus.

3. What acid-base and electrolyte disorder can be caused by prolonged vomiting? How does it develop?

Hypochloremic metabolic alkalosis may be caused by prolonged vomiting. Because gastric parietal cells secrete hydrochloric acid into the lumen of the stomach, prolonged vomiting can

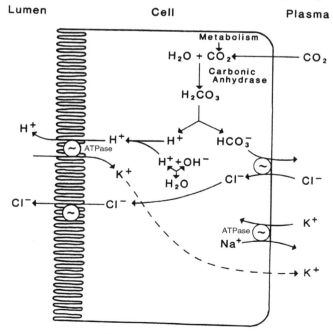

Intracellular mechanism of gastric acid secretion. (From Granger, Barryman, Kvietys: Clinical Gastrointestinal Physiology. Philadelphia, W.B. Saunders, 1985, p 75, with permission.)

deplete the body of both hydrogen and chloride ions. The alkalosis that develops is caused by the loss of hydrochloric acid and the simultaneous retention of the bicarbonate that is generated when the parietal cells make hydrochloric acid.

4. Why might an improperly functioning pyloric sphincter after surgery cause dumping syndrome?

Dumping syndrome is caused by the delivery of excessive amounts of hyperosmotic chyme from the stomach to the small intestine. This condition may occur with a dysfunctional pyloric sphincter. The intestine is unable to "process" such a large quantity of chyme, resulting in an osmotic diarrhea, which may cause dizziness, weakness, and tachycardia after meals.

5. Which congenital pancreatic disease causes projectile vomiting in the first few days of life?

Annular pancreas, which is caused by abnormal rotation of the ventral pancreatic bud around the second part of the duodenum during embryologic development. The result is fusion of the ventral and dorsal pancreatic buds, which can cause duodenal obstruction.

6. What abnormalities of intestinal development might be suspected if a baby begins coughing and becomes cyanotic immediately after his first breast-feeding?

Tracheoesophageal fistula, an abnormal communication between the esophagus and the trachea. In this condition, the breast milk can enter the trachea through the fistula, causing cough and cyanosis. Tracheoesophageal fistulas typically develop at the mid level of the esophagus because during embryologic development the lungs bud from the foregut at this point.

Note: Esophageal atresia, in which the esophagus ends in a blind pouch, is another disorder of embryologic esophageal development. In this condition, food may accumulate in the esophagus and then reflux into the airway, also causing coughing and cyanosis.

7. When may duodenal atresia cause bilious vomiting?

When the atresia is at a location distal to the point where the common bile duct enters the second part of the duodenum.

8. What congenital gastrointestinal disorder presents with constipation and a massively dilated colon? What is the cause?

Hirschsprung's disease, also known as congenital megacolon or aganglionic megacolon. In Hirschsprung's disease the neural crest cells that form the myenteric plexus fail to migrate to the colon.

9. Another cause of bowel obstruction is ileocecal intussusception. What does the term *intussusception* imply?

Intussusception occurs when a proximal section of intestine invaginates into a section of bowel immediately distal. This condition occurs most commonly in infants at the ileocecal valve. An ileoileal intussusception can also occur as a complication of Meckel's diverticulum. Infarction and perforation of the intussuscepted bowel can occur as a result of poor blood supply. Therefore, surgery is usually required immediately.

CASE 7

A 33-year-old woman complains of a long history of diarrhea, flatus, and abdominal pain. More recently she has experienced weight loss and weakness. A complete blood count and peripheral blood smear reveal a macrocytic anemia with hypersegmented neutrophils. A pathology report from a small intestinal biopsy describes an intestinal mucosa significant for "villous atrophy, lymphocytic infiltration of the lamina propria, and hyperplastic crypts." The woman is told that she has a malabsorption syndrome and is put on a special diet devoid of wheat, barley, and rice. Weeks later, a repeat biopsy shows complete resolution of mucosal damage to the small intestines. The patient is encouraged to stay on her diet.

1. What is the diagnosis?

Celiac disease (also called celiac sprue or nontropical sprue). The diagnosis is established by resolution of mucosal damage after a gluten-free diet.

2. What causes celiac disease?

Hypersensitivity to the gliadin in gluten, which is present in wheat, barley, and rice.

3. How does celiac disease differ from tropical sprue?

Both diseases have the same symptoms and intestinal biopsy findings, but tropical sprue does not respond to a gluten-free diet. In addition, tropical sprue is most commonly found, of all places, in the tropics. Although an infectious organism is suspected, the precise etiology of tropical sprue remains unknown.

4. How do signs, symptoms, and intestinal biopsy findings differ in Whipple's disease and celiac disease?

The signs and symptoms are fairly similar, but intestinal biopsy shows lipid vacuolation with infiltration of periodic acid-Schiff (PAS)-positive macrophages with small bacilli in Whipple's disease. *Note:* Whipple's disease is due to infection with *Torphyrema whippelii*.

5. What dermatologic condition is associated with celiac sprue?

Dermatitis herpetiformis, which manifests as pruritic erythematous papules on the extensor surfaces of the limbs. The lesions are arranged in groups, like the vesicles in herpes simplex (hence herpetiformis).

6. What most likely explains the macrocytic anemia and hypersegmented neutrophils on peripheral blood smear?

The patient has a megaloblastic anemia secondary to vitamin B12 and/or folate deficiency. The presence of hypersegmented neutrophils confirms the diagnosis of megaloblastic anemia.

7. What are the three most common physiologic causes of malabsorption? Give an example of a disease in which each process is impaired.

1. Reduced secretion of digestive enzymes (chronic pancreatitis, cystic fibrosis)
2. Insufficient production or delivery of bile to the intestine, which impairs emulsification and digestion of fats (cholestasis)
3. Reduced surface area available for absorption (celiac sprue, tropical sprue)

8. What are the two primary classifications of diarrhea?

Diarrhea can be broadly classified into two types: osmotic diarrhea and secretory diarrhea. **Osmotic** diarrhea is characterized by malabsorption (e.g., lactose intolerance), resulting in the accumulation of osmotically active substances within the lumen of the gut, which causes net transudation of water and electrolytes from the blood into the gut lumen. **Secretory** diarrhea is characterized by excess of active fluid secretion by the intestinal mucosa, as seen in diseases such as cholera.

CASE 8

A 32-year-old woman complains of a long history of abdominal pain and diarrhea. She has lost 15 pounds and has experienced several episodes of bloody diarrhea in the past few weeks. She denies any pain with bowel movements (tenesmus) but does complain of abdominal pain after meals. Physical exam is significant for mild fever as well as tenderness in the right lower quadrant of the abdomen. Lab studies show an elevated erythrocyte sedimentation rate (ESR) as well as decreased plasma levels of vitamins B12, D, and K. Lower endoscopy reveals a "cobblestone" appearance and the presence of "skip" lesions. Biopsy of the terminal ileum reveals infiltration of the lamina propria with inflammatory cells. A diagnosis of inflammatory bowel disease is made, and sulfasalazine is prescribed.

1. What is the diagnosis?

Crohn's disease.

2. Why are the findings in this patient more consistent with Crohn's disease than with ulcerative colitis?

This patient most likely has Crohn's disease due to involvement of the terminal ileum and the classic findings on endoscopy ("cobblestone" pattern and presence of "skip" lesions). Ulcerative colitis does not involve the small bowel, and involvement is continuous without skipping areas. ~~Ulcerative colitis~~, however, spares the rectum.

Crohn's disease

3. In some cases of Crohn's disease stool can be found in the urine. What mechanism explains this finding?

Crohn's disease is characterized by transmural inflammation involving all layers of the gut wall. This inflammation predisposes to fistula formation, in which an abnormal passage is created from one epithelialized surface to another. If a fistula develops between the colon and the bladder, both air (pneumaturia) and stool (fecaluria) can enter the urine. In contrast, the inflammatory process in ulcerative colitis is typically restricted to the mucosal and submucosal layers of the gut wall, explaining why fistulas are rarely seen with ulcerative colitis.

4. In what special situation does transmural inflammation of the colon occur in ulcerative colitis?

Toxic megacolon, which is a medical emergency. Surgery (usually a colectomy) is required to prevent peritonitis and sepsis.

5. How can Crohn's disease cause deficiencies of vitamins A, B12, D, E, and K?

Crohn's disease commonly involves the terminal ileum, where vitamin B12 is absorbed. The terminal ileum is also the site at which bile salts are reabsorbed, and since most of the bile salts secreted into the intestine are from enterohepatic recirculation, a deficiency of bile salt secretion develops. This deficiency can impair the absorption of fats and fat-soluble vitamins. Surgical resection of the ileum can also cause these vitamin deficiencies.

Note: The fat-soluble vitamins are A, D, E, and K.

6. What pharmacokinetic properties of sulfasalazine make it particularly well suited to treating inflammatory bowel disease? *NSAID — not really*

Sulfasalazine is a precursor for the active compound 5-aminosalicylic acid, a nonsteroidal anti-inflammatory agent that can reduce inflammation in the bowel. However, if 5-aminosalicylic acid is given orally in sufficient quantities to reduce inflammation in the large bowel, significant gastric irritation will develop. Sulfasalazine avoids this problem because it is not broken down into 5-aminosalicylic acid until it reaches the distal ileum and colon. Sulfasalazine is also poorly absorbed from the GI tract; thus, the concentration of active drug that reaches the large bowel is increased.

7. What extraintestinal complication of ulcerative colitis should be suspected in a patient who presents with signs of obstructive jaundice?

Primary sclerosing cholangitis, which is caused by fibrosis of the large bile ducts. This complication is more commonly associated with ulcerative colitis than Crohn's disease.

8. What extraintestinal complication of inflammatory bowel disease should you suspect if the patient complains of lower back pain in the morning and x-rays reveal bilateral sacroiliitis?

Ankylosing spondylitis, which is more commonly associated with ulcerative colitis than Crohn's disease and is usually seen in male patients.

9. Will a total colectomy alleviate the extraintestinal complications of inflammatory bowel disease?

Not necessarily. The extraintestinal manifestations (i.e., arthritis, sclerosing cholangitis) often persist.

CASE 9

peritoneum   *visceral*

An 11-year-old girl is brought to the emergency department because of severe abdominal pain. Several hours earlier she begins to experience pain in the periumbilical region. She now complains of pain in her lower right abdomen, nausea, and anorexia. She has positive psoas, obturator, and Rovsing's signs on exam and experiences acute pain with palpation at McBurney's point. Her temperature is 100.2°F. Lab tests show leukocytosis with a left shift and a negative pregnancy test. A computed tomography (CT) scan reveals a thickened and inflamed appendix.

1. Pain   1. Anorexia
2. Anorexia   2. Pain

1. What is the diagnosis?
Acute appendicitis.

Appy   Gastritis

2. What is the most common cause of appendicitis?
Obstruction of the lumen of the appendix, most commonly by a fecalith. Obstruction can also be caused by lymphoid hyperplasia, tumors, and/or an intestinal stricture.

3. What conditions can be mistaken for acute appendicitis?
- Infectious: *Yersinia* enterocolitis, mesenteric lymphadenitis
- Inflammatory: acute onset of Crohn's disease   *elderly*
- Congenital: Meckel's diverticulitis, diverticulitis of the ascending colon
- Gynecologic: pelvic inflammatory disease (PID), ectopic pregnancy, ruptured ovarian cyst

most common appendiceal tumor

4. What type of cancer of the appendix is occasionally seen as an incidental finding during an appendectomy? What substance do these tumors secrete?
Carcinoid tumors, which secrete large quantities of serotonin, resulting in elevated levels of 5-hydroxyindolacetic acid (5-HIAA), which can be easily detected in the urine.   *Rx: octreotide*
Note: The appendix is the most common site of gut carcinoid tumor.

5. Explain the neuroanatomic basis for the pain pattern of appendicitis, which begins around the umbilicus and migrates to the right lower quadrant (RLQ).
The initial pain from appendicitis is due to activation of visceral pain receptors in the inflamed appendix and visceral peritoneum. The sensory nerves that carry this information synapse on spinal neurons that also receive sensory signals from the anterior abdominal wall in the periumbilical area. Because the origin of the signal cannot be discerned, the brain misinterprets the visceral pain as a poorly localized pain arising from the periumbilical area (T10 dermatome). Later, when the parietal peritoneum adjacent to the appendix becomes inflamed, the pain becomes sharper and is more accurately localized to the RLQ by somatic pain fibers.

6. What is the location of McBurney's point?
One-third the distance from the anterior superior iliac spine to the umbilicus.

7. What is the principal danger if appendicitis remains untreated?
Perforation and peritonitis as well as abdominal abscess formation.

8. Of what is Meckel's diverticulum an embryologic remnant?
The vitelline duct, which connects the lumen of the developing gut to the yolk sac.

*Vitelline Duct
(gut to yolk sac)*

ischial spine = pudendal n. block

9. Describe the pathophysiology of Meckel's diverticulitis.

Most Meckel's diverticula are asymptomatic. About 50% are lined with heterotopic gastric or pancreatic tissue. The gastric mucosa can secrete acid and eventually create adjacent intestinal ulcerations that can bleed and cause pain that mimics acute appendicitis. Alternatively, the diverticulum can cause symptoms because of intussusception, incarceration, or perforation.

Note: Recall the law of the three "2s" pertaining to Meckel's diverticulum: it affects about 2% of the population, is about 2 inches long, and is located about 2 feet from the ileocecal valve.

CASE 10

∅ clotting factors (2,7,9,10)

A man known locally as drunken Duncan comes to the emergency department vomiting blood (hematemesis). Physical examination reveals jaundice, scleral icterus, spider angiomata on the face and thorax, gynecomastia, and a periumbilical caput medusae. The abdomen is distended and the spleen enlarged. The patient also has pedal and periorbital edema, and his breath has a sweet, ammoniacal odor (fetor hepaticus). When an IV line is started to give him fluids, a fairly large hematoma develops at the IV site. Lab tests reveal elevations in direct bilirubin, indirect bilirubin, and prothrombin time; an abnormally low blood urea nitrotgen (BUN) level; and a normal creatinine level. Serologic tests for hepatitis B and C and antimitochondrial antibodies are negative. Serum iron, transferrin, percent iron saturation, ferritin, and ceruloplasmin are within normal limits.

1. What is the most likely cause of the hematemesis? Describe its pathogenesis.

The patient most likely has ruptured esophageal varices. Portal hypertension secondary to alcoholic cirrhosis creates portacaval anastamoses, in which the pressure in the portal venous system diverts blood from the portal system into the systemic circulation at sites of anastomoses. In this patient, blood from the gastric veins backed up into their esophageal tributaries, which became distended and eventually ruptured. Hemorrhoids may result from a portacaval anastomosis between the superior rectal vein and inferior rectal vein, and a caput medusae can result from diversion of blood from the portal vein into the paraumbilical veins that run along the round ligament of the liver to the anterior abdominal wall.

Note: The round ligament of the liver (ligamentum teres hepatis) is an embryologic remnant of the umbilical vein. The major morphologic characteristics of cirrhosis are extensive fibrosis with nodules of regenerating hepatocytes.

(L) ; (R) umbilical v. atrophies

2. Why should a Mallory-Weiss tear be included in the differential diagnosis?

Mallory Weiss tears are seen most commonly in alcoholics and are due to excessive vomiting that causes lacerations extending through the gastroesophageal junction. It is another common cause of hematemesis in alcoholics or people with conditions causing excessive vomiting (e.g., bulimia).

3. What is the value of the hepatitis serology tests, serum iron tests, ceruloplasmin levels, and antimitochondrial antibody tests?

These tests identify different causes of liver cirrhosis. Hepatitis B and C can cause liver cirrhosis, as can hemochromatosis (too much iron), Wilson's disease (too much copper) and primary biliary cirrhosis (antimitochondrial antibodies).

Note: All of the above listed causes of liver cirrhosis increase the risk for hepatocellular carcinoma, as do alpha-1 antitrypsin deficiency and aflatoxin.

4. Assuming that the patient is not taking anticoagulants, what is the most likely reason that he developed a large hematoma at the IV site?

The liver is where most of the clotting factors are produced, and some of these factors (II, VII, IX, and X) are modified after translation. Severe liver disease impairs their production and maturation, causing a coagulopathy. Note that the prothrombin time (PT) was elevated as result.

5. Describe the pathophysiology of the patient's ascites and pedal and periorbital edema.

Severe liver disease is associated with inadequate production of serum albumin, which is the major determinant of plasma oncotic pressure. Consequently, fluid resorption from the interstitium back into the capillary beds is reduced. This reduction explains the pedal and periorbital edema. In addition to the reduced capillary oncotic pressure, the increased venous pressure in the portal system from portal hypertension causes greater intracapillary hydrostatic pressure, which opposes movement of fluid from the interstitium into the capillaries; hence the ascites.

Note: Because the splenic vein drains into the portal vein, portal hypertension can also cause congestive splenomegaly.

6. Why would you expect the ascitic fluid to be a transudate instead of an exudate?

Ascites is caused by lowered oncotic pressure (secondary to hypoalbuminemia) and portal hypertension, both of which alter hemodynamic forces but not vessel permeability, resulting in a transudate.

Note: A transudate develops when fluid moves across a membrane as a result of changes in hemodynamic forces. Because there is no alteration in the permeability of the membranes, the fluid that accumulates has a low protein content. In contrast, exudates are fluid collections that develop because of alterations in membrane/vessel permeability; thus, proteins and cells accumulate in the fluid collections.

7. How does liver cirrhosis cause unconjugated and conjugated hyperbilirubinemia?

Because there are fewer functional hepatocytes, a reduced ability to take up and conjugate bilirubin results in an unconjugated hyperbilirubinemia. Because of the hepatocyte damage in cirrhosis, bilirubin that is conjugated leaks back into the bloodstream, causing a conjugated hyperbilirubinemia.

8. How does liver cirrhosis cause gynecomastia and spider angiomata?

The liver's impaired ability to metabolize estrogen results in gynecomastia and testicular atrophy. Because estrogen weakens vascular walls, the patient has spider angiomata. Note that the spider angiomata are not in the same place as the portacaval anastomoses.

9. How does liver cirrhois cause reduced BUN levels, fetor hepaticus, and mental status abnormalities?

The liver is a major site of amino acid metabolism and is the only site of the urea cycle. Reduced output of the urea cycle due to hepatocyte destruction results in a lower BUN level. Because the urea cycle is also the major site of ammonia detoxification, elevated blood ammonia levels become detectable as a sweet odor on the breath (fetor hepaticus). The elevated blood ammonia, which can enter the brain, may alter cerebral metabolism and produce what is called hepatic encephalopathy.

10. How can an acute alcohol binge cause development of fatty liver?

Fatty liver, also called hepatic steatosis, results from shunting substrates to lipid biosynthesis, impaired secretion of lipoproteins from the liver, and increased peripheral catabolism of fat. The condition is reversible.

11. How does chronic alcohol consumption lead to more rapid catabolism of ingested alcohol?

Alcohol can be degraded by two separate metabolic pathways. The pathway that begins with alcohol dehydrogenase (ADH), which is found in the cytosol of most tissues, is constitutively active and can metabolize only a fixed amount of alcohol. People who do not abuse alcohol rely principally on this pathway for metabolism. In contrast, the microsomal ethanol oxidizing system (MEOS) begins in liver microsomes with enzymes that are induced by alcohol and other drugs. Such induction enhances the capacity to metabolize ethanol. In alcoholics, both the ADH and the MEOS pathways metabolize ethanol, resulting in lower blood levels after alcohol consumption.

cirrhosis = #1
cause of Portal HTN
+ ascites in US.

#1 sign of portal HTN =
asympt. splenomegaly

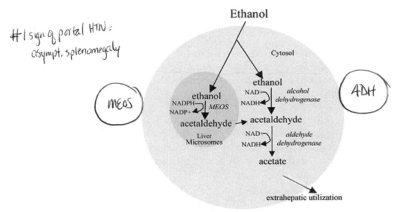

The two pathways for alcohol metabolism. (Courtesy of Gloria Yueh, Ph.D., Midwestern University.)

12. Why are ethanol and/or fomepizole used to treat methanol poisoning and ethylene glycol poisoning?

Methanol and ethylene glycol are metabolized through the same pathway as ethanol, and the intermediates that are formed in this process (formaldehyde from methanol and oxalic acid from ethylene glycol) are highly toxic. Alcohol competes with both methanol and ethylene glycol for metabolism by alcohol dehydrogenase, thereby reducing the rate of formation of the toxic metabolites. Fomepizole further inhibits conversion of methanol or ethylene glycol to their toxic intermediates by directly inhibiting alcohol dehydrogenase.

13. Why should alcoholics avoid acetaminophen?

Acetaminophen is metabolized to a free radical that is hepatotoxic and can make an already bad liver worse. In addition, alcoholics are more susceptible to the hepatotoxic effects of acetaminophen because of increased metabolism to toxic intermediates.

Note: Drugs that are metabolized or eliminated by the liver or biliary system should be used with particular caution in people with liver or biliary disease because of alterations in pharmacokinetics. An acetaminophen overdose is treated with N-acetylcysteine.

14. By what mechanism can an elevated hematocrit lead to Budd-Chiari syndrome and portal hypertension?

An elevated hematocrit (polycythemia) increases blood viscosity and predisposes to thrombosis. One possible consequence is thrombosis of the hepatic veins, which is known as Budd-Chiari syndrome. The occlusion of the hepatic veins, which provide the venous outflow from the liver, can cause blood to back up in the portal system.

CASE 11

A 47-year-old man complains of joint pain and general malaise for the past year. Physical exam is significant for hepatosplenomegaly, ascites, tender swollen joints, and testicular atrophy. His skin appears "bronzed" even though he denies significant sun exposure. He and his wife have been trying unsuccessfully for the past 2 years to have children. His father died of liver and cardiac complications at the age of 55, and his mother died in a car accident at age 60. Lab studies show nonfasting plasma glucose of 200 mg/dl and significantly elevated levels of serum iron and ferritin. A liver biopsy shows markedly elevated hepatic iron content. He is told that he has a rare disease and will have to undergo phlebotomy once a week for the next 1–2 years.

1. What is the diagnosis?

Hemochromatosis, which can be either hereditary (autosomal-recessive) or acquired.

2. What is the source of excessive iron in the hereditary form of hemochromatosis?

The genetic defect causes increased intestinal absorption of iron in excess of daily iron loss. Because only a few extra milligrams of iron are absorbed per day, the symptoms of iron overload can take several decades to manifest.

3. What is the source of excessive iron in the acquired forms of hemochromatosis?

The acquired form of hemochromatosis usually develops in the setting of a hemolytic anemia, such as the thalessemias. Such patients receive excessive iron from repeated blood transfusions. In addition, the ineffective erythropoiesis in certain types of anemias stimulates excessive intestinal absorption of iron.

4. What are the normal cellular storage sites for iron?

Iron is transported in the blood bound to transferrin, endocytosed into almost all cells, and stored intracellularly in the form of ferritin. When ferritin is saturated, it is degraded to hemosiderin.

5. Why are women less susceptible to the effects of hemochromatosis?

Menstruation and its attendant iron loss explain why symptoms frequently do not occur in woman until they are postmenopausal. Although autosomal recessive disorders typically occur with equal frequency in males and females, hemochromatosis is an example of a sex-influenced disorder that has a lower incidence of pathologic consequences in females (one tenth the incidence in males). Another factor that can influence the development of hemochromatosis is daily iron consumption.

6. What is the treatment for hemochromatosis? How does it work?

Repeated phlebotomy is used to reduce total body iron stores. If patients are anemic, the iron chelator deferoxamine is used instead to avoid exacerbating the anemia.

Note: Deferoxamine is also used to treat acute iron poisoning.

7. How can hemochromatosis cause ascites and/or pulmonary edema?

Deposition of excessive iron within the liver causes cirrhosis of the liver, resulting in both portal hypertension and hypoalbuminemia, both of which contribute to ascites. Iron deposition in the heart can lead to a restrictive cardiomyopathy, which causes pulmonary edema because of impaired cardiac output.

Note: Patients with hemochromatosis can develop esophageal varices, much like alcoholics, and are occasionally mistaken for alcoholics by physicians.

8. Why is hyperglycemia often observed in hemochromatosis?

Deposition of iron in the pancreas may lead to destruction of the islet cells, resulting in diabetes mellitus. Impaired hepatic uptake of glucose in patients with cirrhosis may also contribute to hyperglycemia.

9. How can excessive iron deposition in the hypothalamus and/or pituitary cause the testicular atrophy observed in hemochromatosis?

Deposition of iron in the hypothalamus can cause hypothalamic hypogonadotrophic hypogonadism. This disorder is due to decreased secretion of gonadotropin-releasing hormone (GnRH), which results in insufficient pituitary secretion of luteinizing hormone (LH) and follicle-stmulating hormone (FSH). Deposition of excessive iron in the pituitary can directly reduce LH and FSH secretion. The reduced gonadotropin levels lead to hypogonadism, which manifests in males as loss of libido, testicular atrophy, and impotence.

Note: In women with hemochromatosis, the hypogonadism can cause amenorrhea.

10. Why does the patient's skin appear "bronzed"?

Deposition of iron (in the form of hemosiderin) in the skin gives it a bronzed appearance. Patients also have increased melanin production.

11. Why do patients with hemochromatosis tend to develop a thyroid abnormality?

Iron deposition in the thyroid gland can cause primary hypothyroidism. In addition, iron deposition in the pituitary may reduce secretion of thyroid-stimulating hormone (TSH) and cause secondary hypothyroidism.

CASE 12

An 18-year-old man seen for an annual physical exam complains of slight malaise and anorexia but says that he feels fine otherwise. He appears jaundiced, and slit-lamp examination of his eyes reveals yellow-brown deposits at the limbus of the cornea. Lab studies reveal elevated levels of aspartate aminotrasferase (AST) and alanine aminostransferase (ALT), decreased plasma ceruloplasmin, decreased total serum copper but increased free copper, and increased urinary excretion of copper. A liver biopsy confirms the suspected diagnosis.

1. What is the diagnosis?

Wilson's disease (hepatolenticular degeneration).

2. Explain the cause and genetics of Wilson's disease.

Insufficient synthesis of ceruloplasmin and impaired biliary excretion of copper result in abnormal copper deposition in the liver, lenticular nuclei, cornea, and other sites throughout the body. The disorder is inherited in autosomal recessive manner and usually manifests initially between the ages of 6 and 20 years.

3. If the patient remains untreated, what neurologic manifestations may develop?

Because of the degeneration of the lenticular nuclei (putamen and globus pallidus) in the basal ganglia, a Parkinson-like syndrome, characterized by tremors, dysarthria, and spasticity, can develop.

4. What is liver biopsy likely to show?

Elevated copper content, piecemeal necrosis, and lymphocytosis, which can evolve to cirrhosis.

5. What are the yellow-brown corneal deposits seen with slit-lamp examination of the eyes?

The deposits, called Kayser-Fleischer rings, result from copper deposition in the corneal limbus.

6. How can the patient have low levels of total serum copper but high levels of free serum copper?

A deficiency in ceruloplasmin, which normally functions to bind plasma copper, results in low total plasma copper but elevated free plasma copper. It is the elevated free plasma copper that causes pathology, resulting in deposition of copper in the lenticular nuclei (neurologic symptoms), cornea (Kayser-Fleischer rings), liver (cirrhosis), and other organs throughout the body.

7. What is the treatment for Wilson's disease? How does it work?

Copper chelation therapy with lifelong use of D-penicillamine or trientine hydrochloride, drugs that help remove copper from tissue. Extra oral zinc, which competes with copper for intestinal absorption, is commonly used in combination with copper chelation therapy.

CASE 13

While vacationing in a third-world country, not-so-sanitary Steve decided to eat some shell-fish that were harvested from a bay in which sewage enters. A few weeks later, when he re-turned to the U.S., he developed fever, nausea, vomiting, malaise, anorexia, and abdominal pain; he also mentions that his urine is dark. He thinks that mosquito bites during his travel may have infected him with malaria. On physical exam he is jaundiced and has tender he-patomegaly. Lab studies reveal a peripheral smear negative for malaria, marked elevations of AST (aspartate aminotransferase) and ALT (alanine aminotransferase), mildly elevated ALK (alkaline phosphatase), and elevated direct and indirect bilirubin. A hepatitis profile tests positive for anti-HAV IgM, negative for anti-HAV IgG, and negative for HBsAg.

1. What is the diagnosis?

Acute hepatitis A infection.

2. Why does he have an elevation of both direct and indirect bilirubin?

In viral hepatitis, elevated indirect bilirubin is caused by a decrease in serum unconjugated bilirubin uptake into the liver, resulting in indirect hyperbilirubinemia. Elevated direct bilirubin is a result of leakage of conjugated bilirubin from damaged hepatocytes into the systemic circula-tion, resulting in direct hyperbilirubinemia.

3. Explain how the hepatitis profile results facilitate the diagnosis of acute infection, rather than chronic one.

IgM is the first antibody isotype produced in response to a new infectious agent and remains in the circulation for about 12 weeks in hepatitis A infection. A previous infection would have been negative for anti-HAV IgM and positive for anti-HAV IgG, since the IgG isotype is pro-duced later in the infection and memory B cells do not make IgM; generally they make IgG.

Note: In the vast majority of cases, hepatitis A does not develop into a chronic state.

4. How do liver function test patterns (AST, ALT, ALK, GGT) differ between viral hepa-titis and cholestatic diseases?

Generally, in diseases that primarily affect the liver parenchyma both AST and ALT are ele-vated to a greater extent than ALK and gamma-glutamyl transferase (GGT). In cholestatic dis-ease, the converse is generally the case, with ALK and GGT elevated to a greater extent than AST and ALT.

5. Why does cholestasis cause a disproportionate rise in ALK and GGT?

If hepatocytes are exposed to lipophilic agents prior to being damaged, such as bile from cholestasis, the lipophilic agents cause an upregulation of ALK and GGT expression. This upreg-ulation results in a more marked elevation of ALK and GGT when the cholestasis eventually causes hepatocyte damage. AST and ALT also are released from hepatocyte damage, but far from the extent seen in viral hepatitis, which is associated with widespread hepatocyte damage.

6. Summarize characteristic features of the different hepatitis viruses.

HEPATITIS VIRUS	TYPE OF VIRUS	TRANS-MISSION	CHRON-ICITY	CIRRHOSIS	HEPATOCELLULAR CARCINOMA RISK	COMMENTS
A	ssRNA	Fecal-oral	No	No	No	
B	dsDNA	Parenteral	Yes	Yes	Yes	
C	ssRNA	Parenteral	Yes	Yes	Yes	Most common cause of post-transfusion hepatitis

(Cont'd.)

HEPATITIS VIRUS	TYPE OF VIRUS	TRANS-MISSION	CHRON-ICITY	CIRRHOSIS	HEPATOCELLULAR CARCINOMA RISK	COMMENTS
D	?					Requires hepatitis B to replicate
E	ssRNA	Fecal-oral	No	No	No	20% mortality in pregnant women

CASE 14

A 3-day-old, full-term baby presents with jaundice that started on his face and spread to his body. Physical examination reveals no hematomas. Lab tests show elevated indirect bilirubin, a negative Coombs test, normal reticulocyte count (for his age), and normal complete blood count (CBC). Enzyme assays for glucuronyl transferase activity are also within normal limits.

1. **What is the most likely diagnosis?**
Physiologic jaundice of the newborn.

2. **Why does physiologic jaundice develop?**
In the process of converting from red blood cells (RBCs) with fetal hemoglobin to RBCs with adult hemoglobin, there is an approximate six-fold increase in the amount of unconjugated bilirubin presented to the liver. The neonatal liver often does not have the capacity (because it is not sufficiently mature) to take up and conjugate this amount of bilirubin. The result is transient physiologic jaundice.

3. **Why did the physician check for hematomas on physical exam?**
Breakdown of RBCs in hematomas and the attendant bilirubin formation can be a cause of jaundice.

4. **Why are a normal reticulocyte count and a normal CBC important in the diagnostic work-up for this neonate?**
Hemolytic anemias can cause jaundice and generally show elevated reticulocyte counts in the presence of anemia.

5. **What is the most serious complication of neonatal jaundice? How does it develop?**
Kernicterus, which is deposition of insoluble unconjugated bilirubin in the brain. It is dangerous because it can lead to brain damage.

6. **Would you expect physiologic jaundice to be exacerbated or attenuated by Gilbert's syndrome?**
In Gilbert's syndrome, uridine diphosphate (UDP)-glucuronyl transferase activity is mildly decreased, resulting in increased unconjugated bilirubin levels.Therefore, the disease would exacerbate physiologic jaundice.

7. **What hereditary syndrome is associated with a more serious deficiency of UDP-glucuronyl transferase than Gilbert's syndrome?**
Crigler-Najjar syndrome. This disease also causes an unconjugated hyperbilirubinemia.

8. **Why is phenobarbital used to treat Crigler-Najjar syndrome?**
Phenobarbital induces hepatic enzymes, including UDP-glucuronyl transferase, which increases the capacity of the liver to conjugate bilirubin.

9. What are the two hereditary forms of conjugated hyperbilirubinemia? What is the major morphologic difference between them?

Dubin-Johnson and Rotor syndromes. Dubin-Johnson syndrome is associated with a black-pigmented liver, whereas Rotor syndrome is not. To remember this distinction, think of the liver as smoking a "Duby" after being "conjugated" and becoming charred with black pigment.

CASE 15

A 41-year-old obese woman complains of nausea, vomiting, fever, and right upper quadrant (RUQ) abdominal pain. She has a temperature of 100.5°F and experiences sharp pain on inspiration when pressure is provided to the lower edge of the right costal cartilage (positive Murphy's sign). Lab tests show leukocytosis with a left shift. Ultrasound of the RUQ reveals an inflamed gallbladder with a gallstone located in the neck of the gallbladder. She is placed on antibiotics and scheduled for surgery.

1. What is the diagnosis?

Cholecystitis (inflammation of the gallbladder), which is usually due to obstruction of the gallbladder neck or cystic duct by a gallstone.

2. What are the most common types of gallstones?

Cholesterol monohydrate (about 80%) and calcium bilirubinate (about 20%).

3. Why does an obstructing stone in the common bile duct predispose to jaundice whereas a stone in the cystic duct generally does not?

A stone in the common bile duct (choledocholithiasis) can completely prevent the flow of bile to the intestines (cholestasis), causing biliary backpressure that damages the liver and results in hyperbilirubinemia and jaundice. However, a stone in the cystic duct only prevents bile from flowing into or out of the gallbladder, leaving bile flow into the intestines unimpeded.

4. What is cholangitis?

Infection of the biliary tree, usually as a result of a stone in the common bile duct. It is a serious condition.

5. What is Charcot's triad for cholangitis?

Charcot's triad consists of fever, RUQ pain, and jaundice and is present in approximately 50% of patients with cholangitis. The fever is due to the response to infection, the jaundice is due to obstruction of the common bile duct (or other bile ducts).

6. Why do patients with gallstones experience pain particularly after eating a high-fat meal?

Entry of fatty acids into the duodenum stimulates the release of CCK, which causes gallbladder contraction and creates pain by increasing biliary pressure.

7. Where in the pancreas would a neoplasm causing obstructive jaundice most likely be located? Why?

In the head of the pancreas. The common bile duct runs through the head of the pancreas on its way to the second part of the duodenum and can become obstructed along the way.

8. How can cholestasis cause pale stools?

Conjugated bilirubin is normally metabolized to urobilinogen (clear color) by colonic bacteria and ultimately to stercobilin (brown color) via auto-oxidation, which causes the normal stool color. Neither of these processes occurs if bile does not reach the intestines.

9. Define steatorrhea. How can it develop from complete obstruction of the common bile duct?

Steatorrhea is the presence of significant amounts of fat in stool. Bile acids emulsify fats so that they can be digested by pancreatic lipases, then form micelles of the digested fatty acids and deliver them to the intestinal mucosa for absorption. Consequently, impaired delivery of bile to the intestines impairs all of these processes and causes steatorrhea.

10. What prevents the formation of cholesterol stones in the normal physiologic setting?

Bile salts and phospholipids solubilize cholesterol and prevent it from precipitating out of solution. In fact, for patients with small stones who are poor surgical candidates, oral bile acids are given to facilitate dissolution of the stone.

11. Why are people with Crohn's disease predisposed to the development of cholesterol stones?

Crohn's disease often involves the terminal ileum, where bile salts are reabsorbed. Because these salts are important in the solubilization of cholesterol, reduced reabsorption facilitates stone formation.

12. Which cholesterol-lowering drugs bind bile acids in the intestine, causing reduced hepatic excretion? Explain how these drugs lower serum cholesterol.

Cholestyramine and cholestipol, which are nonabsorbable ionic resins, bind bile acids in the intestine and are eliminated in the feces, promoting the excretion of bile salts. As a result, more bile acids need to be produced de novo. Because serum cholesterol is used as a precursor for bile acids, this process results in a lower serum cholesterol level. Recall that formation of bile salts is the only method available to the body for elimination of cholesterol.

13. How can primary infection with *Clonorchis sinensis* also lead to obstructive jaundice?

This trematode infects the hepatobiliary tree. Chronic inflammation from this infection can cause fibrotic strictures within the bile ducts that impede the egress of bile. This infection is most commonly seen in Southeast Asia.

2. NEUROLOGY

Dave Brown and Thomas Brown

BASIC CONCEPTS

1. How do upper motor neurons (UMNs) differ from lower motor neurons (LMNs)?

The cell bodies of UMNs are supraspinal in location, and the axons of these neurons synapse either directly or indirectly, via interneurons, on lower motor neurons located in the ventral horn of the spinal cord or brainstem motor nuclei (e.g., facial nerve motor nucleus). The axons of LMNs (alpha and gamma motor neurons) project directly to skeletal muscle fibers.

Note: The corticobulbar tract, like the corticospinal tract, conveys axons of UMNs, but it conveys them to brainstem motor nuclei such as the oculomotor nucleus and facial motor nucleus.

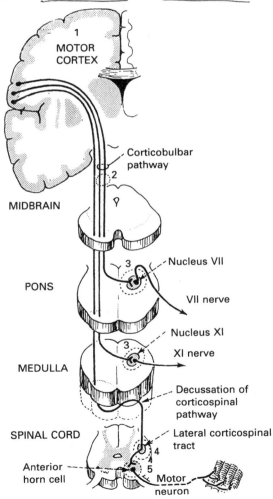

Corticobulbar and corticospinal tracts. (From Lindsay KW, Bone I, Callander R (eds): Neurology and Neurosurgery Illustrated, 3rd ed. Edinburgh, Churchill Livingstone, 2002, p 535, with permission.)

2. What is a motor unit? Do most alpha motor neurons innervate a few or many fibers in a large muscle such as the gluteus maximus?

A motor unit is a group of muscle fibers all of which are innervated by a single alpha motor neuron. In the large muscles, alpha motor neurons innervate many muscle fibers, which explains why there is little fine motor control in these muscles. On the other hand, in the smaller muscles (e.g., extraocular muscles or muscles of the hand), a given alpha motor neuron innervates only a few muscle fibers, resulting in much finer control of movement. In both types of muscle, the strength of muscle contraction is increased primarily by *recruitment* of additional motor units.

3. What is the primary function of the cerebellum in movement?

The cerebellum fine-tunes movement. It does so by comparing commands sent by the motor cortex to the muscular system with proprioceptive feedback about actual movements (via the spinocerebellar tracts). The cerebellum uses this feedback to influence and fine-tune output from the motor cortex (if differences in the planned movement and the actual movement exist).

4. Why do cerebellar lesions classically produce ipsilateral symptoms?

The cerebellar hemispheres influence motor activity by their projections to the contralateral motor cortices (via the motor thalamus) and to the contralateral red nuclei. In turn, both the corticospinal tract and the rubrospinal tract arising from these structures cross back over en route to their target motor neurons, thereby producing symptoms on the same side of the body as the lesion.

5. What are the two ascending sensory pathways? What information does each convey?

The **anterolateral system,** also called the spinothalamic tract, conveys sensations of pain, temperature, crude (nondiscriminative) touch, and pressure. The **dorsal columns** convey the sensations of fine touch, vibration, and conscious proprioception.

Note: Unconscious proprioception is transmitted by the spinocerebellar pathways.

6. What are the two anatomic divisions of the dorsal columns? From which anatomic structures do they relay sensory information?

The **fasciculus gracilis** relays information from the lower extremities and lower thorax. It is located most medially in the dorsal columns, just as the gracilis muscle is the most medial muscle of the thigh.

The **fasciculus cuneatus** relays information from the upper thorax and upper extremities. It is immediately lateral to the fasciculus gracilis.

Note: Both fasciculi carry fibers that synapse on their respective nuclei in the medulla: the nucleus gracilis and nucleus cuneatus.

7. At what neuroanatomic locations do the corticospinal tract, dorsal columns, and anterolateral system (spinothalamic system) cross over?

The corticospinal tract crosses over (i.e., decussates) as it descends through the inferior aspect of the medulla through the medullary pyramids. The dorsal columns cross over between their nuclei in the brainstem and the thalamus via the arcuate fibers of the medial lemniscus. The axons of the anterolateral system cross over almost immediately after their first-order neurons synapse in the dorsal horn of the spinal cord. (See figure on next page.)

8. Based on where the major motor and sensory pathways cross over, identify and explain the neurologic deficits that occur in Brown-Sequard syndrome.

Brown-Sequard syndrome is caused by a lateral hemisection of the spinal cord. Motor loss is on the same side as the lesion, because the corticospinal tract has already crossed superior to the lesion (in the medulla) and in the spinal cord innervates only motor neurons on the same side as it courses. Fine touch, vibration, and proprioception (modalities of the dorsal columns) are lost on the same side as the lesion because the sensory information of the dorsal columns does not cross

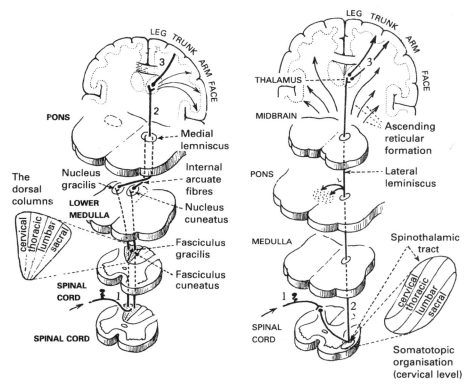

Divisions of the ascending sensory pathways. **Left,** Dorsal columns. **Right,** Anterolateral system (spinothalamic tract). (From Lindsay KW, Bone I, Callander R (eds): Neurology and Neurosurgery Illustrated, 3rd ed. Edinburgh, Churchill Livingstone, 2002, p 196, with permission.)

over until it passes more superiorly (between the brainstem nuclei and the thalamus). The loss of pain and temperature sensation (anterolateral system), however, will be contralateral to the side of the lesion, because the fibers of the anterolateral system cross over and ascend shortly after entering the spinal cord.

Note: There may be some loss of all modalities at the level at which the lesion occurs.

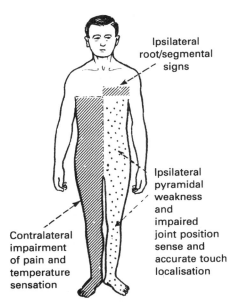

Brown-Sequard syndrome. (From Lindsay KW, Bone I, Callander R (eds): Neurology and Neurosurgery Illustrated, 3rd ed. Edinburgh, Churchill Livingstone, 2002, p 198, with permission.)

9. Where (below the head) do the motor and sensory deficits manifest in patients with a lesion of the internal capsule?

The corticospinal tract, dorsal columns, and anterolateral system travel to or from the cerebral cortex through the posterior limb of the internal capsule. Because these three tracts either originated from or eventually cross over to the contralateral side, the patient will have contralateral hemiplegia due to effects on the corticospinal tract and contralateral sensory loss from both ascending sensory systems.

10. How do opioids reduce pain transmission in the spinothalamic system?

The mechanisms by which opioids are thought to reduce pain transmission in the spinothalamic tract are complicated and probably beyond the level of detail required for step 1. However, students should understand that opioids provide analgesic relief primarily via inhibition of the spinothalamic tract. For students who are curious about the mechanisms of this inhibition, it is thought to involve:

1. Inhibition of voltage-gated calcium channels in the presynaptic terminal of primary afferent neurons, thereby reducing the amount of neurotransmitter released by these neurons, and

2. Facilitation of potassium conductance in postsynaptic spinothalamic neurons in the dorsal horn, which hyperpolarizes these cells and makes them less excitable, and

3. Increasing activity of descending cortical pathways that modulate pain transmission by the spinothalamic system.

CASE 1

A 45-year-old retired baseball player presents with a 6-month history of unexplained weight loss, difficulty with swallowing, and weakness so severe that he has difficulty with walking. Physical exam reveals a strange combination of flaccid paralysis and spastic paralysis as well as hyporeflexia and hyperreflexia in both upper and lower extremities. He has significant, diffuse muscle wasting, and fasciculations can occasionally be observed. Sensation is intact to all modalities in all areas tested. A mental status examination is within normal limits for the patient's age and cultural background, although he does have difficulty with articulation. Cerebrospinal fluid analysis is negative for oligoclonal bands (of immunoglobulins), elevated protein, or white blood cells. MRI scans of the brain and spinal cord appear normal. Muscle biopsy shows groups of atrophied and angulated muscle fibers (grouped atrophy).

1. What is the most likely diagnosis?

Amyotrophic lateral sclerosis (ALS), or Lou Gehrig's disease.

2. What are the principal pathologic findings in ALS?

Loss of pyramidal cells in the cerebral motor cortex leads to fibrosis of the lateral corticospinal tracts. In addition, loss of ventral horn neurons up and down the spinal cord result in loss of ventral nerve roots. However, sensory tracts and cognitive function usually are spared, which explains why the patient's mental status and sensory function are completely normal.

Note: Both UMNs and LMNs are damaged in ALS.

3. What are the signs of UMN lesions? Which are present in this patient?

Signs of UMN lesions include spastic paralysis (the muscles have an increased resistance to passive movement or manipulation), hyperactive deep tendon reflexes (hyperreflexia), and clonus (alternating contraction and relaxation of a muscle in rapid succession in response to sudden stretching of the muscle). This patient has spastic paralysis and hyperreflexia.

Note: Muscle atrophy with UMN lesions may occur secondary to muscle disuse but does not result from muscle denervation.

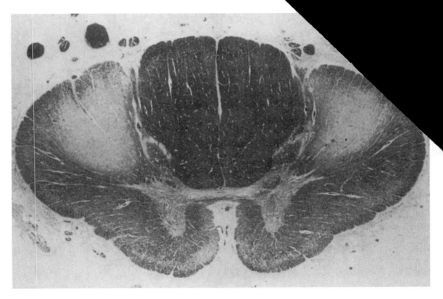

Transverse section of the spinal cord in ALS showing degeneration of corticospinal tract with loss of myelinated fibers (lack of stain). (From Cotran RS, Kumar V, Collins T (eds): Robbins Pathologic Basis of Disease, 6th ed. Philadelphia, W.B. Saunders, 1999, p 1339, with permission.)

4. Why are the signs and symptoms of hyperreflexia, spastic paralysis, and clonus seen with a UMN lesion?

The most widely accepted theory is that UMNs are tonically inhibitory to LMNs. Thus, disruption of UMNs *disinhibits* (i.e., activates) LMNs, making the motor component of the deep tendon reflexes (DTRs) more active and increasing baseline muscle tone, which increases resistance to passive movement.

5. What LMN signs are present in this patient?

When a lower motor neuron is damaged, the muscle that it innervates does not receive stimulation; as a result, it atrophies and has less muscle tone (hypotonia). The denervated muscle also has flaccid paralysis (decreased resistance to passive movement or manipulation), and the efferent part of the DTRs is abolished so that the DTRs are weak or absent (hyporeflexia). Fibrillations (invisible contractions of single muscle fibers, seen only on electromyography [EMG]) and fasciculations (involuntary contraction of one or more muscle units, which is often visible) may also be present in LMN lesions. This patient had hyporeflexia, fasciculations, and flaccid paralysis.

6. Is ALS more commonly inherited or acquired?

ALS is more commonly acquired (about 80%) rather than inherited (about 20%). The precise cause of the acquired form remains unknown. However, one of the familial forms has been associated with mutations in the zinc/copper superoxide dismutase gene, which plays an important role in scavenging free radicals in metabolically active cells such as neurons.

7. Why is the absence of both periventricular plaques on MRI and oligoclonal bands in the cerebrospinal fluid significant in the diagnosis of this patient?

The absence of these findings makes the diagnosis of multiple sclerosis improbable. Another important distinction between multiple sclerosis and ALS is that ALS affects only the motor system, whereas multiple sclerosis affects both motor and sensory neurons.

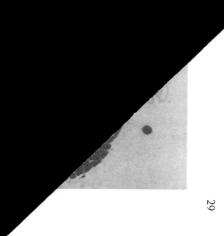

g resting tremor that resolves with movement,
ovements (akinesia), and his movements are
expressionless face (masked facies) and a for-
wide-based gait, and his muscles demonstrate
ives way in a series of successive jerks when it

ιg, of course, that the patient is not taking any
opramide?
osis of Parkinson's disease (PD), the pathophysi-
ιergic activity within the brain. In making the di-
h PD from *parkinsonism*, which can present with
similar symptoms and is caused by drugs that decrease dopaminergic activity in the brain (e.g.,
metoclopramide, antipsychotics).

2. What neurologic structures are affected in PD? How does this pattern affect the motor symptoms?

Dopaminergic neurons in the substantia nigra are selectively destroyed in PD. These neurons normally modulate motor behavior through dopaminergic input to the basal ganglia via the ni-grostriatal tract. The destruction of these dopamine-producing cells produces a deficiency of stri-atal dopamine and a relative excess of striatal acetylcholine, explaining why both dopamine agonists and anticholinergics are used in treating PD.

Note: The striatum consists of the caudate nucleus and putamen, both of which are part of the basal ganglia.

3. Why does this patient have difficulty with initiating voluntary movements?

Basal ganglia function is important in regulating voluntary movements. Before a voluntary movement is performed, the motor cortex sends a copy of the planned movement to the basal ganglia, essentially asking for "permission." In the case of PD, permission is not granted, and ini-tiating voluntary movements becomes difficult. In contrast, if permission is granted too readily or even when it is not requested by the cortex, involuntary movements may occur (e.g., as in Huntington's chorea)

4. Why is levodopa used to treat PD instead of dopamine?

Dopamine cannot cross the blood-brain barrier. However, levodopa, a lipid soluble precursor to dopamine, can cross the blood-brain barrier and increases dopamine levels in the central ner-vous system (CNS).

5. Why is levodopa typically administered along with carbidopa?

Carbidopa inhibits the peripheral metabolism of levodopa to dopamine, thereby increasing the delivery of levodopa to the brain and minimizing the peripheral side effects of levo-dopa/dopamine (which include arrhythmias and gastrointestinal symptoms).

6. Drugs such as bromocriptine and pergolide are also used to treat PD. How do they exert their effects?

These drugs are dopamine receptor agonists and increase central dopaminergic activity with-out increasing dopamine levels. This effect, of course, is beneficial in PD.

7. What is the mechanism of action of selegeline in treating PD?

Selegeline selectively inhibits monoamine oxidase B (MAO-B), an enzyme that degrades dopamine.

8. Why is it preferable to selectively inhibit MAO-B rather than both MAO-A and MAO-B in patients with PD?

MAO-A principally degrades norepinephrine and serotonin, whereas MAO-B is more selective for dopamine degradation. Because MAO-A inhibitors increase serotonin and norepinephrine levels, they have been used for treating depression, but they are not expected to be as effective in treating the motor symptoms of PD.

9. What is benztropine? Why is it useful in Parkinson's disease?

Benztropine is an anticholinergic drug (like atropine) that crosses the blood-brain barrier. Recall that there is a *relative* excess of striatal acetylcholine in PD because of the deficiency of dopamine. Thus, anticholinergics that can enter the CNS are also useful in treating the motor symptoms of PD.

10. Which antiviral medication is also effective in treating PD?

Amantadine, which is effective against influenza and was incidentally discovered to be effective in PD. Its mechanism of action is uncertain, but it probably acts by increasing dopaminergic output by the substantia nigra.

11. How does the drug MPTP cause parkinsonism? Is this process reversible?

MPTP (1-methyl-4-phenyl-1,2,3,6-tetrahydropyridine) is an analog of the opioid meperidine and is occasionally present as a contaminant in certain illicit drugs. It causes parkinsonism by selectively destroying neurons in the substantia nigra. Unfortunately, the effect is not reversible.

12. Why should you be suspicious of a diagnosis of PD in a patient treated for schizophrenia?

Antipsychotic drugs that block dopamine receptors in the mesolimbic system to achieve their effect can also block dopaminergic activity in the nigrostriatal tract and cause symptoms similar to PD (pseudoparkinsonism, which is often reversible with discontinuation of the antipsychotics). However, the motor disorders that develop after long-term use of antipsychotics (e.g., tardive dyskinesia) may prove irreversible.

13. How does a pathologist establish the diagnosis of PD in evaluation of the brain at autopsy?

Bilateral depigmentation of the midbrain substantia nigra and the presence of neuronal Lewy bodies (eosinophilic cytoplasmic inclusions).

14. The present patient has a tremor resulting from basal ganglia dysfunction. How does it differ from the tremor typically associated with cerebellar dysfunction?

A cerebellar lesion produces tremor during volitional movements (when the cerebellum normally functions), whereas a basal ganglia lesion, as in PD or Huntington's disease, produces tremor at rest.

CASE 3

A 40-year-old man has become notably demented and has developed involuntary and spastic (choreiform) movements. MRI of the head is notable for significant atrophy of the basal ganglia, especially the caudate nucleus. He had known for a while that this process would eventually occur, because he had tested positive for the gene that caused his father to have similar problems. However, the patient is upset because the disease has developed several years earlier in his life than in his father's.

1. What is the most likely diagnosis? What is the mode of inheritance?

Huntington's disease (HD) or chorea, which is inherited in an autosomal dominant manner with 100% penetrance.

2. What neurotransmitter is reduced in the basal ganglia in HD? How does its reduction relate to the hyperkinetic motor abnormalities?

Gamma-aminobutyric acid (GABA), the major inhibitory neurotransmitter of the CNS, is reduced in HD. Loss of inhibitory signals within the basal ganglia results in *disinhibition* of the motor thalamus, explaining the hyperkinetic motor abnormalities seen in HD. This deficiency in GABA within the basal ganglia has the opposite effect (i.e., hyperkinesia) to that seen with the deficiency of dopamine associated with PD (i.e., hypokinesia).

3. What does the term *penetrance* imply with respect to genetic diseases? Is the penetrance of HD high or low?

Penetrance is the frequency with which a pathologic phenotype is observed in the presence of the disease genotype. In HD, which has a penetrance of 100%, every person with the gene defect eventually develops the disease. Hence the patient was certain that he was going to develop HD. Fortunately, most genetic diseases have incomplete penetrance.

4. What type of gene mutation gives rise to HD?

A trinucleotide (CAG) repeat expansion in the huntingtin gene located on chromosome 4, which translates into insertion of a polyglutamate tract in the huntingtin protein. Insertion of this polyglutamate tract appears to disrupt the normal function of the huntingtin protein in a dominant negative manner; hence, the autosomal dominant mode of inheritance.

5. What is the meaning of anticipation with respect to genetic diseases? What is the cause of anticipation in HD?

Anticipation is the expression of a hereditary disease at an earlier age and in a more severe form throughout succeeding generations. In HD (i.e., in this patient), it is caused by an increase in the number of trinucleotide repeats within the gene responsible for the disease.

6. How is it possible for someone with a negative family history of HD to develop the disease?

Because HD exhibits 100% penetrance and is inherited in an autosomal dominant manner, its appearance in a person with a negative family history is most likely due to a new mutation.

7. Why might it make sense to measure levels of serum ceruloplasmin in patients who present with similar motor abnormalities and a similar family history?

Serum ceruloplasmin is a screening test for Wilson's disease (hepatolenticular degeneration), which is also hereditary and causes movement abnormalities. In this disease, serum levels of copper are abnormally high and serum levels of ceruloplasmin, a copper transport protein, are abnormally low. Copper deposition in the lenticular nuclei (globus pallidus and putamen) results in motor abnormalities.

CASE 4

A 30-year-old woman complains of a long history of double vision (diplopia) and some difficulty with swallowing solid foods. Recently, she has become quite fatigued following even mild exercise. These symptoms become worse throughout the day. Her physical appearance is remarkable only for ptosis and perhaps slight atrophy of facial muscles. When asked to look upward for 1 minute without closing her eyes, she closes her eyes after only 15 seconds due to muscle exhaustion. Muscle strength improves markedly in response to administration of edrophonium (positive Tensilon test). An MRI of the thorax indicates the presence of a thymoma.

1. What is the most likely diagnosis?

Myasthenia gravis (MG).

Note: MG is often associated with thymoma, and a thymectomy frequently improves the symptoms.

2. Describe the pathophysiology of the motor weakness in MG.

MG is an autoimmune disorder characterized by the production of antibodies to the post-synaptic nicotinic acetylcholine receptors on skeletal muscle fibers. These autoantibodies reduce the number of acetylcholine receptors on the motor endplate, making it less responsive to acetylcholine.

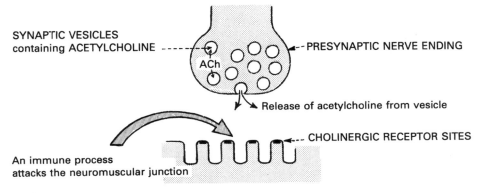

Pathophysiology of myasthenia gravis. (From Lindsay KW, Bone I, Callander R (eds): Neurology and Neurosurgery Illustrated, 3rd ed. Edinburgh, Churchill Livingstone, 2002, p 463, with permission.)

3. Describe the normal mechanism by which an action potential is generated in skeletal muscle cells.

Nicotinic acetylcholine receptors are ligand-gated sodium channels, and binding of acetylcholine to nicotinic receptors produces an endplate potential in skeletal muscle cells. This endplate potential has to be above a certain threshold value for activation of fast voltage-gated sodium channels to open and generate an action potential, which causes muscle contraction by triggering release of calcium from the sarcoplasmic reticulum. In MG, there are not enough acetylcholine receptors to respond to the synaptic acetylcholine and depolarize the cell to reach the threshold for action potential formation.

4. To what class of drugs does edrophonium belong? How does it resolve the weakness of MG?

Edrophonium is a short-acting cholinesterase inhibitor. The function of cholinesterase is to degrade synaptic acetylcholine. By antagonizing cholinesterase, edrophonium increases the concentration of acetylcholine in the synaptic cleft, thereby overcoming the deficiency of available acetylcholine receptors by activating a higher percentage of receptors that are present.

Note: For long-term management of MG, the long-acting cholinesterase inhibitors pyridostigmine and neostigmine are used.

5. If a patient treated for MG overdoses on one of the cholinesterase inhibitors, what side effects may occur?

The side-effect profile of an overdose of cholinesterase inhibitors mimics excessive stimulation of the parasympathetic nervous system (i.e., excessive cholinergic activity), resulting in diarrhea, miosis, bronchospasm, excessive urination, bradycardia, salivation, and lacrimation. In addition, because the sympathetic nervous system stimulates sweating via the release of acetylcholine from postganglionic sympathetic fibers, excessive sweating may also occur.

Note: If someone is poisoned with organophosphates (e.g., parathion), which are *irreversible* cholinesterase inhibitors, treatment is aimed at reducing total cholinergic activity. This goal is accomplished with pralidoxine, which regenerates active cholinesterase, and with the anticholinergic atropine.

6. Describe the mechanism of action of the nondepolarizing neuromuscular blockers. Why are these drugs particularly dangerous in patients with MG?

These agents (e.g. pancuronium, tubocurarine) are analogs or derivates of curare and work by antagonizing the nicotinic acetylcholine receptor on the neuromuscular endplate. They are often used as an adjunct in surgical anesthesia to achieve muscle relaxation. These drugs exacerbate muscle weakness in MG and may even produce respiratory failure due to diaphragmatic dysfunction.

7. How is Lambert-Eaton syndrome (LES) similar to MG? What causes LES?

LES is also an autoimmune diseases caused by the abnormal production of self-reactive antibodies. Antibodies to voltage-gated calcium channels located in the terminal bouton of presynaptic neurons result in impaired neurotransmitter (acetylcholine) release.

Note: LES is often associated with paraneoplastic syndromes, particularly small-cell carcinoma of the lung.

CASE 5

A 35-year-old man presents with bilateral loss of pain and temperature sensation in the arms and upper thorax as well as several painless ulcers on his fingers from burning his hands repeatedly while cooking. Fine touch, vibration, and proprioception remain intact in all areas, although pain and temperature sensation is severely compromised in both arms and upper thorax. An MRI reveals a fluid-filled cavity within the cervical spinal cord.

1. What is the diagnosis? Which ascending sensory system is affected?

This patient has syringomyelia, which is an expanded fluid-filled cavity in the spinal cord. The spinothalamic system, which is also called the anterolateral system, is affected. This system conveys modalities of pain, temperature, crude touch, and pressure.

Note: Syringobulbia is a variant of syringomyelia in which fluid-filled, slit-like cavities are located in the medulla. Remember that *myelo* = spinal cord and *bulbo* = brainstem.

2. How can this disease progress to cause atrophy of the muscles of the hands and hypoactive reflexes of the upper extremities?

Expansion of the syrinx to compress the ventral horns of the spinal cord produces the lower motor neuron signs of muscle atrophy and hyporeflexia.

Note: If the interossei and lumbrical muscles of the hand are primarily affected, suspect involvement of the C8-T1 segments.

3. How does this fluid-filled cavity cause the bilateral loss of temperature and pain sensation?

The anterolateral system crosses over shortly after its first order neuron synapses in the dorsal horn of the spinal cord. The site of crossing is directly adjacent to the central canal of the spinal cord; thus, expansion of a fluid-filled cavity in the central cord can compress and compromise these fibers. The sensory deficit arises from areas that send fibers across at the level of the fluid-filled cavity.

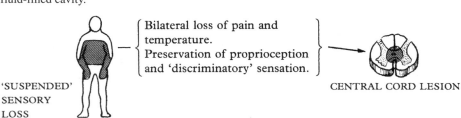

'SUSPENDED' SENSORY LOSS — { Bilateral loss of pain and temperature. Preservation of proprioception and 'discriminatory' sensation. } → CENTRAL CORD LESION

Syringomyelia. (From Lindsay KW, Bone I, Callander R (eds): Neurology and Neurosurgery Illustrated, 3rd ed. Edinburgh, Churchill Livingstone, 2002, p 198, with permission.)

CASE 6

A 65-year-old woman complains of intermittent episodes of lancinating pain in her right lower jaw. She is occasionally wakened at night by this pain. An extensive work-up reveals no dental pathology, and an MRI reveals no mass lesions in the posterior fossa.

1. What is the most likely diagnosis?
Trigeminal neuralgia (tic douloureux)

2. What is the value of examining the posterior fossa for masses?
The trigeminal nerve courses through the posterior fossa, and its nuclei are in the pons and medulla. Compression anywhere along this pathway may cause similar symptoms.

3. Which division of the trigeminal nerve is affected in this patient? What is the anatomic distribution of the other divisions?
In this woman the mandibular division (V3), which innervates the lower jaw, is affected. The maxillary division (V2) innervates the upper jaw and cheek, and the ophthalmic division (V1) innervates the region of the eyes and forehead.

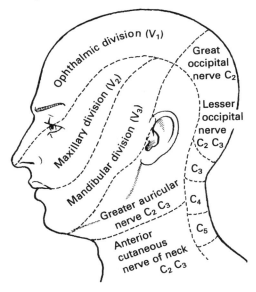

Divisions of the trigeminal nerve. (From Lindsay KW, Bone I, Callander R (eds): Neurology and Neurosurgery Illustrated, 3rd ed. Edinburgh, Churchill Livingstone, 2002, p 14, with permission.)

4. If surgical sectioning of the involved branch were performed, what modalities of sensation would we expect to be impaired?
All modalities of sensation would be lost in the distribution of the mandibular division because the trigeminal nerve conveys all sensory information from the face (i.e., pain, temperature, fine touch, vibration, and proprioception).

5. Why might therapy with carbamazepine (Tegretol) make sense for this patient?
Carbamazepine is an anticonvulsant medication that is also used for trigeminal neuralgia and is prescribed for treating neuropathic pain of almost any etiology. It reduces the rate of nerve transmission by inhibiting voltage-gated sodium channels of neurons.

CASE 7

A woman previously diagnosed with megaloblastic anemia and treated only with folic acid supplements presents with complaints of confusion, memory difficulties, depression, and a feeling of pins and needles (paresthesias) in her extremities for the past few months. Physical exam is notable for atrophic glossitis, positive Romberg's sign, and positive Babinski signs bilaterally. Lab tests reveal a normal complete blood count, elevated methy-malonic acid, and normal fasting plasma glucose. An MRI of the brain appears normal.

1. What is the probable diagnosis? Justify your answer.

The patient most likely has a neuropathy due to vitamin B12 deficiency (subacute combined degeneration). Vitamin B12 deficiency can cause megaloblastic anemia, which can be corrected with folic acid supplementation. However, folic acid supplementation does not prevent the neurologic manifestations of B12 deficiency. Therefore, in a patient with megaloblastic anemia, serum levels of both folic acid and B12 should be tested, and both vitamins should be supplemented.

Note: Vitamin B12 neuropathy is called subacute *combined* degeneration because it can cause degeneration of both the corticospinal tracts and the dorsal columns. Vitamin B12 deficiency is commonly seen in pernicious anemia (autoimmune gastritis) and in patients who have undergone surgical resection of the terminal ileum (e.g., patients with Crohn's disease).

2. How is a positive Romberg sign elicited on exam? Why may vitamin B12 deficiency give rise to a positive Romberg sign?

A positive Romberg sign is defined as swaying of the body or falling when the patient stands with the feet close together and the eyes closed. A positive sign indicates vestibular dysfunction, cerebellar dysfunction, or proprioceptive sensory loss (i.e., sensory ataxia). In this patient, the positive Romberg sign is caused by proprioceptive sensory loss, most likely caused by damage to the dorsal columns.

3. What is a positive Babinski sign? What does it indicate?

A positive Babinski sign is spontaneous dorsiflexion of the big toe upon stroking the plantar surface of the foot with a solid object. It indicates an UMN lesion and in this patient probably represents demyelination of the corticospinal tracts.

Note: Positive Babinski signs are normal in infants (up to 12 months). Suppression of the Babinski reflex by higher brain centers is a prerequisite for learning to walk; otherwise we would be jumping every time we touched the ground!

4. What was the value of obtaining a fasting plasma glucose level in this patient?

Many of the symptoms of diabetic neuropathy are similar to those of B12 deficiency and generally present in a "stocking-glove" pattern (i.e., the symptoms commonly first appear in the hands and feet).

CASE 8

A 32-year-old woman complains of a puzzling array of symptoms, including numbness and tingling (paresthesias) in her right arm, weakness of her left leg, clumsiness, and vertigo. She mentions that these symptoms seem to "come and go" every several months and last for a few weeks. She also had a recent episode of visual impairment in which she was temporarily unable to see out of her right eye. On ocular exam, convergence is intact, but medial rectus palsy is noted on attempted lateral conjugate gaze (internuclear ophthalmoplegia). An MRI reveals periventricular plaques in the brain. Cerebrospinal fluid analysis reveals the presence of oligoclonal immunoglobulin bands (absent in the serum), elevated IgG, and myelin basic protein.

1. What is the most likely diagnosis?

Multiple sclerosis (MS), a disease that involves demyelination of various white matter areas of the central nervous system (CNS). It can have a relapsing and remitting course (as in this patient) or a chronically progressive course. The various neurologic manifestations that develop are due to demyelination in different sites within the CNS. An MRI classically shows multiple plaques in different areas of white matter, most notably in the periventricular areas.

2. Why is a diagnosis of Guillain-Barré syndrome unlikely in this patient?

The symptoms are not consistent with Guillain-Barré syndrome, which classically presents as an ascending paralysis, typically following an acute infectious process. Although Guillain-Barré syndrome is similar to MS in being an *inflammatory demyelinating disease*, it does not involve alterations in the CNS, such as plaques in the brain. Rather, it is due to demyelination of the peripheral nerves. In addition, Guillain-Barré syndrome is an acute illness; it does not relapse and remit as MS typically does.

3. What cell type is attacked and destroyed during an exacerbation of MS?

The oligodendrocytes, which provide the myelination in the CNS. Schwann cells provide myelination in the peripheral nervous system, but peripheral nerves are spared in MS.

Note: The peripheral Schwann cells are attacked in Guillain-Barré syndrome.

4. Would an EMG reveal slow, fast, or normal peripheral nerve conduction velocity in this patient?

Myelinated nerve fibers conduct impulses faster than unmyelinated nerve fibers, but since the peripheral nerves are not subject to demyelination in MS, the conduction speed of peripheral nerves would not be altered in this patient. However, in Guillain-Barré syndrome nerve conduction velocity may be reduced because of the demyelination.

5. Would you expect patients with MS to show signs of upper or lower motor neuron lesions when the motor system is involved?

They show upper motor neuron signs, because MS involves white matter in the brain and spinal cord (i.e., the CNS), and does not affect lower motor neurons.

CASE 9

A 70-year-old man presents with acute onset of paralysis and loss of sensation in his left leg and left flank, with slight weakness in the left arm. His past medical history is notable for hypertension, hyperlipidemia, and a 40-pack-year history of cigarette smoking. Urgent CT of the brain reveals no intracranial bleeding. Cerebral angiography is subsequently performed, and the site of arterial occlusion is identified. The patient is examined and questioned for contraindications (e.g., severe hypertension, recent GI bleeding, intracranial bleeding, recent surgery) to treatment with tissue plasminogen activator (tPA) and is cleared for thrombolytic therapy.

1. What is the diagnosis?

Ischemic stroke.

2. What are the two classifications of stroke? Which is more common? How do their etiologies differ?

The two major classifications of stroke are ischemic and hemorrhagic. Ischemic stroke is the more common of the two. **Ischemic strokes** result predominantly from atherosclerosis and subsequent thrombosis/embolism or from hypercoagulability in the left atrium (e.g., atrial fibrillation) or ventricle (after myocardial infarction) with subsequent embolus. **Hemorrhagic strokes** result predominantly from trauma, ruptured arteriovenous malformation, ruptured aneurysm, or vessel rupture due to hypertension. The distinction between the two types is important because hemorrhagic strokes are ruled out with CT before administration of tPA to restore perfusion in patients with ischemic stroke who are suitable candidates.

3. How does atrial fibrillation predispose to stroke?

Atrial fibrillation makes it easier for blood to pool and clot within the atria, and the clots can then embolize to the brain. For this reason patients with atrial fibrillation are routinely given the anticoagulant warfarin.

4. What artery was probably occluded in this patient? Explain.

The right anterior cerebral artery (or branches thereof) was probably occluded since it serves the motor and sensory cortex devoted to the contralateral (left) leg.

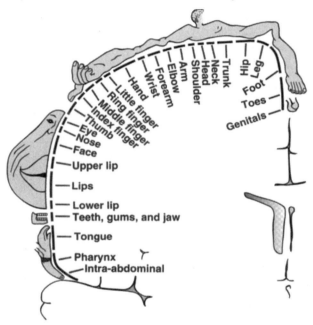

Coronal view of the brain showing body representation of different areas of motor and somatosensory cortex. (From Guyton AC, Hall JE: Textbook of Medical Physiology, 10th ed. Philadelphia, W.B. Saunders, 2000, with permission.)

5. What motor and sensory abnormalities may develop from occlusion of the middle cerebral artery or its branches?

The middle cerebral artery supplies the motor and sensory cortex for the contralateral upper extremity, head, neck and face. Occlusion can cause abnormalities in this distribution.

6. If a patient suddenly develops difficulty with understanding or articulating speech due to an ischemic stroke, branches of which major cerebral artery are most likely occluded?

The middle cerebral artery, typically on the left (dominant) side that controls speech. Difficulty with understanding speech (receptive aphasia) results from lesions in Wernicke's area and is called Wernicke's aphasia. Although people with this lesion can articulate, their speech is devoid of logical structure and often amounts to what is called a "word salad." Difficulty with articulating speech (expressive aphasia) without impaired comprehension is due to a lesion in Broca's area and is called Broca's aphasia. In this disorder it requires extreme effort to utter a single word.

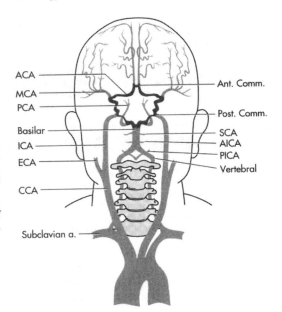

Coronal view of the extracranial and intracranial arterial supply to the the brain. ACA = anterior cerebral artery, AICA = anterior inferior cerebellar artery, Ant. Comm. = anterior communicating artery, CCA = common carotid artery, ECA = external carotid artery, ICA = internal carotid artery, MCA = middle cerebral artery, PCA = posterior cerebral artery, PICA = posterior inferior cerebral artery, Post. Comm. = posterior communicating artery, SCA = superior cerebellar artery. (From Andreoli TE (ed): Cecil Essentials of Medicine, 5th ed. Philadelphia, W.B. Saunders, 2001, with permission.)

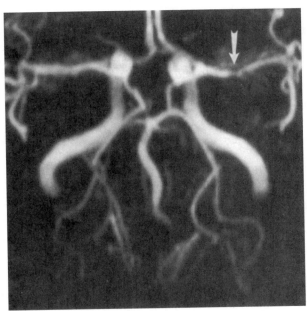

Stenosis resulting in partial occlusion of the left middle cerebral artery. (From Waclawik AJ, Sutula TP : Neurology Pearls. Philadelphia, Hanley & Belfus, 2000, p 177, with permission.)

7. How may occlusion of the right <u>posterior cerebral artery</u> or its branches cause loss of the left <u>visual</u> field of each eye (left homonymous hemianopsia)?

1. The posterior cerebral artery supplies the visual cortex in the occipital lobe. The visual cortex on the right receives sensory input from the nasal retina of the left eye and the temporal retina of the right eye, each of which receives sensory information from the left visual field.

2. A branch of each posterior cerebral artery also supplies the lateral geniculate nucleus on the same side, which is the major relay center from the optic tract to the visual cortex.

8. Occlusion of the most proximal segment of the anterior cerebral artery typically does not cause symptoms of stroke. Explain.

If the occlusion is proximal to the anterior communicating artery, collateral blood flow from the contralateral anterior cerebral artery through the communicating artery can prevent a perfusion deficit.

9. In a sudden hypotensive episode, what regions of cerebral circulation are particularly susceptible to infarction. Why?

The watershed areas—for example, the bordering zones between the regions of the brain that are supplied exclusively by the anterior cerebral artery or the middle cerebral artery.

10. What mechanism protects the brain tissue from inadequate perfusion during systemic hypotension?

The cerebral circulation is "autoregulated." By activating either vasodilation or vasoconstriction, the cerebral blood flow remains constant at mean arterial pressures ranging from 60 mmHg to 140 mmHg. This autoregulatory mechanism also protects the brain from excessive arterial pressure, which can cause vascular rupture and hemorrhage.

CASE 10

A 37-year-old man presents to the emergency department complaining of the "worst headache of my life." On questioning, he also complains of nausea and vomiting and states that bright lights bother him (photophobia). Physical examination reveals a stiff neck (nuchal rigidity). CT shows blood in the basal cisterns. Subsequently, cerebral angiography is performed and localizes the site of bleeding.

1. What is the diagnosis?

Subarachnoid hemorrhage.

Note: The basal cisterns are areas of expansion of the subarachnoid space.

2. If a CT scan does not reveal any characteristic bleeding into the subarachnoid space, what other diagnostic test can be done to establish the diagnosis?

A spinal tap. Blood in the cerebrospinal fluid (not due to a traumatic puncture) supports a diagnosis of subarachnoid hemorrhage.

Note: Because the spinal cord terminates at the level of L1–L2 in adults, spinal taps are performed at the level of the L3–L4 or L4–L5 interspace. An external landmark that helps to locate the L4 spinous process is the iliac crest.

3. What are the common causes of subarachnoid hemorrhage?

Ruptured berry aneurysm, ruptured arteriovenous malformation (AVM), and head trauma. Although we often associate ruptured aneurysms with subarachnoid hemorrhage, head trauma is actually the most common cause.

4. Why is a patient who presents with hematuria, bitemporal hemianopsia, and impaired renal function at increased risk for subarachnoid hemorrhage?

The patient may have polycystic kidney disease, which is associated with berry aneurysms, most commonly at the bifurcation of the anterior communicating artery. Berry aneurysms of the anterior communicating artery can compress the optic chiasm and cause visual deficits.

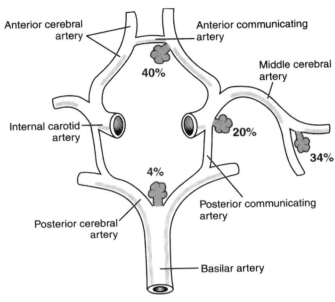

Frequency of aneurysmal sites. (From Cotran RS, Kumar V, Collins T (eds): Robbins Pathologic Basis of Disease, 6th ed. Philadelphia, W.B. Saunders, 1999, p 1131, with permission.)

CASE 11

The patient in the previous vignette managed to survive the subarachnoid hemorrhage after heroic neurosurgical procedures. However, several months later he develops severe headaches and difficulty with walking. In addition, his wife now complains that his memory has become very poor and that he has difficulty with paying attention to anything. Ophthalmic exam shows papilledema, and a CT of the brain is shown below.

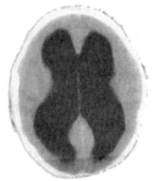

Massively dilated lateral ventricles. (From Lindsay KW, Bone I, Callander R (eds): Neurology and Neurosurgery Illustrated, 3rd ed. Edinburgh, Churchill Livingstone, 2002, p 362, with permission.)

1. **What is the diagnosis?**
   Hydrocephalus, most likely secondary to the previous subarachnoid hemorrhage.
   Note: About one-half of all cases of hydrocephalus are idiopathic; the other half develops after meningitis, subarachnoid hemorrhage, or intracranial surgery. Occasionally, hydrocephalus is produced by tumors of the CNS that obstruct cerebrospinal fluid flow (e.g., by compressing the cerebral aqueduct).

2. How is cerebrospinal fluid (CSF) produced? What is its function?

CSF is produced by an active secretory process (rather than mere filtration of plasma) in the choroid plexus of the lateral ventricles, third ventricle, and fourth ventricle.

3. Describe the pathway of CSF flow.

CSF flows from the lateral ventricles into the third ventricle via the foramen of Monroe (interventricular foramen). From the third ventricle it flows through the cerebral aqueduct (aqueduct of Sylvius) to the fourth ventricle. From the fourth ventricle it flows into the subarachnoid space via the lateral foramens of Lushka and the medial foramen of Magendie.

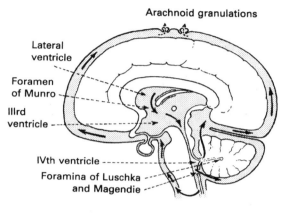

Pathway of cerebrospinal fluid flow. (From Lindsay KW, Bone I, Callander R (eds): Neurology and Neurosurgery Illustrated, 3rd ed. Edinburgh, Churchill Livingstone, 2002, p 360, with permission.)

4. What happens if the cerebral aqueduct is blocked?

Blockage of the cerebral aqueduct creates a backup of CSF in the ventricles, enlarging them. This process is called a noncommunicating hydrocephalus, because the CSF does not communicate with the subarachnoid space. On CT or MRI, the lateral and third ventricles are enlarged, but the fourth ventricle is not, because its outflow is not typically obstructed.

5. How is CSF reabsorbed?

CSF empties into the dural venous sinuses via arachnoid granulations.

6. What causes a communicating hydrocephalus?

If outflow of CSF from the subarachnoid space to the venous sinuses is obstructed (e.g., by fibrosis of the arachnoid granulations after a bout of meningitis), a communicating hydrocephalus develops.

CASE 12

A boy playing baseball is hit on the left side of the head by a pitch and falls unconscious. He quickly recovers consciousness and refuses to be taken to the hospital but agrees to sit out the rest of the game. After a few minutes he appears to act confused, lethargic, and disoriented, and an ambulance is called to take him to the hospital. Examination at the hospital shows a dilated left pupil, and a rapidly expanding mass between the dura and skull is seen on CT scan.

1. From what type of injury did the boy most likely suffer?

An epidural (extradural) hematoma, which is a result of intracranial bleeding that dissects the periosteal dura away from the skull.

Note: The dura mater is composed of a periosteal layer adherent to bone and a meningeal layer continuous with the arachnoid mater.

2. What vascular structures are typically involved in an epidural hematoma?

An epidural hematoma occurs when a blood vessel, usually an artery, ruptures between the outer membrane covering of the brain (the dura mater) and the skull. The middle meningeal artery is most commonly involved.

3. What are the three different layers of the meninges?

The outermost layer is the dura mater (*dura* = tough or durable), which is made of a fibrous connective tissue. The next layer is the arachnoid layer, which contains the subarachnoid space through which CSF flows through and blood vessels course. The innermost layer is the pia mater, which is attached directly to the brain parenchyma.

4. Would CSF analysis in this patient show multiple red blood cells? Explain your answer.

No, because blood from an epidural bleed does not reach the subarachnoid space, where CSF is located.

5. What vascular structures are typically involved in a subdural hematoma?

The bridging veins that interconnect the subarachnoid space and the dural (venous) sinuses. Subdural hematomas are more common in elderly people whose brains have atrophied. Since the atrophied brain can move around more freely in the skull, mild trauma, such as falling down, can tear the bridging veins more easily.

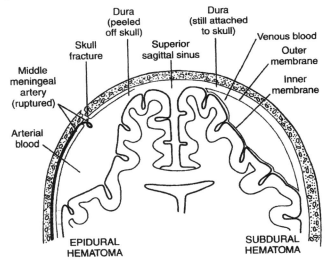

Vascular structures typically involved in a subdural hematoma. (From Cotran RS, Kumar V, Collins T (eds): Robbins Pathologic Basis of Disease, 6th ed. Philadelphia, W.B. Saunders, 1999, p 1305, with permission.)

6. Why do the symptoms of subdural hematomas typically develop slowly?

Because subdural hematomas result from tearing of the low-pressure bridging veins, it takes a while for blood to accumulate and cause compressive symptoms.

CASE 13

On awakening one morning, a 40-year-old woman realizes that she cannot grimace or blink her eye on the right side of her face. Her husband's voice seems particularly loud and is somewhat painful (hyperacusis) to listen to. He takes her to the emergency department, where specialized testing reveals an absent corneal reflex on the right side and a lack of taste sensation from the anterior two-thirds of the right side of her tongue.

1. What is the diagnosis?

Bell's palsy (facial paralysis), which is caused by paralysis of the facial nerve (generally due to inflammation within the facial canal). The facial nerve controls the muscles of facial expression, including blinking (orbicularis oculi) and grimacing (platysma).

2. Why does a mumps infection produce symptoms similar to those seen in Bell's palsy?

The parotid gland, through which the facial nerve travels, becomes inflamed (parotitis) in mumps.

3. Why does an acoustic neuroma (schwannoma) produce symptoms similar to those seen in Bell's palsy?

Acoustic neuromas (tumors of the Schwann cells of the eighth cranial nerve) commonly arise adjacent to the point where the facial nerve exits the pons. These tumors can compress the facial nerve at this location and should be suspected if a patient also presents with hearing loss or difficulties with balance.

4. Why is taste sensation absent from the anterior two-thirds of the right side of the tongue?

A branch of the facial nerve (technically, a branch of the trigeminal nerve that then joins with the facial nerve), the chorda tympani, provides taste sensation to this part of the tongue.

5. What causes the hyperacusis?

The hyperacusis is due to paralysis of the stapedius muscle, which functions to dampen the oscillations of the stapes against the oval window. The facial nerve innervates the stapedius.

6. Why is the corneal reflex absent?

The corneal reflex is blinking of the eye when the cornea is touched. Touch sensation from the cornea is carried by the ophthalmic division (V1) of the trigeminal nerve (afferent loop of reflex). The efferent part of the reflex is carried by the facial nerve and causes contraction of the orbicularis oculi, which closes the eyelid (blinking). Because the facial nerve is paralyzed, the efferent part of the reflex is defective.

7. If instead the patient could blink but had lower facial paralysis on the same side, where would the lesion be? Why?

She would have a lesion of the contralateral facial area of the motor cortex or its associated corticobulbar tract (i.e., an UMN lesion). The facial motor cortex with its upper motor neurons that send fibers through the corticobulbar tract to the facial motor nucleus provides the *only* motor input from the motor cortex to the contralateral lower face. Thus, disruption of this tract causes paralysis of the lower face. In contrast, the lower motor neurons in the facial motor nucleus that control the muscles of the upper face receive innervation from upper motor neurons in both cerebral hemispheres. Therefore, if one hemisphere with its facial motor cortex or corticobulbar tract is disrupted, the other hemisphere can still provide adequate innervation and motor control.

CASE 14

After hearing about how he failed the boards (because he did not use *USMLE Step 1 Secrets*) "Seizin' Steven" lost consciousness and wet his pants. His whole body became rigid. After a minute he started having rhythmic whole body jerks, while at the same time he was frothing at the mouth. After he quit seizing he was confused and lethargic for about an hour (postictal state). When he came to his senses, he decided to use a different review book the next time around.

1. What kind of seizure did Seizin' Steven have?

A generalized tonic-clonic seizure (previously called a grand-mal seizure). In this type of seizure both cerebral hemispheres initiate the process, with loss of consciousness and whole-body rigidity (tonic phase) followed by whole-body jerks (clonic phase).

2. What is the principal difference between a partial and a generalized seizure?

A partial seizure begins focally, within one cerebral hemisphere. It may secondarily become generalized, but it begins in one hemisphere. In contrast, a generalized seizure has its focus of onset diffusely throughout both hemispheres.

3. Differentiate the following seizure types in terms of origin in the brain and alteration in consciousness.

SEIZURE TYPE	SEIZURE ORIGIN	ALTERATION OF CONSCIOUSNESS
Partial	Focal (one cerebral hemisphere)	Yes or no
Simple partial	Focal	No
Complex partial	Focal	Yes
Generalized	Diffuse (both hemispheres)	Yes
Absence seizure	Diffuse	Yes
Tonic-clonic	Diffuse	Yes

4. Match the side effect with the anticonvulsants best known for causing them.

SIDE EFFECT	CAUSATIVE ANTICONVULSANT
Gingival hyperplasia, nystagmus, ataxia	Phenytoin
Hepatotoxicity, thrombocytopenia	Valproic acid
Stevens-Johnson syndrome	Lamotrigine, ethosuximide
Respiratory depression	Phenobarbital, diazepam
Agranulocytosis	Carbamazepine
Tremor	Gabapentin

Note: Ethosuximide is the first-line treatment for absence seizures and blocks calcium channels.

5. If this is Seizin' Steven's first seizure, can he be diagnosed with epilepsy?

No. Epilepsy indicates *recurrent unprovoked seizures*. "Unprovoked" means that the seizure is not secondary to medical illness (meningitis), toxic conditions (uremia), drug withdrawal (delirium tremens), fever (febrile seizures), head trauma, hyperventilation, or sleep deprivation. A diagnosis of epilepsy can be made only after he experiences another seizure and other possible causes have been ruled out.

6. What is an atonic seizure?

A seizure associated with sudden loss of muscle tone (i.e., *a*-tonic).

7. What effects do most anticonvulsants have on neuronal discharge?

They decrease the frequency of neuronal discharge by increasing the threshold required for neuronal discharge (i.e., they stabilize neuronal membranes). Most anticonvulsants achieve this goal by blocking sodium or calcium channels, but the benzodiazepines activate chloride channels to hyperpolarize neurons.

CASE 15

An 80-year-old woman has become increasingly demented over the past 10 years. She has difficulty with short-term memory (e.g., where she put her keys, recent conversations), but her long-term memory (e.g., of her earlier years) is good. When relating events that have happened to her recently she makes things up to fill the gaps in her memory but is unaware that she is doing so (confabulation). She has never had a stroke, and physical exam reveals no focal neurologic signs or other finding. A mini-mental status examination reveals that she is moderately demented.

1. What is the probable diagnosis?
Alzheimer's disease (AD), the most common cause of dementia in the elderly.

2. What specific pathologic microscopic findings are characteristic of this disease at autopsy?
Neurofibrillary tangles and neuritic senile plaques. Deposition of beta-amyloid proteins (amyloid angiopathy) may also be seen.

3. How would the pattern of cortical atrophy differ if the patient had Pick's disease?
Pick's disease is characterized by selective atrophy of the frontal and temporal lobes as opposed to the diffuse cerebral atrophy of AD.

4. What is the pathophysiologic rationale for treating AD with cholinesterase inhibitors?
AD is associated with selective destruction of cholinergic neurons (although other transmitter systems are variably affected). Cholinesterase inhibitors are believed to compensate for this destruction to some degree by increasing the concentration and prolonging the action of acetylcholine in the synaptic cleft.
Note: Donepezil is a new anticholinesterase used in AD that does not have the hepatotoxic effects of tacrine.

5. If the patient also suffered from depression, as many patients with AD do, why should we avoid prescribing tricyclic antidepressants?
Tricyclic antidepressants have powerful anticholinergic side effects that may exacerbate the cognitive decline due to AD. The newer selective serotonin reuptake inhibitors (SSRIs), therefore, are a much better choice for treating her depression.

6. Based on what you know about the regions of the brain that are selectively destroyed in AD, why would you expect long-term potentiation to be affected?
Long-term potentiation, which occurs in the hippocampus (among other locations), is currently believed to be the mechanism by which short-term memory is consolidated into long-term memory. The hippocampus is an early site of degeneration in AD, and this degeneration is believed to be one of the causes of memory loss.

7. What is the second most common cause of dementia in the elderly? How does it develop?
Multi-infarct dementia, which occurs because of the cumulative effect of multiple small or large infarcts. It often presents with focal neurologic deficits because of the infarcts. Such findings help to differentiate it from AD on clinical grounds.

CASE 16

A homeless alcoholic decides to check himself into a hospital to get something to eat. He enters the emergency department (ED) and uses his usual trick of complaining about "pain all over." However, he also honestly admits that his memory is getting increasingly worse and that he has difficulty standing up when sober. After sitting in the ED for a few hours, he appears to be confused and irritable and complains of a headache. A quick blood glucose test reveals hypoglycemia.

1. The patient is given intravenous glucose to relieve his hypoglycemic condition. Why should thiamine be administered immediately before glucose?

Thiamine deficiency is common in alcoholics. Thiamine is a necessary cofactor for pyruvate dehydrogenase, which catalyzes the conversion of pyruvate (from glucose breakdown) to acetyl CoA. In the absence of thiamine, pyruvate is converted to lactic acid by lactate dehydrogenase, causing lactic acidosis within the CNS, which is detrimental to neuronal cells.

Note: Acute CNS changes due to thiamine deficiency are called Wernicke's encephalopathy. However, *chronic* CNS changes due to thiamine deficiency, such as the longstanding memory impairment and unsteady gait of this patient, are part of what is termed Wernicke-Korsakov syndrome.

2. In the hospital the patient becomes agitated and develops anxiety, muscle cramps, tremors, delusions, and hallucinations. What is happening? What drugs may have prevented or may relieve these symptoms?

He is going through alcoholic withdrawal, the most severe manifestations of which are called delirium tremens. A long-acting benzodiazepine or barbiturate may have prevented withdrawal symptoms.

3. Explain why benzodiazepines and barbiturates are useful in treating alcoholic withdrawal.

Alcohol, benzodiazepines, and barbiturates bind to and activate the same receptor type, GABAa. When activated, this receptor opens a chloride channel, resulting in hyperpolarization. The net effect of this hyperpolarization is reduced neuronal excitability. However, if given for prolonged times or in large doses, any of these pharmacologic agents can cause desensitization of the GABA-ergic system. If these substances are then acutely withdrawn, the CNS becomes hyperexcitable, causing manifestations similar to what this patient experienced. Consequently, the benzodiazepines and barbiturates are effective in treating withdrawal because they are essentially "alcohol substitutes."

Note: The longer-acting benzodiazepines and barbiturates cause significantly milder withdrawal symptoms than the short-acting agents. The benzodiazepine antagonist flumazenil can be used for benzodiazepine overdoses.

4. Why do alcoholics often require a larger dose of benzodiazepines than healthy nonalcoholics to achieve the same pharmacologic effect?

Because they have developed cross-tolerance to other GABAa agonists. Alcohol consumption causes downregulation of the GABAa receptor, which makes GABAa agonists such as the benzodiazepines and barbiturates less effective.

5. Why is it dangerous to discharge this patient with a benzodiazapine or barbiturate prescription?

Because he is expected to resume alcohol abuse, the interactions of the benzodiazepines or barbiturates with alcohol can lead to respiratory depression and possibly even respiratory failure.

CASE 17

A 48-year-old woman complains of a new-onset headache that is worse in the morning. She also complains of nausea and has vomited several times in the past few weeks. Fundoscopic exam reveals papilledema, and neurologic exam reveals focal deficits with strength and sensory loss in her left arm. An MRI reveals a brain tumor in the right cerebral hemisphere. An extensive work-up does not reveal any primary tumor outside the CNS. A biopsy reveals the diagnosis of astrocytoma.

1. Before biopsy, why is a presumptive diagnosis of astrocytoma reasonable?

Astrocytoma is the most common *primary* brain tumor, although metastases are the most common sources of brain tumor overall. Biopsy must be done to distinguish between the two possibilities.

2. What is the worst grade of astrocytoma?

Gliobastoma multiforme. Lower grades of astrocytoma, such as juvenile pilocytic astrocytoma or anaplastic astrocytoma, may evolve into a glioblastoma multiforme.

Note: Glioblastoma multiforme has a characteristic *pseudopalisading arrangement* of tumor cells under the microscope and often crosses over into both hemispheres.

3. What pharmacologic property of drugs such as lomustine and carmustine make them more suitable for treatment of brain tumors?

These drugs belong to a class of alkylating agents called nitrosoureas and can effectively penetrate the blood-brain barrier.

4. What does the clinical finding of papilledema represent?

Edema of the optic disc, which is most commonly due to increased intracranial pressure, malignant hypertension, or central retinal vein occlusion. In this woman the papilledema is secondary to increased intracranial pressure.

5. What is a meningioma? How does it typically cause cognitive symptoms?

A meningioma is a benign tumor that arises from the arachnoid cells of the meninges. It often causes cognitive symptoms by compressing the underlying parenchyma. Because meningiomas are external to the brain, usually they can be surgically resected.

6. What is a medulloblastoma?

A malignant tumor of the cerebellum that most commonly occurs in young children.

7. What is the most common location of primary brain tumors in children? In adults?

Children: infratentorial (below the tentorium cerebelli)
Adults: supratentorial (above the tentorium cerebelli)

3. OPHTHALMOLOGY

Dave Brown and Thomas Brown

BASIC CONCEPTS

1. Describe the course of sensory information arriving from the left and right visual fields.

Sensory information from the **left visual field** initially hits the nasal retina (right side) of the left eye and temporal retina (right side) of the right eye. The fibers from the nasal retina of the left eye then traverse through the left optic nerve to the optic chiasm, and in the optic chiasm they cross over to the right optic tract, in which they traverse to the lateral geniculate nucleus on the right, and onward to the visual cortex in the occipital lobe on the right. The fibers from the temporal retina of the right eye run through the right optic nerve but do not cross over in the optic chiasm; instead, they continue along the right optic tract to the right lateral geniculate nucleus and on to the right visual cortext. Obviously, visual information coming from the **right visual field** will do exactly the opposite.

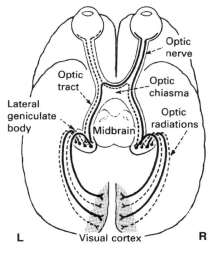

The left side (**L**) shows the course of sensory information from the left visual field. The right side (**R**) shows the course of sensory information from the right visual field. (From Lindsay KW, Bone I, Callander R (eds): Neurology and Neurosurgery Illustrated, 3rd ed. Edinburgh, Churchill Livingstone, 2002, p 129, with permission.)

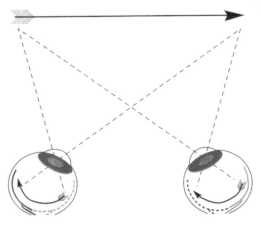

The temporal visual field is received by the nasal retina, and the nasal visual field is received by the temporal retina. (From Nolte J (ed): The Human Brain, 4th ed. St. Louis, Mosby, 1999, p 417, with permission.

49

2. What visual field defect results from midline sectioning of the optic chiasm? Explain.

Bitemporal hemianopsia, a loss of the temporal (lateral) field of vision in both eyes. Fibers from the nasal retina, which receive visual input from the lateral (temporal) fields of vision, cross over in the optic chiasm and are severed by a midline section of this structure.

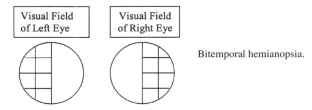

Bitemporal hemianopsia.

3. What visual field deficit results from sectioning of the left optic tract? Why?

Loss of the right field of vision in both eyes (right homonymous hemianopsia). The left optic tract receives input from the right nasal retina and left temporal retina, both of which receive their input from the right visual field of their respective eyes. (See figures in question 1).

4. In patients with a lesion in the left optic nerve, what is the pupillary response to shining a light in the left eye? In the right eye?

Left eye: no pupillary response by either eye, because no signal is transmitted to activate the reflex arc.

Right eye: pupillary constriction of both eyes, because the signal is transmitted and the efferent part of the reflex arc (oculomotor nerve) is intact for both eyes.

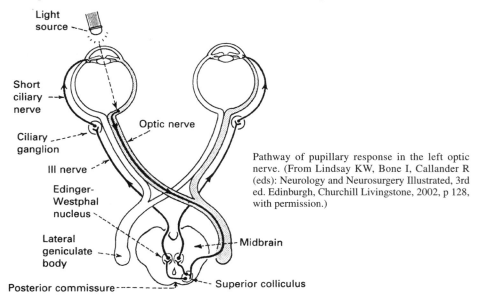

Pathway of pupillary response in the left optic nerve. (From Lindsay KW, Bone I, Callander R (eds): Neurology and Neurosurgery Illustrated, 3rd ed. Edinburgh, Churchill Livingstone, 2002, p 128, with permission.)

5. What will the pupillary response be to shining a light in either eye of patients with a lesion in the left oculomotor nerve?

Because both optic nerves and tracts and all the remainder of the afferent pathways are intact, the right pupil will constrict, but because of the lesion of the left oculomotor nerve, the left pupil will not constrict. If there is a lesion only in the right oculomotor nerve, the opposite would be true. (See figure above.)

6. If the oculomotor nerve is paralyzed on one side, why is the eyeball on that side rotated laterally and inferiorly?

The oculomotor nerve innervates all of the extraocular muscles but the lateral rectus (LR) and superior oblique (SO), which are innervated by the abducens nerve (CN VI) and trochlear nerve (CNIV), respectively (e.g., LR6SO4). The lateral rectus rotates the eyeball laterally, and the superior oblique rotates it inferiorly, giving the "down-and-out" position in oculomotor palsy. Note in the figure that the pupil is dilated also, as would be expected in oculomotor nerve palsy.

Eyeball (*left*) in a patient with oculomotor nerve palsy. (From Lindsay KW, Bone I, Callander R (eds): Neurology and Neurosurgery Illustrated, 3rd ed. Edinburgh, Churchill Livingstone, 2002, p 138, with permission.)

7. Why does retinoblastoma usually occur bilaterally in familial cases as opposed to unilaterally in sporadic cases?

For retinoblastoma to occur, the Rb gene on both chromosomes must mutate in a single cell. In familial cases, the Rb gene on the chromosome from the maternal or paternal side is already mutated in every cell. Therefore, all that is required is one mutation on the other chromosome in any cell of either retina for a tumor to develop in that retina. Because this event is highly probable, tumors commonly develop in both retinas. However, in sporadic cases it is quite unlikely that both chromosomes will be mutated in a single cell in both retinas.

CASE 1

A patient presents with gradually deteriorating vision and pain in both eyes. Fundoscopic exam reveals cupping of the optic nerve, and a tonometer measurement indicates significant elevation of the intraocular pressure.

1. What is the most likely diagnosis?

Glaucoma, a group of diseases associated with elevated intraocular pressures.

2. What is the difference between open-angle glaucoma and closed-angle glaucoma?

The "angle" refers to the junction of the cornea and the iris, where the aqueous humor drains out through the canal of Schlemm. In closed-angle glaucoma, outflow through the canal of Schlemm is obstructed; this obstruction increases the intraocular pressure. In open-angle glaucoma, the angle appears open, but drainage is still compromised. The precise reason for this functional obstruction remains unclear.

3. What is the mechanism by which beta blockers reduce intraocular pressure in glaucoma?

Beta blockers inhibit the secretion of aqueous humor, thereby lowering the intraocular pressure.

4. Describe the mechanism of action by which topical carbonic anhydrase agents (e.g., acetazolamide) can be used to treat glaucoma.

Carbonic anhydrase inhibitors also inhibit the production of aqueous humor, thereby lowering intraocular pressure, much like beta blockers.

5. Why are cholinomimetics such as carbachol and physostigmine useful for closed-angle glaucoma?

The sphincter pupillae is stimulated to constrict by parasympathetic cholinergic nerves. By causing the sphincter pupillae to constrict, cholinomimetics open the angle between the pupil and the cornea, allowing better drainage.

4. ENDOCRINE SYSTEM

Thomas Brown and Dave Brown

BASIC CONCEPTS

1. Describe the cellular mechanism of action of the steroid hormones.

Steroid hormones diffuse across the plasma membrane and form complexes with cytosolic or nuclear receptors (Fig. 1, next page). The bound complexes then activate transcription of various genes. Because steroid hormones rely on the intermediary process of gene expression and protein translation, it can take hours to days for their effects to manifest.

Note: Examples of steroid hormones include testosterone, estrogen, progesterone cortisol, and aldosterone. Cholesterol is the precursor to all steroid hormones. Although thyroid hormone is not a steroid hormone, it uses the same cellular mechanism as the steroids.

2. Describe the cellular mechanism of action of the peptide hormones and catecholamines.

The peptide hormones and catecholamines bind to cell surface receptors, which can then initiate a great diversity of biochemical events, including activating or inhibiting enzymes, altering membrane proteins, and affecting cellular trafficking (Fig. 2). These processes can occur rapidly, within seconds to minutes. Nevertheless, several peptide hormones can stimulate gene expression as well. This effect is delayed, as it is with the steroid hormones.

Note: Examples of peptide hormones include insulin, parathyroid hormone, vasopressin, and oxytocin.

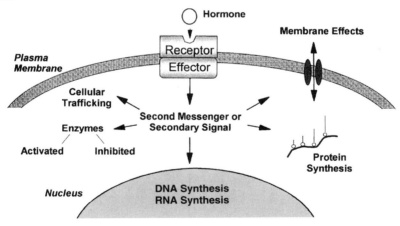

FIGURE 2. A general model for the action of peptide hormones, catecholamines, and other membrane-active hormones. The hormone in the extracellular fluid interacts with the receptor and activates an associated effector system (which may or may not be in the same molecule). This activation results in generation of an intracellular signal or second messenger that, through a variety of common and branched pathways, produces the final effects of the hormone on metabolic enzyme activity, protein synthesis, membrane transport, cellular trafficking, DNA and RNA synthesis, and cellular growth and differentiation. (From Williams Textbook of Endocrinology, 9th ed. Philadelphia, W.B. Saunders, 1998, p 96, with permission.)

3. Why is the total serum hormone level not an accurate reflection of hormone activity?

Many of the hormones in the serum are inactive because they are attached to serum binding proteins. Only the *free* hormone is biologically active. Another important factor that affects

53

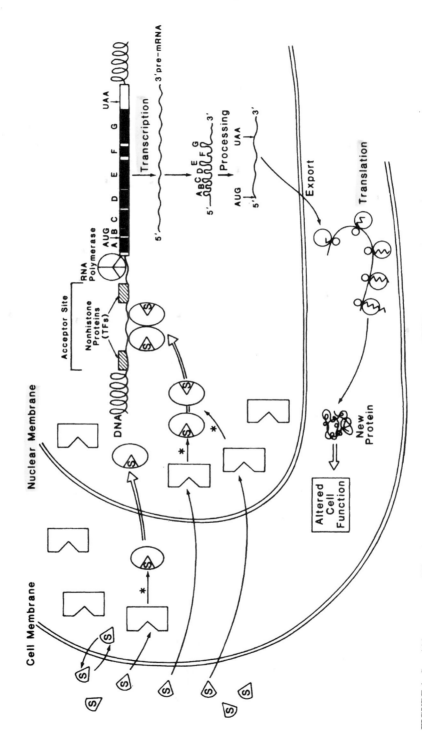

FIGURE 1. Steroid hormones can diffuse freely across the cell membrane because they are lipophilic. They then bind to cytosolic or nuclear receptors, forming complexes that can activate transcription various genes. (From Williams Textbook of Endocrinology. 9th ed. Philadelphia, W.B. Saunders, 1998, p 56, with permission.)

hormone activity is the concentration of cellular hormone receptors available for binding and mediating the action of a specific hormone.

4. How does a hormone binding to the same type of receptor have different effects in different cell types?

Different tissues are different because they express different genes (i.e., differential transcription). Therefore, although different target tissues may express the same hormone receptor, they may also express entirely different downstream protein targets. For example, by binding the same beta$_2$-adrenergic receptors, epinephrine is able to elicit a host of different physiologic responses depending on the tissue location of that receptor (e.g., glycogenolysis in the liver, lipolysis in adipose tissue).

5. List the primary classes of receptors to which peptide hormones bind.

The four primary classes of membrane-spanning receptors to which peptide hormones bind are (1) tyrosine and serine kinase receptors, (2) receptor-linked kinases, (3) G-protein-coupled receptors, and (4) ligand-gated ion channels (Fig. 3). As a gross simplification, the "prototypical" agonists for these receptor types can be considered as growth factors, growth hormones, peptide hormones, and neurotransmitters, respectively.

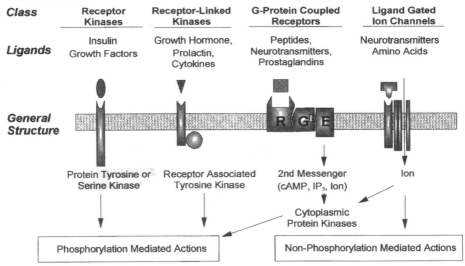

FIGURE 3. The four major classes of membrane receptors for hormones and neurotransmitters. Many growth factors, including insulin, bind to cell-surface receptors that act as protein tyrosine kinases, stimulating the phosphorylation of proteins on tyrosine residues. Growth hormone, prolactin, and many cytokines act on receptors that associate with cytoplasmic tyrosine kinases. A third class of agonists binds to receptors (R) that are coupled to separate effector (E) molecules by G proteins (G). The fourth major class of receptors includes ligand-gated ion channels. Some of these are self-contained; in others, the receptor and the ion channel are coupled by G proteins.

6. How do the receptor kinases and receptor-linked kinases transduce their messages?

As depicted in the diagram above, signal transduction via activation of these receptors involves phosphorylation of downstream target proteins, which are thereby activated or inhibited. A kinase is an enzyme that phosphorylates other proteins.

7. How do the ligand gated ion channels work?

Activation of ligand-gated ion channels results in an influx (or efflux) of ions into (or out of) the cell. The nicotinic receptor on skeletal muscle is an example of such a receptor. Binding of acetylcholine to this receptor results in an influx of principally sodium ions into the cell.

8. How do the G-proteins transduce their signals?

Binding of hormone/agonist to G-protein-coupled receptors causes an alpha-beta-gamma subunit complex to exchange guanosine diphosphate (GDP) for guanosine triphosphate (GTP) (Fig. 4). Once GTP is bound to the subunit complex, it dissociates into the alpha subunit and a separate beta-gamma subunit. These dissociated subunits then activate or inhibit enzymes (adenylate cyclase, phospholipase) and ion channels (Ca^{2+} channels).

Note: Adenylate cyclase synthesizes cyclic adenosine monophosphate (cAMP) from adenosine triphosphate (ATP), and the cAMP activates various target proteins. Gs receptors stimulate adenylate cyclase, whereas Gi receptors inhibit adenylate cyclase.

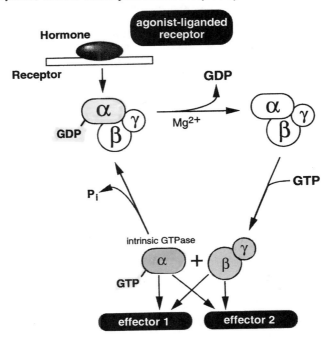

FIGURE 4. G protein signal transduction. In the absence of ligand binding to the receptor, the heterotrimer G protein ($\alpha\beta\gamma$) binds GDP via its alpha subunit but apparently without interaction with receptor effectors. Formation of the hormone receptor or agonist-liganded receptor complex results in interaction of the receptor and G protein and subsequent replacement of GDP with GTP in the presence of magnesium. At this point, the GTP-bound activated alpha subunit dissociates from the beta-gamma subunit. Then either one or both contact effectors and modulate their activities. Simultaneously, the intrinsic GTPase activity of the alpha subunit hyrodlyzes GTP to GDP, which terminates peptide hormone signaling. (From Williams Textbook of Endocrinology, 9th ed. Philadelphia, W.B. Saunders, 1998, p 117, with permission.)

9. How do endocrine, paracrine, and autocrine mechanisms of cell communication differ?

Endocrine secretions (i.e., hormones) affect their target organs at considerable distance from their site of secretion; thus, they must be carried by the bloodstream. Paracrine secretions act locally on adjacent cells and tissues. Paracrine communication seems particularly important in endocrine tissues, such as the pancreatic islets, where constant communication between adjacent cells (e.g., alpha and delta cells) is critical for optimal functioning. Autocrine secretions are secretions from a cell that bind to receptors on the same cell and exert regulatory actions on that cell.

Note: Neuroendocrine secretions involve the secretion of peptides into the blood from specialized neurons (hence the term neuroendocrine). Hypothalamic peptides released into the blood from the terminal boutons of axons located in the posterior pituitary are one example of this mechanism of regulation.

CASE 1

A 38-year-old woman developed a massive postpartum hemorrhage, for which she was eventually stabilized with multiple blood transfusions and crystalloids. A few weeks later she complains that she has not been able to lactate since delivering her baby. She also feels lethargic and weak and often gets dizzy when she stands up. Physical exam is unremarkable except for the fact that her axillary and pubic hairs seem a little sparser than before. Injection of corticotropin-releasing hormone (CRH) causes only a blunted elevation of serum levels of adenocorticotropic hormone (ACTH). Similarly, injection of a gonadotropin-releasing hormone (GnRH) analog causes only a blunted elevation of follicle-stimulating hormone (FSH) and luteinizing hormone (LH). Serum prolactin was abnormally low as well. A magnetic resonance imaging (MRI) study of the brain reveals necrosis of the anterior pituitary.

1. What is the diagnosis?

Sheehan's syndrome (or postpartum necrosis), which is an infarction of the anterior pituitary.

2. Why is the pituitary more susceptible to infarction in postpartum hemorrhage than in hemorrhagic shock unrelated to pregnancy?

Pregnancy is associated with hyperplasia of the lactotrophs (prolactin-secreting cells) in the anterior pituitary (adenohypophysis), which increases this tissue's minimal perfusion needs. In postpartum hemorrhage, the blood supply to the anterior pituitary may become inadequate to meet this increased need; the result is infarction.

3. Why is the posterior pituitary typically spared in Sheehan's syndrome?

The posterior pituitary (neurohypophysis) has a different embryologic origin from the anterior pituitary and therefore has a different blood supply. The embryologic origin of the anterior pituitary is Rathke's pouch (an endodermal evagination from the roof of the mouth), whereas the posterior pituitary is derived from a ventral outgrowth from the primitive hypothalamus.

Note: Because both vasopressin and oxytocin are secreted by the posterior pituitary, these hormones are rarely affected in Sheehan's syndrome. Craniopharyngiomas are thought to arise from remnants of Rathke's pouch.

4. Secretion of which pituitary hormones may be affected in this patient?

The hormones secreted by the anterior pituitary include FSH, LH, thyroid-stimulating hormone (TSH), growth hormone (GH), ACTH, and prolactin (Fig. 5, next page). Depending on the extent of the infarction, all may be affected. The patient's inability to lactate is consistent with decreased prolactin secretion; sparse axillary and pubic hairs are consistent with decreased gonadotropin (FSH, LH) secretion; and weakness and lethargy are consistent with decreased secretion of ACTH, which causes hypocortisolism.

5. Why may infarction of the anterior pituitary result in increased secretion of hypothalamic-releasing hormones?

The loss of pituitary hormone secretion decreases negative feedback on the hypothalamic hormones both from low pituitary hormone levels and from low target organ hormone production. These releasing hormones include corticotropin-releasing hormone (CRH), growth hormone-releasing hormone (GHRH), thyrotropin-releasing hormone (TRH), and gonadotropin-releasing hormone (GnRH).

6. True or false: An anterior pituitary infarction also leads to increased secretion of hypothalamic dopamine. Explain.

False. In contrast to the other hypothalamic hormones, dopamine is inhibitory in nature and reduces the secretion of prolactin by the lactotrophs. Because serum prolactin normally stimulates dopamine secretion from the hypothalamus, in a setting of hypoprolactinemia secondary to pituitary infarction, we would expect decreased secretion of hypothalamic dopamine.

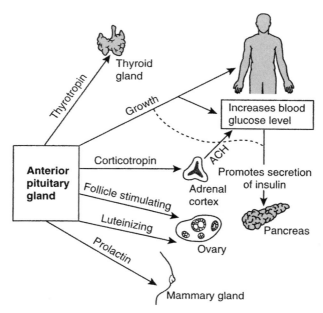

FIGURE 5. Metabolic functions of the anterior pituitary hormones. (From Textbook of Medical Physiology, 10th ed. Philadelphia, W.B. Saunders, 200, p 847, with permission.)

CASE 2

A 32-year-old woman complains of recent visual problems and slight breast discharge (galactorrhea). She has not had her period for the past 6 months (amenorrhea). She is upset that she has been unable to become pregnant, despite trying for the past year with her husband. She denies any history of schizophrenia or treatment with phenothiazines. A pregnancy test is negative. Levels of thyroxine (T$_4$) and TSH are normal, but significantly elevated levels of prolactin are found. Subsequently, an MRI of the head shows enlargement of the structure located in the sella turcica.

1. **What is the most likely diagnosis?**
   Prolactinoma (a pituitary adenoma caused by abnormal proliferation of lactotrophs).
   Note: The pituitary is situated in the sella turcica.

2. **What are the normal physiologic functions of prolactin during and after pregnancy?**
   Prolactin functions primarily to stimulate breast maturation and milk production. Following delivery prolactin levels increase further only in response to suckling by the baby. Suckling stimulates prolactin secretion, which stimulates milk production by the breasts in preparation for the next feeding. In addition, prolactin secretion in the breast-feeding mother helps prevent future pregnancies.

3. **Why does the patient have galactorrhea, whereas pregnant women with a similar level of serum prolactin generally do not?**
   Although prolactin stimulates milk production, the high concentrations of estrogen and progesterone that are present during pregnancy inhibit this effect. In contrast, this patient has hyperprolactinemia in the absence of elevated levels of estrogen and progesterone, which causes galactorrhea.

Note: Milk letdown occurs after childbirth because during pregnancy the placenta makes most of the estrogen and progesterone. Levels of both hormones decrease after this structure is expelled in delivery. In addition, oxytocin is secreted in response to suckling and stimulates contraction of myoepithelial cells around the glandular tissue of the breast, causing milk ejection.

4. How does an elevated prolactin level prevent pregnancy? In other words, what is the mechanism of infertility and amenorrhea in this patient?

Prolactin inhibits the hypothalamic release of GnRH, which is a stimulus for FSH and LH secretion. The consequent reduction of FSH and LH eliminates the ovulatory cycle, resulting in infertility and amenorrhea.

Note: Elevated prolactin levels in men can cause impotence and infertility through a similar mechanism, except in this case testosterone is lowered as a result of the decreased LH.

5. Why are questions about a history of schizophrenia and use of antipsychotic medications relevant to the diagnostic work-up of this patient?

Many antipsychotics (particularly the typical antipsychotics) can cause hyperprolactinemia. This effect makes sense if it is recalled that antipsychotics are dopamine antagonists and that hypothalamic dopamine is the major inhibitor of pituitary prolactin secretion.

6. What is the mechanistic basis for using bromocriptine (an antiparkinson agent) in the medical treatment of prolactinoma?

Bromocriptine is a dopamine agonist that inhibits prolactin secretion by the anterior pituitary. Recall that Parkinson's disease is caused by a lack of striatal dopamine.

7. How can head trauma with a severed pituitary stalk cause a similar increase in prolactin (assuming that the anterior pituitary itself was not damaged)?

This effect is due to disruption of the tuberoinfundibular tract, which runs from the hypothalamus through the pituitary stalk and is the source of dopamine that inhibits prolactin release.

Note: Plasma levels of all other anterior pituitary hormones (e.g., TSH, ACTH) decrease with a severed pituitary stalk.

8. Why was hypothyroidism ruled out in this woman before making a diagnosis of prolactinoma?

Hypothalamic TRH stimulates secretion of both prolactin and TSH by the anterior pituitary. Hypothyroidism causes elevated levels of TRH and should be ruled out as a cause of hyperprolactinemia.

CASE 3

A 38-year-old man complains of gradually enlarging hands and feet over the past several years. He shows a picture of himself 10 years ago, and in comparison his facial features have become obviously coarsened. Lab studies show fasting hyperglycemia and a significantly elevated serum level of insulin growth factor-1 (IGF-1). In addition, an oral glucose load does not cause the usual suppression of growth hormone secretion. An MRI of the brain reveals a pituitary adenoma.

1. What is the diagnosis?

Acromegaly, caused by a growth hormone-secreting tumor.

2. Why is hyperglycemia commonly associated with this disease?

Growth hormone secretion increases serum glucose levels and is one of the body's mechanisms for preventing serious hypoglycemia. The elevation of blood glucose can be significant enough in acromegaly that many of these patients will have clinical diabetes. For normal individuals, a glucose load will cause almost complete suppression of growth hormone secretion, but it will not suppress growth hormone secretion as much or at all by an independently functioning pituitary adenoma that is secreting growth hormone.

3. What causes the elevated levels of IGF-1 in this patient?

Growth hormone stimulates the secretion of IGF-1 from the liver, and this hormone mediates many of the effects of growth hormone (Fig. 6).

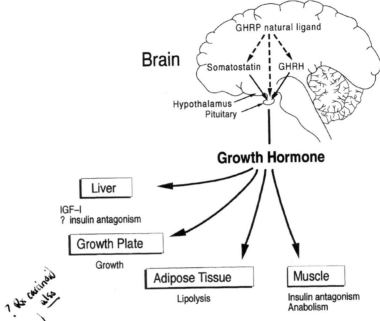

FIGURE 6. Multiple sites of growth hormone action. ((From Williams Textbook of Endocrinology, 9th ed. Philadelphia, W.B. Saunders, 1998, p 262, with permission.)

4. Why is octreotide, a somatostatin analog, useful in the treatment of acromegaly?

Somatostatin is an endogenous inhibitor of growth hormone secretion that is secreted by the hypothalamus (Fig. 7, next page), and its analog is effective in reducing GH levels. Of interest, somatostatin is also synthesized by pancreatic islets and gastric mucosa and has an inhibitory effect on intestinal activity and gastrointestinal motility.

5. If this patient developed a growth hormone-secreting tumor in his early teens, how might the clinical manifestations differ?

Growth hormone stimulates bone growth, and if the epiphyseal plates have not yet closed, excessive growth hormone can result in extremes of body height. When this effect occurs, the disease is called gigantism.

6. What growth abnormality results from deficient secretion of growth hormone during the growing years?

Dwarfism. The most common cause is deficient growth hormone secretion.

Note: The dwarfism caused by deficient growth hormone secretion is proportional (the limbs and trunk are of normal relative proportions), as opposed to the comparatively shorter limbs that are found in dwarfism caused by achondroplasia.

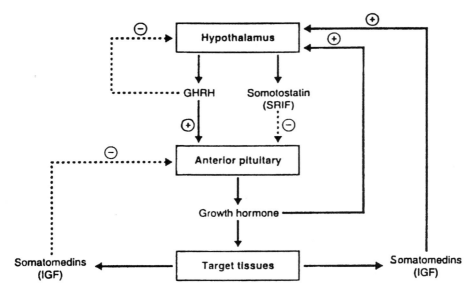

FIGURE 7. Regulation of growth hormone secretion. Somatostatin, which inhibits growth hormone secretion, is secreted by the hypothalamus in response to elevated levels of growth hormone and insulin growth fact, creating a negative feedback loop. Elevated serum levels of insulin growth factor also inhibit anterior pituitary secretion of growth hormone. (From STARS Physiology. {Philadelphia, W.B. Saunders, 1998, p 352, with permission.)

CASE 4

A 35-year-old woman, is seen for a pre-employment physical exam. She has not seen a doctor in several years and complains of fatigue, weakness, hip pain, and amenorrhea for the past 6 months. On exam, the physician notes muscle wasting in her extremities, central obesity, a moon-like facies and dorsocervical fat pad ("buffalo hump"), purple cutaneous striae on the abdomen, hypertension, and hirsutism. Lab tests show hyperglycemia, elevated morning levels of plasma cortisol, elevated levels of ACTH at 5 AM, hypokalemia, and an elevated 24-hour urinary free cortisol (UFC). Radiographs of her hip demonstrate marked osteoporosis. She is referred to an endocrinologist, who orders a dexamethasone suppression test. The results show that morning plasma levels of cortisol decrease negligibly in response to low-dose dexamethasone but significantly in response to high-dose dexamethasone.

1. What is the diagnosis?

Cushing's syndrome, which results from hypercortisolism of any cause. More specifically, this patient's hypercortisolism is from Cushing's disease, which is due to pituitary hypersecretion of ACTH from a pituitary adenoma or corticotroph hyperplasia.

Note: The most common cause of Cushing's syndrome is prescription of corticosteroids (iatrogenic).

2. Explain why the patient has Cushing's disease as opposed to excessive cortisol production by an autonomous adrenal tumor or ectopic production of ACTH by a different tumor (e.g., small cell carcinoma).

Because an elevated level of ACTH is the cause of her hypercortisolism, she cannot have an adrenal adenoma or carcinoma. The excessive cortisol produced by the adrenal gland in such cases would cause reduced pituitary ACTH secretion by negative feedback. In addition, dexamethasone (a synthetic corticosteroid) would not suppress the cortisol production by an autonomous adrenal tumor. High doses of dexamethasone would also have no effect on ectopic production of ACTH by tumors because no negative feedback mechanism is available. High-dose dexamethasone, however, can suppress ACTH production by the pituitary in Cushing's disease, as observed in this patient.

CAUSE OF CUSHING'S SYNDROME	ACTH	CORTISOL	EFFECTS OF DEXAMETHASONE SUPPRESSION TEST ON PLASMA CORTISOL
Cushing's disease	High	High	High dose lowers cortisol
Ectopic ACTH production	High	High	No effect
Adrenal adenoma/carcinoma	Low	High	No effect
Iatrogenic	Low	High	No effect

Note: Dexamethasone is a synthetic glucocorticoid that is approximately 30 times more potent than cortisol. The small-cell (oat-cell) type of bronchogenic carcinoma is one of the most common causes of ectopic ACTH production.   *and ADH*

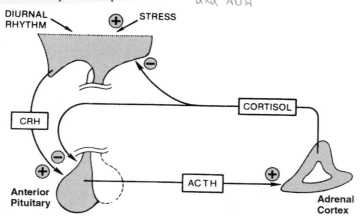

FIGURE 8. Circadian regulation of the hypothalamic-pituitary-adrenal axis. The plus sign (+) indicates that stress stimulates corticotropin-releasing hormone (CRH), that CRH stimulates adrenocorticotropin hormone (ACTH), and that ACTH stimulates cortisol (feedforward control). The minus sign (–) indicates the cortisol inhibits CRH and ACTH release (negative feedback). (From Hedge GA, Colby HD, Goodman RL: Clinical Endocrine Physiology. Philadelphia, W. B. Saunders, 1987, with permission.)

3. Why are the results of a dexamethasone suppression test read at a specific time of day?

Cortisol secretion has a wide circadian rhythm, with plasma levels varying several-fold throughout a 24-hour period (normal range: 5–20 mg/dl) and peaking in the morning hours. The morning upsurge is necessarily preceded by an upsurge in ACTH; thus, ACTH levels should also be measured at a specific time (usually 5 AM).

4. Why has hirsutism developed in this patient?

Hirsutism is the presence of excessive facial and body hair in women, especially in a male pattern, and typically reflects elevated androgen levels in women. Elevated androgen levels in this patient resulted from elevated levels of plasma ACTH, which, in addition to stimulating cortisol synthesis by the adrenals, also stimulates the synthesis and secretion of androgens by the adrenals.

5. Why is hyperaldosteronism not typically seen in Cushing's disease?

Although aldosterone is secreted by the adrenal cortex, its synthesis and secretion are influenced only minimally by ACTH levels. Rather, the principal stimulators of aldosterone secretion are angiotensin II and serum potassium.

6. What morphologic feature of the adrenal glands would you expect to see in this patient?

Bilateral adrenal hyperplasia is typically seen because ACTH is trophic for the adrenal glands. This finding is also present with ectopic production of ACTH.

7. How does hypercortisolism contribute to hyperglycemia?

Cortisol causes hyperglycemia by stimulating hepatic gluconeogenesis and inhibiting the peripheral utilization of glucose. The increase in gluconeogenesis is due to the fact that cortisol stimulates the synthesis of gluconeogenic enzymes and also to greater mobilization of amino acids from skeletal muscle to participate in gluconeogenesis (hence the muscle wasting).

8 How does hypercortisolism contribute to hypertension and hypokalemia?

At higher plasma levels, cortisol exerts mineralocorticoid effects similar to those of aldosterone. The results are sodium retention and an ensuing plasma volume expansion that contributes to hypertension. The sodium is retained in exchange for secreting more potassium, which explains the patient's hypokalemia. Another contributing factor to the patient's hypertension is that cortisol stimulates the expression of adrenergic receptors in vascular smooth muscle.

9. Why doesn't cortisol have mineralocorticoid actions in the normal physiologic setting?

Cortisol can bind mineralocorticoid receptors with an affinity similar to that of aldosterone, but cells in mineralocorticoid-sensitive tissues (kidneys, colon, salivary glands) produce enzymes that inactivate cortisol. When the plasma cortisol is significantly elevated, these enzymes become saturated, thereby allowing intracellular cortisol to exert its mineralocorticoid effects. This process explains the plasma volume expansion and hypertension discussed above.

10. How does hypercortisolism contribute to osteoporosis?

Cortisol inhibits osteoblasts and stimulates osteoclasts—a double whammy.

11. What are the three layers of the adrenal cortex? Which layer is responsible for the excess production of cortisol in this patient?

Think of the mnemonic **GFR:** the zona **g**lomerulosa, zona **f**asciculata, and zona **r**eticularis, which secrete mineralocorticoids (e.g., aldosterone), glucocorticoids (e.g., cortisol), and androgens (e.g., dehydroepiandrosterone [DHEA]), respectively.

CASE 5

An 18-year-old man complains of extreme fatigue and weakness that developed gradually over the past 6 months. His blood pressure is 90/55 mmHg, and he has hyperpigmentation of the skin and buccal mucosa. His morning plasma cortisol level is depressed, the 5 AM ACTH level is increased, and injection of ACTH elicits only a blunted increase in plasma cortisol. He also has hyponatremia, hyperkalemia, and hypoglycemia. He is started on routine hydrocortisol and fludrocortisone.

1. What is the diagnosis?

Addison's disease, or primary adrenocortical insufficiency.

Note: Addison's disease is most commonly caused by autoimmune destruction of the adrenal cortices.

2. Why can adrenocortical insufficiency cause hypotension?

Aldosterone and cortisol, both of which are adrenal corticosteroids, contribute to blood pressure maintenance. Aldosterone stimulates sodium retention and with it plasma volume expansion. At higher doses, cortisol has mineralocorticoid activities like aldosterone and in addition stimulates alpha-1 receptor expression in smooth muscle.

3. Why is ACTH increased?

Loss of negative feedback due to the low plasma cortisol levels.

4. Why do both the previous patient (with Cushing's disease) and this patient (with Addison's disease) have hyperpigmentation?

The common denominator for both diseases is elevated ACTH production. The elevated ACTH may lead to hyperpigmentation by two potential mechanisms. First, the gene product from which ACTH is made also contains melanocyte-stimulating hormone (MSH); whenever more ACTH is produced, more MSH is produced, thus enhancing skin pigmentation. Second, elevated ACTH itself may cause direct stimulation of melanocyte receptors.

5. What adrenal disease should be suspected in a young patient with bacterial meningitis due to *Neisseria meningitidis* who also becomes acutely hypotensive?

Waterhouse-Friderichsen syndrome, typically caused by hemorrhagic destruction of the adrenals by *N. meningitidis*.

6. How would we expect plasma aldosterone levels to be affected in a patient with adrenal insufficiency secondary to decreased pituitary ACTH secretion (secondary adrenal insufficiency)?

Because aldosterone secretion is primarily stimulated by angiotensin II and serum potassium and because ACTH has little influence, aldosterone continues to be secreted at essentially normal levels.

CASE 6

A 21-year-old man complains of intermittent episodes in which he experiences severe headaches, dizziness, forceful heartbeats (palpitations), and sweating. He describes experiencing a fear of "impending death" during these episodes. He denies any history of cocaine or amphetamine abuse. Blood pressure measured at the beginning of the patient encounter was 120/70 mmHg, but he developed symptoms 30 minutes later, during which his blood pressure increased to 200/120 mmHg. Blood work reveals hyperglycemia, and a 24-hour urine sample shows elevated levels of vanillylmandelic acid (VMA). Positron emission tomography (PET) shows a highly vascular mass above the left kidney. He is prescribed antihypertensive therapy that includes prazosin and propranolol and informed that surgical correction can offer a cure.

1. What is the diagnosis?

Pheochromocytoma, a tumor that generally arises from chromaffin cells of the adrenal medulla.

2. What does the elevated urinary VMA indicate?

VMA is a product of catecholamine metabolism. Elevated 24-hour urinary levels indicate increased daily production of catecholamines. Metanephrine, another catecholamine metabolite, is also commonly increased in the urine of patients with pheochromocytoma, as are free catecholamines.

3. How can administration of clonidine be used to differentiate a pheochromocytoma from excessive cathecholamine production due simply to increased sympathoadrenal stimulation?

Clonidine is a centrally acting alpha-2 agonist that inhibits sympathetic outflow from the central nervous system, and its administration results in reduced production of epinephrine and norepinephrine by the sympathoadrenal system. In contrast, the catecholamine production of a pheochromocytoma is unaffected by this maneuver.

4. Norepinephrine and epinephrine increase the rate and force of cardiac contraction by binding to what type of receptors on the heart?

$Beta_1$-adrenergic receptors on nodal cells (positive chronotropic effect) and cardiac myocytes (positive inotropic effect). For this reason, a beta blocker, such as propranolol, is used as part of the management of hypertension in patients with pheochromocytoma.

(Zosins) : α_1 = periph vasc. sm m. constr d
β_2 = sk m. vasc. sm. m. dilation

5. How do elevated levels of epinephrine cause hyperglycemia?

In the liver, epinephrine stimulates hepatic glycogenolysis and gluconeogenesis. In the pancreas, it inhibits the release of insulin and stimulates the release of glucagon. In muscle, it inhibits cellular glucose uptake but activates glycolysis to generate lactate and alanine as gluconeogenic precursors. Finally, in fatty tissue it stimulates lipolysis, and the liberated fatty acids can be used as a substitute in many tissues for serum glucose.

6. The patient's blood pressure was normalized with phenoxybenzamine before surgery for tumor removal. How does this drug work?

Phenoxybenzamine is an irreversible, noncompetitive antagonist of $alpha_1$-adrenergic receptors. Because of its irreversible binding of $alpha_1$-adrenergic receptors, it is preferred over other $alpha_1$ blockers in preoperative preparation. It minimizes the hypertensive effects of catecholamines released during surgery.

7. Which antihypertensive drugs competitively antagonize $alpha_1$ receptors? Where do they exhibit their effect?

The "osins", which include doxazosin, terazosin, and prazosin, are $alpha_1$ receptor antagonists. These receptors are located predominantly on vascular smooth muscle.

8. Why might treatment with nonselective beta blockers precipitate a hypertensive crisis in this patient?

In addition to blocking the $beta_1$ receptors on the heart, nonselective beta blockers antagonize the effects of epinephrine on the vasodilatory $beta_2$-adrenergic receptors located in the vascular beds of skeletal muscle. Consequently, plasma epinephrine will not affect these $beta_2$ receptors, because they are blocked. Instead, it will bind primarily to the vasoconstrictor $alpha_1$-adrenergic receptors, thereby raising the blood pressure.

9. Why was this patient given propranolol, a nonselective beta blocker, if it can cause a hypertensive crisis?

He was also given prazosin, which is an $alpha_1$ receptor antagonist and can prevent this problem. In fact, it is important to achieve alpha blockade first with a drug such as prazosin before beta blockers are even started in order to avoid such a hypertensive crisis.

10. On a related note, what class of antihypertensive agents, if given prior to epinephrine, would make it so that epinephrine actually lowered the blood pressure?

Questions such as this one are board favorites because they stress a broad conceptual understanding of physiology and pharmacology. In this case, the initial administration of $alpha_1$ blockers (e.g., prazosin) will "block" all of the $alpha_1$ receptors, leaving only beta-adrenergic receptors available for binding to subsequently administered epinephrine. Stimulation of $beta_2$-adrenergic receptors results in vasodilation, which lowers peripheral vascular resistance and causes a drop in blood pressure.

CASE 7

A 40-year-old woman complains of easy fatigability, heat intolerance, excessive sweating, and palpitations. Her history is significant for a recent 20-lb weight loss, although she states that her appetite has actually increased. She admits to an increased frequency of bowel movements and occasional bouts of diarrhea. Physical exam is significant for blood pressure of 165/75 mmHg, a systolic ejection murmur, and tachycardia as well as diffuse nontender enlargement of the thyroid, slight resting tremor, fine hair, separation of the fingernail plate from the nail bed (onycholysis), and brisk reflexes. Lab tests reveal elevated free plasma T_4 and reduced TSH.

1. What is the diagnosis?

Hyperthyroidism.

2. What is the difference between primary and secondary hyperthyroidism? Which does this patient have?

Primary hyperthyroidism results from excessive production of thyroid hormones by the thyroid gland, which in turn suppresses pituitary TSH production. In contrast, secondary hyperthyroidism results from excessive pituitary secretion of TSH.

3. What additional laboratory and physical findings would you expect in the most common cause of hyperthyroidism?

Graves' disease is the most common cause and is additionally characterized by exophthalmos, pretibial myxedema, and antibodies to the TSH receptor in the thyroid. The antibodies presumably stimulate the thyroid in the same way as TSH does. Note that this patient had a diffusely enlarged thyroid, which is consistent with TSH receptor stimulation causing diffuse thyroid gland enlargement.

Note: Pretibial myxedema is a nonpitting edema caused by accumulation of interstitial glycosaminoglycans (GAGs) within the dermis. Paradoxically, myxedema can also be seen in severe hypothyroidism. Toxic multinodular goiter and toxic adenoma are the other common causes of hyperthyroidism.

4. Why has the patient experienced weight loss?

The thyroid hormones increase the basal metabolic rate (BMR), principally through increasing the production and insertion of the sodium/potassium adenosine triphosphatase (Na/K ATPase) pumps in various cell types. The increased metabolic rate also contributes to heat intolerance.

5. Assuming that plasma levels of catecholamines are normal in this patient, what explains the tachycardia, tremors, and palpitations?

Thyroid hormones increase the expression of adrenergic receptors in target tissues, resulting in increased sensitivity to circulating catecholamines. Thyroid hormone also has a direct stimulating effect on the heart, independent of the sympathetic nervous system.

Note: Beta blockers are often given to alleviate the sympathomimetic effects of hyperthyroidism.

6. What is pulse pressure? Why is pulse pressure increased in this patient?

Pulse pressure is the difference between systolic and diastolic blood pressure. A patient with a blood pressure of 120/80 mmHg has a pulse pressure of 40 mmHg. As mentioned, upregulation of adrenergic receptors on the heart and the direct effects of thyroid hormone on the heart cause positive chronotropic and inotropic cardiac effects. As stroke volume increases, so, too, does the pulse pressure. In addition, because thyroid hormones stimulate metabolism and increase tissue oxygen needs, they consequently cause vasodilation due to local metabolism, which reduces diastolic pressure. To summarize, the systolic pressure is increased because cardiac contractility increases the stroke volume, and the diastolic pressure is reduced because of widespread vasodilation, resulting in an increased pulse pressure.

7. What are the two thyroid hormones? Which is more potent?

Thyroxine (T_4) and triiodothyronine (T_3). T_3 is much more potent than T_4 (approximately 5 times more so) and is primarily produced by the peripheral conversion of T_4 to T_3 (which is catalyzed by the intracellular enzyme 5′-monodeiodinase), although as much as 20% of T_3 can be secreted from the thyroid gland.

8. What is thyroglobulin?

It is a protein that serves as a site of synthesis of thyroid hormones and also as the site on which synthesized thyroid hormones are stored in the follicular lumen of the thyroid gland. The follicular lumen is a storage space enclosed by a circle of thyroid follicular cells.

9. How are the thyroid hormones synthesized?

Ultimately, four iodine residues have to be attached to two tyrosine residues to form T_4, or three iodine residues must be attached to form T_3. The first step in the synthesis is the uptake of iodide ion (I^-) from plasma into follicular cells and eventually the follicular lumen via the iodide "pump." Within the lumen, the enzyme thyroid peroxidase then catalyzes the next two steps, in which iodide is oxidized to iodine (I_2) and iodine molecules are attached to tyrosine residues on thyroglobulin (organification step). Iodinated tyrosine residues are then coupled together to form either T_4 or T_3. Endocytosis of this modified thyroglobulin protein into the follicular cells and its subsequent hydrolysis yields T_4 and T_3, which diffuse across the plasma membrane into the circulation (Fig. 9).

Note: Of interest, excessive iodide appears to inhibit the synthesis of thyroid hormones and their release from the thyroid gland (the so-called Wolff-Chaikoff effect), which may be an intrinsic mechanism to protect against hyperthyroidism in a setting of iodine excess.

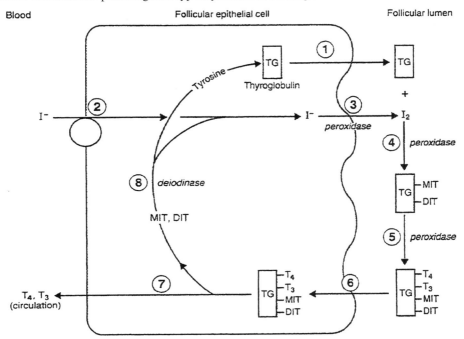

FIGURE 9. Synthesis of thyroid hormones (see text for explanation). (From STARS Physiology. Philadelphia, W.B. Saunders, 1998, p 359, with permission.)

10. Why might a physician prescribe propylthiouracil or methimazole to this patient?

Both propylthiouracil and methimazole are largely concentrated in the thyroid and inhibit thyroid hormone synthesis. Propylthiouracil also acts by preventing the peripheral deiodination of thyroxine (T_4) to triiodothyronine (T_3) to some extent.

Note: Both propylthiouracil and methimazole freely cross the placenta but can be used in pregnancy (although there are some risks), whereas radioactive iodide is clearly contraindicated in pregnancy because it permanently destroys thyroid function.

11. Why is iodide therapy generally initiated 2 weeks before thyroidectomy in hyperthyroid patients?

By an unknown mechanism, administration of a large amount of iodide decreases the vascularity of the thyroid gland, which reduces bleeding complications during surgery. By inhibiting thyroid hormone synthesis and release, excessive iodide also helps prevent thyroid storm.

12. What is thyroid storm? Why is propylthiouracil (PTU) used for this condition instead of methimazole?

Thyroid storm results from excessive levels of thyroid hormone, which cause a substantial elevation in basal metabolic rate and extreme fever (patients can literally "burn up right in front of you"). Thyroid storm is potentially fatal. Both PTU and methimazole inhibit thyroid hormone synthesis, but because the thyroid has an abundant store of thyroid hormone it may take weeks for this effect to manifest. However, because at higher doses PTU also inhibits the conversion of T_4 to T_3 in the peripheral tissues and T_3 is the more active form of thyroid hormone, PTU can have a fairly rapid effect.

Note: Both of these drugs can cause a fatal agranulocytosis, often preceded by a sore throat. Therefore, periodic monitoring is required.

13. Describe the typical clinical presentation of a patient with hyperthyroidism secondary to de Quervain's thyroiditis (subacute granulomatous thyroiditis).

In patients with de Quervain's thyroiditis, the thyroid gland is exquisitely sensitive to palpation. Patients also generally have signs of infection (e.g., fever).

14. How can a teratoma produce hyperthyroidism? / monolayer teratoma

In women, a rare form of teratoma called *struma ovarii* is made exclusively of thyroid tissue, which can produce enough thyroid hormone to cause clinical hyperthyroidism.

CASE 8

A 42-year-old woman complains of recent weight gain, heavy periods (menorrhagia), fatigue, cold intolerance, and constipation. She has a rough voice, and her rate of speech is slow. Physical exam is significant for an enlarged thyroid, slow reflexes, and the presence of brittle and coarse hair. She denies any history of bipolar disorder or treatment with lithium. Lab tests show elevated TSH and low free T_4.

1. What is the diagnosis?

Hypothyroidism.

2. Does the patient have primary, secondary, or tertiary hypothyroidism? Distinguish among the three.

She has primary hypothyroidism, which results from inadequate secretion of thyroid hormones by a dysfunctional thyroid gland. Inadequate secretion reduces negative feedback to the pituitary, thereby elevating plasma TSH levels. Secondary hypothyroidism is due to deficient pituitary secretion of TSH, and tertiary hypothyroidism is due to deficient hypothalamic secretion of TRH.

FORM OF HYPOTHYROIDISM	T_4/T_3	TSH	TRH
Primary	Low	High	High
Secondary	Low	Low	High
Tertiary	Low	Low	Low

Note: To complicate matters further, subclinical hypothyroidism is characterized by elevated TSH but normal levels of T_4 and T_3.

3. What is the most common cause of primary hypothyroidism? Describe the characteristic laboratory and pathologic findings.

Hashimoto's thyroiditis, an autoimmune disease, is the most common cause of primary hypothyroidism. Characteristic findings include plasma antimicrosomal (antiperoxidase) antibodies and biopsy showing lymphocytic infiltration of the thyroid gland.

4. Why are serum B12 levels routinely evaluated in patients with Hashimoto's thyroiditis?

This disease is frequently associated with pernicious anemia, a manifestation of autoimmune gastritis in which decreased secretion of intrinsic factor impairs vitamin B12 absorption.

Note: Autoimmune diseases are frequently associated with one another.

5. For seriously depressed patients, why are the thyroid hormones routinely evaluated?

Hypothyroidism is an organic cause of depression (as well as memory loss and dementia).

6. Why was asking about lithium use relevant in the diagnostic work-up of this patient?

Lithium inhibits the uptake and organification of iodine by the thyroid gland and also inhibits the peripheral conversion of T_4 to T_3 by 5'-monodeiodinase, thereby causing hypothyroidism. Amiodarone, an antiarrythmic agent, is also known to cause hypothyroidism.

7. What is the most serious manifestation of untreated (and severe) hypothyroidism?

Myxedema coma, which manifests as profound lethargy or coma, weakness, hypothermia, hypoventilation, hypoglycemia, and hyponatremia.

8. If the patient's history had been significant for a recent upper respiratory infection and the thyroid was tender to palpation, what would be the probable diagnosis?

Subacute thyroiditis (de Quervain's thyroiditis), which initially results in *hyper*thyroidism because the inflammation causes release of stored thyroid hormones. It then may progress to *hypo*thyroidism. Subacute thyroiditis is thought to involve viral infection of the thyroid gland and classically follows an upper respiratory infection. It usually resolves on its own.

9. If a patient has the same symptoms as the woman in the vignette but normal T_4 and TSH levels, what test should be ordered? Why?

Serum free T_3 should be assessed, because the patient may have sick euthyroid syndrome, caused by decreased peripheral conversion of T_4 to T_3. Recall again that, because it is normally present in much larger amounts, T_4 is the primary inhibitor of pituitary TSH secretion; therefore, TSH secretion is not significantly affected by reduced levels of T_3.

10. How can a thyroidectomy cause muscle cramps and paresthesias?

Through accidental removal of the parathyroid glands, resulting in hypocalcemia.

11. How is it possible for a thyroid gland to develop at the back of the tongue?

The thyroid begins its development at the back of the tongue and then migrates to its position below the thyroid cartilage in the neck. Failure to migrate along the thyroglossal duct, therefore, may result in a thyroid gland at the back of the tongue!

Note: Persistence of the thyroglossal duct that facilitates the migration of the thyroid can cause a thyroglossal duct cyst.

12. Why are thyroid hormone levels routinely evaluated in newborns?

Hypothyroidism is one of the preventable causes of mental retardation.

13. What is cretinism?

Hypothyroidism that develops in infancy or childhood. It impairs the maturation of the skeletal system and central nervous system, resulting in short stature, coarse facial features, and severe mental retardation.

14. Cover the left side of the chart and list the manifestations of hypothyroidism and hyperthyroidism in each organ/category.

See chart on next page.

	HYPOTHYROIDISM	HYPERTHYROIDISM
Metabolic rate	Decreased	Increased
Body weight	Gain	Loss
Intestinal activity	Constipation	Diarrhea
Mental status	Memory loss/dementia	Psychosis
Body temperature	Cold intolerance	Heat intolerance
Deep tendon reflexes	Hypoactive	Hyperactive
Most severe complication	Myxedema coma	Thyroid storm

CASE 9

A previously healthy 12-year-old boy complains of fatigue and excessive thirst (polydipsia). His mother mentions that he uses the bathroom quite frequently (polyuria), and friends at school tease him about this behavior. His mother is also concerned because he has lost 10 pounds despite eating "everything in sight." A nonfasting blood glucose test shows a plasma glucose of 220 mg/dl, and serum insulin levels are substantially reduced. To confirm the diagnosis, an oral glucose tolerance test (OGTT) is performed and shows a plasma glucose level of 225 mg/dl 2 hours after the administration of a 75-gram glucose load.

1. **What is the diagnosis?**
   Type 1 diabetes mellitus.

2. **Does this patient have normal beta-cell function? Will measurement of plasma C-peptide reveal low, normal, or high levels?**
   Type 1 diabetes mellitus is caused by autoimmune destruction of beta cells of the endocrine pancreas. Because C-peptide is cosecreted with insulin, plasma levels of C-peptide are also low.

3. **What is the short-term value of controlling blood sugar levels in this patient?**
   To prevent the symptoms of hyperglycemia, such as polyuria, polydypsia, and polyphagia, as well as weight loss. In addition, in type 1 diabetes, the correction of insulin deficiency prevents diabetic ketoacidosis.

4. **What is the long-term value of glycemic control in this patient?**
   Tight glycemic control has been proved to reduce the incidence of microvascular complications, including retinopathy, neuropathy, and nephropathy. However, it has not yet been shown to reduce macrovascular events such as heart attack and stroke, although future long-term studies may show such an effect.

5. **What is the value of routine measurements of hemoglobin A1c levels in this patient?**
   Hemoglobin A1c represents glycated hemoglobin, and the levels of hemoglobin A1c are directly associated with levels of plasma glucose. It is an effective measure of long-term diabetes control because the life span of hemoglobin-laden red blood cells is approximately 120 days in the circulation. Moreover, reduced HbA1c levels have been shown to correlate with better clinical outcomes.

6. **Why should blood pressure be closely scrutinized as the boy ages and treated aggressively with angiotensin-converting enzyme (ACE) inhibitors if it develops?**
   Blood pressure reduction substantially reduces the incidence of nephropathy, and the ACE inhibitors are most effective for this purpose.

7. Why is administration of beta blockers relatively contraindicated in this patient?

Beta blockers mask the warning signs of hypoglycemia, such as tremors, shakes, and tachycardia. In addition, by antagonizing hepatic beta receptors, these drugs make it more difficult for the liver to respond to epinephrine, a counterregulatory hormone that elevates the blood glucose by stimulating glycogenolysis and gluconeogenesis. In type 1 diabetes, hypoglycemia is predominantly due to insulin overdosing.

8. Why may this patient experience hyperglycemia in the morning if he administers too much insulin the previous night?

Insulin-induced hypoglycemia during the night triggers release of "stress" hormones (e.g., cortisol, growth hormone, glucagon, catecholamines), which cause a compensatory increase in plasma glucose. If diabetic patients are not educated about this possibility, they may mistakenly increase the nighttime dose of insulin to reduce morning blood sugar levels and cause hypoglycemic coma or even death during the night.

9. Explain the mechanism by which the major metabolic pathways behave as though the body is in the fasting state during insulin deficiency. In other words, why has the patient lost weight?

After consuming a high carbohydrate meal, insulin secretion is stimulated, which in turn activates glycolysis, glycogenesis, fatty acid synthesis, and protein synthesis. In the setting of insulin deficiency, all of these pathways shut down (become less active), and the opposing pathways are activated, including gluconeogenesis (which depends on protein catabolism), glycogenolysis, and fatty acid catabolism. In essence, insulin deficiency causes a hypercatabolic state.

10. What rate-limiting enzyme does insulin stimulate in the following anabolic pathways?

Glycolysis	Phosphofructokinase 1 (PFK-1)
Fatty acid synthesis	Acetyl-CoA carboxylase
Glycogenesis	Glycogen synthase
Pentose phosphate pathway	Glucose-6-phosphate dehydrogenase
Cholesterol synthesis	HMG-CoA reductase

11. What is the biochemical mechanism by which diabetic ketoacidosis develops in the setting of insulin deficiency?

Ordinarily, insulin stimulates fatty acid uptake by adipocytes through stimulation of lipoprotein lipase. In the absence of insulin (or significant insulin deficiency) fewer fatty acids are taken up by the adipocytes, and more fatty acids are delivered to the liver, where they are metabolized, with ketoacids as a byproduct. Further exacerbating this problem is the fact that insulin normally inhibits fatty acid catabolism by the liver; therefore, in the absence of insulin, this pathway is even more active and more ketone bodies are produced. Finally, the acidosis is exacerbated because the corresponding hyperglycemia causes dehydration via an osmotic diuresis, making it more difficult for the kidneys to excrete acid.

12. How can measurements of plasma C-peptide be used to differentiate between factitious hypoglycemia and an insulinoma?

Because plasma C-peptide is cosecreted with endogenous insulin, levels of both substances are high in an insulinoma but very low in factitious hypoglycemia, in which only recombinant insulin is injected.

CASE 10

A middle-aged obese man evaluated for a pre-employment physical exam complains of recent polyuria and polydypsia. His nonfasting plasma glucose is 275 mg/dl. Both of his parents were overweight, had "sugar problems," and died of cardiovascular complications.

You take time to educate him about diabetes and plan a follow-up visit for 2 weeks. Fasting lab tests show a plasma glucose of 180 mg/dl, total cholesterol of 250 mg/dl, low-density-lipoprotein (LDL) cholesterol of 175 mg/dl, and high-density-lipoprotein (HDL) cholesterol of 30 mg/dl. Urinalysis shows microalbuminuria. Pharmacotherapy is initiated with metformin, and the patient is educated about the importance of diet and exercise. Six months later his HgbA1c has decreased from an initial 8.5% to 6.5%.

1. Based on the patient's presentation and pharmacologic treatment, is he more likely to have type 1 or type 2 diabetes mellitus?

The classic presentation for type 2 diabetes is an overweight, middle-aged adult who complains of increased thirst and polyuria (although many cases are detected while asymptomatic by routine screening programs). In addition, oral medications are not adequate to correct the severe insulin deficiency present in type 1 diabetes.

2. What is the likely pathophysiology of diabetes in this patient?

Type 2 diabetes mellitus is typically caused by a combination of insulin resistance and relative insulin deficiency. Although insulin may actually be increased in type 2 diabetes (hyperinsulinemia), plasma levels are clearly deficient to maintain normal plasma glucose (hence, it is described as a relative insulin deficiency, even in the presence of elevated levels!). In the presence of peripheral insulin resistance, plasma glucose increases secondary to reduced uptake of glucose by skeletal muscle and adipose tissue and increased hepatic gluconeogenesis.

Note: Diabetes is thought to be a risk factor for atherosclerosis. This increased risk may be partly explained by the fact that in the setting of insulin deficiency or insulin resistance, the increased lipolysis in adipose tissue results in elevated levels of plasma fatty acids.

3. What are the mechanisms by which sulfonylureas maintain glycemic control in type 2 diabetes?

Sulfonylureas such as tolbutamide (first generation) and glyburide (second generation) act by stimulating insulin secretion. They do so by closing membrane-spanning potassium channels on pancreatic beta cells. The result is depolarization of the cell, which triggers opening of voltage-gated calcium channels on the plasma membrane. The resultant influx of extracellular calcium stimulates insulin secretion, which lowers plasma glucose.

4. What are the major side effects of sulfonylureas?

Improved glycemic control via increased insulin secretion may result in weight gain, because insulin stimulates fat synthesis. However, the more serious side effect of sulfonylureas is their propensity to cause hypoglycemia due to excessive insulin secretion.

5. Why might therapy with a biguanide such as metformin make sense in this patient? What is the drug's mechanism of action?

Metformin (Glucophage) is a wonder drug for type 2 diabetes mellitus. It normalizes plasma glucose primarily by inhibiting hepatic glucose production and by stimulating peripheral uptake of glucose by adipose and skeletal muscle. Furthermore, it has a beneficial effect on the lipid profile. Finally, and perhaps most importantly to some patients, it has an anorexic effect and results in weight loss in the majority of patients.

Note: In rare cases, metformin can cause a life-threatening lactic acidosis.

6. Why should this patient be educated about the importance of examining his feet periodically?

Long-standing hyperglycemia in diabetes is associated with microvascular disease as well as diabetic neuropathy. The microvascular disease may cause poor perfusion of the feet, so that foot ulcers do not heal well. In addition, the neuropathy allows ulcers to fester without causing noticeable pain.

Note: Diabetic neuropathy typically occurs in a "stocking-glove" distribution, with the distal feet affected before the more distal hands. This "stocking-glove" distribution is seen in other metabolic neuropathies as well, because the longer axons are more susceptible to a metabolic abnormality.

7. What forms of renal damage occur in diabetes?

Diabetic nephropathy results in glomerular lesions, including both diffuse glomerulosclerosis and nodules of sclerosis within the glomeruli (the distinctive Kimmelstiel-Wilson lesion), renal vascular lesions (e.g., arteriolosclerosis), and pyelonephritis (probably because the elevated urine glucose content predisposes to urinary tract infection and neurogenic bladder).

Note: Renal papillary necrosis (necrotizing papillitis) is also found in diabetes and is a complication of pyelonephritis.

8. How can poor glycemic control cause this patient to go into coma?

If he overdoses on sulfonylureas, he can go into a hypoglycemic coma. On the other hand, if sugars run too high, he can develop hyperosmolar nonketotic coma.

Note: Type 2 diabetics rarely go into diabetic ketoacidosis, possibly because sufficient insulin is still present to inhibit ketogenesis from excessive degradation of fatty acids by the liver. Insulin normally inhibits fatty acid degradation.

9. Why do the alpha-glucosidase inhibitors cause frequent gastrointestinal symptoms and annoying flatulence?

These drugs, which include *acarbose* and *miglitol*, work by inhibiting intestinal alpha-glucosidases (e.g., sucrase, maltase, isomaltase), which break down disaccharides into monosaccharides that can be absorbed by the intestines. The nondigested sugars are metabolized by colonic bacteria to generate large volumes of gas.

Note: These drugs do not cause hypoglycemia, but in the event that hypoglycemia results from a different oral hypoglycemic agent while the patient is taking an alpha-glucosidase inhibitor, oral glucose should be given because its intestinal absorption will not be impeded. Clearly, intravenous glucose would be given in a hospital setting.

10. How does binding of insulin to the insulin receptor cause increased glucose uptake into cells?

It causes glucose transporters (GLUT4) to be incorporated into the plasma membrane of cells in skeletal muscle and adipose tissue.

11. What is the primary metabolic fuel in the fasting (between-meal) state?

Fatty acids. A notable exception to this rule is the central nervous system (CNS), which relies exclusively on serum glucose in both fed and fasting states, except in periods of prolonged starvation, during which the CNS also metabolizes ketone bodies.

GESTATIONAL DIABETES

12. What is the value of the relative maternal insulin resistance that develops during pregnancy? How is it valuable to the fetus?

Because glucose moves across the placenta by passive diffusion, this physiologic alteration may facilitate delivery of glucose to the fetus.

Note: Gestational diabetes is defined as diabetes detected for the first time during pregnancy and resolving 6 weeks or more after the pregnancy ends. If the woman was not diabetic before pregnancy, she has a higher risk of developing type 2 diabetes later in life if she develops gestational diabetes.

13. What is the most common undesired effect of maternal diabetes on fetal size? Explain.

Fetal macrosomia (large fetus) is a complication of maternal diabetes. It is a problem because of the increased risk of birth injury when an oversized fetus passes through the birth canal. Fetal size is increased because the maternal hyperglycemia stimulates increased fetal insulin secretion, which in turn stimulates fetal growth and fat deposition.

14. Should hypoglycemia or hyperglycemia be expected immediately after delivery in a baby born to a poorly controlled diabetic mother? Explain.

Hypoglycemia. During in utero life, elevated fetal glucose levels (secondary to high maternal glucose levels) cause chronic fetal hyperinsulinemia. Just after delivery, when the fetus is no longer exposed to the elevated maternal glucose, the residual hyperinsulinemia can cause hypoglycemia.

5. CARDIOVASCULAR SYSTEM

Dave Brown and Thomas Brown

BASIC CONCEPTS

1. What are the mathematical determinants of arterial blood pressure?

The mean arterial blood pressure (MAP) is determined by the amount of blood that the heart pumps into the arterial system in a given time (cardiac output [CO]) and the degree of arterial resistance to this output (total peripheral resistance [TPR]):

$$MAP = CO \times TPR$$

Consequently, all drugs that lower blood pressure work by affecting CO, TPR, or both.

2. What determines CO in the most general sense?

CO is determined by the volume of blood pumped with each beat (stroke volume [SV]) and how frequently the heart beats (heart rate [HR]):

$$CO = HR \times SV$$

HR can be affected by a variety of factors, but is principally under the control of the sympathetic and parasympathetic divisions of the autonomic nervous system. Beta blockers exert part of their antihypertensive effects by decreasing HR, which reduces CO.

Note: The more cardioselective calcium channel blockers (e.g., verapamil, diltiazem) can also reduce HR; they may achieve part of their blood pressure-lowering effect by this mechanism.

3. What are the three main factors that affect stroke volume?

The major players in stroke volume are preload, contractility, and afterload.

4. What is preload? How does it affect stroke volume?

Preload is the volume of blood in the ventricles at the end of diastole. The most widely accepted theory explaining the relationship of preload and stroke volume states that stretching of ventricular muscle fibers (and therefore sarcomeres) occurs with increasing end-diastolic volumes. This stretching causes greater overlap between actin and myosin within sarcomeres, resulting in a stronger ventricular contraction. The relationship between end-diastolic volume and increased force generation is referred to as the Frank-Starling relationship. Diuretics can reduce blood pressure by decreasing intravascular volume, which decreases venous return to the heart and consequently reduces preload.

Increased ventricular output as a function of end-diastolic volume (reflected by atrial pressure). (From Guyton AC, Hall JE: Textbook of Medical Physiology, 10th ed. Philadelphia, W. B. Saunders, 2000, p 104, with permission.)

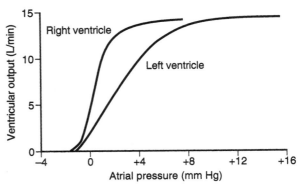

Note: Another theory to explain the Frank-Starling relationship proposes that cardiac troponin becomes increasingly sensitive to cytosolic calcium at greater sarcomere lengths, thereby resulting in increased calcium binding and increased force of muscle contraction.

5. What is contractility? How does it affect stroke volume?

Contractility is a measure of how forcefully the ventricle contracts (at any end-diastolic volume). Naturally, a more forceful contraction ejects a greater fraction of blood from the ventricle, thereby increasing the stroke volume. Normally, contractility is influenced principally by the sympathetic nervous system. Beta blockers exert part of their antihypertensive effects by antagonizing this sympathetic input to the heart and thus reducing contractility. Reduced contractility, in turn, reduces stroke volume and cardiac output.

6. What is afterload? How does it affect stroke volume?

Afterload is the pressure against which the heart must pump blood. It is determined primarily by systemic arterial pressure. For a given preload and contractility, an increase in afterload results in a decrease in stroke volume.

Note: In aortic stenosis, the stenotic aortic valve increases the afterload, thereby reducing stroke volume and cardiac output.

7. What determines the peripheral resistance?

Resistance to blood flow is mediated principally by the diameters of the arterioles, which are modified by arteriolar vasoconstriction and dilation. The sympathetic nervous system increases arteriolar vasoconstriction by stimulating alpha$_1$-adrenergic receptors, which increases calcium influx (via calcium channels) into arteriolar smooth muscle and stimulates their contraction. Consequently, alpha$_1$ receptors and arteriolar calcium channels are selective targets for antihypertensive drugs.

Another major factor that causes arteriolar dilation is local tissue hypoxia and/or metabolic waste products, such as adenosine, that accumulate when oxygen demand exceeds supply. This mechanism is extremely useful during exercise, when increasing tissue oxygen demand causes vasodilation and delivery of more oxygen and nutrients. The vasodilation during exercise can be profound and is necessary because in intense exercise CO can increase by a factor of about six. If there were no decrease in peripheral resistance in this setting, the mean arterial pressure would increase by a factor of six also, creating blood pressures in the range of 500–600 mmHg!

Note: Recall that resistance is inversely proportional to the arteriolar radius to the fourth power (r^4). Two other powerful endogenous mediators of vasoconstriction are angiotensin II and vasopressin. Both are released in response to hypotension (among other stimuli).

Excitation-Contraction Coupling

8. What is the source of cytosolic calcium during ventricular systole?

During the ventricular action potential, calcium influx from the extracellular fluid into the cytosol stimulates calcium release from the sarcoplasmic reticulum, a phenomenon referred to as *calcium-induced calcium release*. In fact, the majority of the cytosolic calcium comes from the sarcoplasmic reticulum, not the extracellular fluid. This mechanism of calcium release is in contrast to skeletal muscle, in which depolarization of the cell membrane triggers sarcoplasmic calcium release without entry of extracellular calcium into the cytosol.

9. What is the function of calcium in cardiac muscle contraction?

Cytosolic calcium binds to cardiac troponin, thereby uncovering myosin-binding sites on troponin to allow the sliding filament mechanism of contraction.

Note: The cardioselective calcium channel blockers (e.g., verapamil, diltiazem), in addition to reducing heart rate, reduce contractility by antagonizing extracellular calcium entry and the subsequent calcium-induced calcium release that occurs in heart muscle.

10. What is the mechanism by which catecholamines increase cardiac contractility?

This mechanism is mostly due to activation of the beta-adrenergic pathway, which causes an increased probability of cell membrane calcium channel opening, thereby increasing calcium influx and increasing the strength of ventricular contractions. Beta-adrenergic activation also increases the activity of myosin adenosine triphosphatase (ATPase), an enzyme that facilitates the interaction of actin and myosin required for contraction.

11. Explain the biochemical mechanism by which sympathetic stimulation of the heart reduces the time required for ventricular relaxation.

In addition to stimulating calcium influx, the beta-adrenergic pathway also stimulates calcium uptake by the ventricular sarcoplasmic reticulum. This removal of cytosolic calcium into the sarcoplasmic reticulum is required for ventricular relaxation; thus, the more rapidly it is removed, the more rapidly the ventricles relax. Such rapid ventricular relaxation at elevated heart rates is important to ensure adequate ventricular filling during the decreased period of diastole.

Note: Calcium uptake into the sarcoplasmic reticulum is an energy-requiring process. In ischemic heart disease, the reduced oxygen delivery makes calcium uptake less efficient, thereby impairing ventricular relaxation and contributing to diastolic dysfunction.

Arrhythmias

12. Describe the relationship between the various phases of the ventricular myocyte action potential and the different ion fluxes across the cell membrane.

In phase 0 of the action potential, the membrane voltage rises sharply due to sodium influx. In phase 1 there is a slight decrease in the membrane potential; the ionic mechanisms responsible for this decrease are fairly complicated. In phase 2, there is a plateau in the action potential due to the balance between calcium influx and potassium efflux. During phase 3, there is rapid repolarization due to unopposed potassium efflux. Phase 4 is the resting membrane potential.

Note: The antiarrythmic agents work by affecting one or more components of the action potential. Class I antiarrhythmics block sodium channels and antagonize phase 0. Class III antiarrhythmics work by blocking potassium channels, which prolongs phase 3 repolarization.

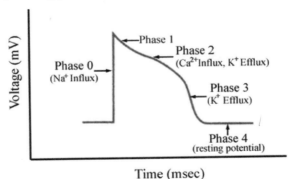

Phases of the ventricular myocyte action potential.

13. What is responsible for the drifting of the resting membrane potential in nodal cells?

Because these cells are more permeable to sodium, sodium influx during the resting potential causes the membrane to depolarize gradually. Eventually, when the membrane depolarizes to its "threshold" value, slow calcium channels are activated and engender an action potential.

Note: The calcium channel blockers verapamil and diltiazem affect heart rate by antagonizing slow calcium channels on the sinoatrial node. They are class IV antiarrhythmics.

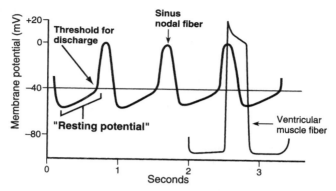

Rhythmic discharge of a sinus nodal fiber. The sinus nodal action potential is also compared with that of ventricular muscle fiber. (From Guyton AC, Hall JE: Textbook of Medical Physiology, 10th ed. Philadelphia, W.B. Saunders, 200, p 108, with permission.)

14. Through what mechanism does sympathetic stimulation increase heart rate?

The release of norepinephrine from sympathetic neurons or epinephrine from the adrenal medulla causes activation of beta$_1$-adrenergic receptors in nodal tissue, which has a positive chronotropic effect on the heart by increasing the cellular influx of sodium ions and decreasing the cellular efflux of potassium ions in these cells (i.e., essentially increasing the slope of the resting membrane potential in the nodal cells). Beta blockers reduce heart rate by antagonizing this effect.

Note: The beta blockers are considered class II antiarrhythmics.

15. What are the classes of antiarrhythmics? How do their mechanisms of action and characteristic side effects vary?

CLASS	MECHANISM OF ACTION	PROTOTYPE(S)	CHARACTERISTIC SIDE EFFECTS
IA	Inhibits Na and K channels, prolongs QRS complex and QT interval, prolongs effective refractory period (ERP)	Quinidine Procainamide	Lupus-like syndrome, torsades de pointes
IB	Inhibit Na+ channels, shortens repolarization, ↓ QT interval	Lidocaine	Neurologic (paresthesias)
IC	Inhibit Na+ channels, prolongs QRS complex	Flecanimide	
II	↑ PR interval, ↓ automaticity (↓ slope of phase 4 depolarization in nodal cells)	Propranolol	Bronchospasm
III	Inhibits K channels	Amiodarone	Pulmonary fibrosis
IV	Inhibits calcium channels, ↑ PR interval, ↓ automaticity	Verapamil Diltiazem	AV block

Note: There is considerable overlap in the mechanisms of action of the antiarrhythmics listed in the above table. For the sake of simplicity, we have classified the above antiarrhythmics according to their *primary* mechanism of action. Virtually all antiarrhythmics may cause arrhythmias themselves.

CASE 1

A 78-year-old woman is evaluated for refractory hypertension. She is taking four different antihypertensives, including a thiazide diuretic, angiotensin-converting enzyme (ACE) inhibitor, beta blocker, and an alpha$_1$ receptor antagonist, but her blood pressure is still

184/105 mmHg. Someone finally auscultates her abdomen and detects a bruit. An angiogram shows 95% atherosclerotic occlusion of the left renal artery. Renal angioplasty is performed to relieve the occlusion, and her blood pressure subsequently normalizes.

1. What disease did this patient have?

Renovascular hypertension, which is most commonly due to atherosclerosis of the renal arteries.

Note: Fibromuscular dysplasia of the renal arteries, a disease that primarily affects middle-aged women, also produces renovascular hypertension by occluding the lumen of the renal arteries.

2. If the kidneys are not well perfused, how is extracellular fluid volume affected?

Underperfused kidneys have a reduced glomerular filtration rate (GFR) and greater tubular reabsorption of salt and water, which expands the extracellular fluid volume. Whereas this effect is an adaptive process in renal hypoperfusion due to dehydration, it causes pathologic fluid volume expansion in hypoperfusion due to other causes.

3. How does the plasma volume affect blood pressure?

Plasma volume affects the blood pressure indirectly by affecting cardiac output. If plasma volume is increased, circulating blood volume is increased. The increase in circulating blood volume increases the venous return to the heart, which in turn increases cardiac output via the Frank-Starling mechanism. If plasma volume decreases, the opposite sequence of events occurs.

4. How do the kidneys regulate blood pressure independently of the renin-angiotensin-aldosterone system?

At higher arterial pressures, the kidneys are better perfused and GFR is increased. This effect increases the volume of urine that is produced, thereby reducing extracellular fluid volume and blood pressure. And, as mentioned, at lower arterial pressures the reduced perfusion reduces GFR and increases tubular reabsorption of salt and water, expanding extracellular fluid volumes and restoring the blood pressure.

5. Describe the physiologic value of the renin-angiotensin-aldosterone system.

This system also serves to restore blood pressure and plasma volume. However, it enables a more rapid and powerful response to hypotension and decreased plasma volume than the mechanism described in question 4. This system is activated when renin is released by the juxtaglomerular cells in response to reduced perfusion pressure of the afferent arteriole. This enzyme quickly catalyzes the conversion of angiotensinogen to angiotensin I, which is then converted to angiotensin II by ACE in the lungs. Angiotensin II then causes widespread vasoconstriction to elevate the blood pressure. This entire process happens quite rapidly. In addition, angiotensin II stimulates adrenal secretion of aldosterone, which further increases renal salt and water reabsorption.

6. How does the renin-angiotensin-aldosterone system contribute to renovascular hypertension?

If one kidney is significantly underperfused because of renal artery narrowing, it will release substantial quantities of the enzyme renin. Renin increases systemic angiotensin II and aldosterone levels, which causes widespread vasoconstriction as well as significant salt and water retention by the normal kidney, both of which increase the blood pressure. In the underperfused kidney, since the renal perfusion is decreased, fractional salt and water reabsorption will be increased as well, further contributing to the hypertension. In essence, because the one kidney is underperfused, it is responding as if the body is in hypovolemic shock, thereby stimulating widespread vasoconstriction as well as significant fluid retention. However, in renovascular hypertension the underperfused kidney is "misinformed" about the blood pressure and volume status of the body.

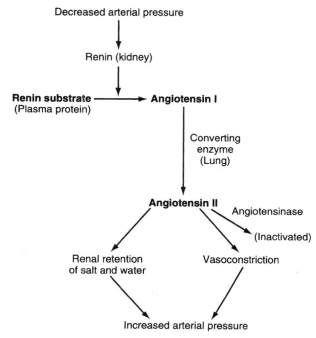

Renin-angiotensin-vasoconstrictor mechanism for arterial pressure control. (From Guyton AC, Hall JE: Textbook of Medical Physiology, 10th ed. Philadelphia, W.B. Saunders, 2000, p 201, with permission.)

7. Does the angiotensin II released during hypovolemic states cause vasoconstriction in the kidney? Wouldn't this reduce GFR and increase the accumulation of toxic metabolites in the blood?

Angiotensin II exploits an elegant mechanism in which it can cause widespread vasoconstriction and reduce renal perfusion, but at the same time maintains GFR. It does this by causing vasoconstriction of the efferent arteriole of the glomerulus. Although this will reduce renal blood flow, it will also increase hydrostatic pressure at the glomerulus, which increases the net filtration pressure and maintains the GFR so toxic metabolites can be excreted.

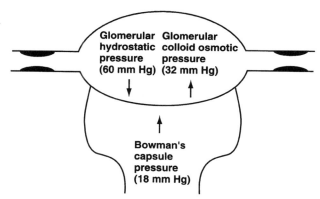

Constriction of the efferent arteriole increases hydrostatic pressure at the glomerulus, which increases filtration fraction. (From Guyton AC, Hall JE: Textbook of Medical Physiology, 10th ed. Philadelphia, W.B. Saunders, 2000, p 487, with permission.)

8. Why should ACE inhibitors be avoided in patients with bilateral renal artery stenosis?

Imagine that perfusion of the kidneys is impaired due to atheromatous occlusion of the renal arteries. The primary mechanism for maintaining adequate GFR in such kidneys is angiotensin II-mediated constriction of the efferent arteriole, which increases the filtration pressure at the glomerulus. This tonic angiotensin-mediated constriction of the efferent arteriole depends on high plasma levels of angiotensin II. If an ACE inhibitor is used in this setting (which is more common than one might suspect), efferent arteriolar vasoconstriction ceases, and GFR may drop precipitously, resulting in acute renal failure.

CASE 2

A 60-year-old man comes in for his third visit in two months. He has had a blood pressure of approximately 155/95 mmHg on each occasion. No abdominal bruits are auscultated on exam. Diet and exercise modifications fail to reduce his blood pressure; therefore, he is started on the beta blocker atenolol.

1. What are the two types of hypertension? Which type does this patient probably have?

Essential (primary, idiopathic) hypertension and secondary hypertension. If causes of secondary hypertension are ruled out (e.g., renal artery stenosis, coarctation of aorta, primary hyperaldosteronism), then the patient has essential hypertension by default.

Note: The vast majority of cases of hypertension (about 90–95%) are classified as essential, whereas about 5–10% are classified as secondary.

2. What is the mechanism by which atenolol reduces blood pressure?

Atenolol is a beta blocker with considerable binding specificity for the beta$_1$-adrenergic receptors located on the heart. By antagonizing these receptors, it decreases heart rate and contractility, both of which reduce cardiac output. Remember, mean arterial pressure is equal to cardiac output multiplied by peripheral resistance.

3. What pharmacologic property makes certain beta blockers more "cardioselective" than others?

Some beta blockers (e.g., atenolol, esmolol, metoprolol) are more specific for the beta$_1$ receptors on the heart and have less effect on the beta$_2$ receptors on bronchiolar smooth muscle cells or on smooth muscle cells within skeletal muscle arterioles. Thus, beta$_1$-specific antagonists are less likely to prevent catecholamine-mediated bronchodilation or vasodilation.

Note: Even beta$_1$-specific antagonists should not be used in asthmatics because they have some effect on beta$_2$ receptors. They should be used only with caution in patients with chronic obstructive pulmonary disease, especially at high doses.

4. Why should beta blockers be given cautiously to a patient with a first-degree atrioventricular (AV) block?

Beta blockers decrease AV conduction and should therefore be used only with great care in patients with first-degree AV block (prolonged PR interval on the EKG). Beta blockers should not be given at all to patients with second- or third-degree AV block. Certain calcium channel blockers (e.g., verapamil and diltiazem) may also reduce AV conduction and, when used in combination with beta blockers, can produce serious AV block.

5. If the patient is taken off the beta blocker, why is it important to wean the drug gradually as opposed to stopping it abruptly?

Beta blockers substantially increase the sensitivity of the heart to catecholamines, in part due to upregulation of beta-adrenergic receptors. Consequently, tachycardia, arrhythmias, anginal pain, and even sudden cardiac death can result from sudden withdrawal.

6. How can beta blockers worsen the manifestations of peripheral arterial disease?

Vasodilation in skeletal muscle arterioles is mediated by $beta_2$-adrenergic receptors on vascular smooth muscle cells. If this vasodilation is inhibited, peripheral ischemia can be exacerbated.

7. How do beta blockers affect the renin-angiotensin system?

The sympathetic nervous system also stimulates the renal production of renin, which effect is mediated by beta receptors on the cells that produce renin (recall the juxtaglomerular apparatus). Beta blockers can antagonize this effect, thereby reducing renin production, which then reduces angiotensin synthesis as well as aldosterone secretion by the adrenals. Thus one can see why beta blockers are more effective in patients with hypertension and high plasma renin activity than in hypertensive patients with low plasma renin activity.

8. What is the mechanism by which the baroreceptors respond to a reduction in blood pressure?

The arterial baroreceptors, whose output tonically inhibits sympathetic outflow, fire less frequently if the blood pressure drops. The result is less inhibition of sympathetic outflow (i.e., increased sympathetic outflow), which helps restore the blood pressure by increasing heart rate and stimulating peripheral vasoconstriction. Conversely, if the blood pressure increases, the baroreceptors fire more frequently because they are being "stretched" more, which causes greater inhibition of the sympathetic outflow.

9. How do the alpha$_1$ receptor antagonists work?

The alpha$_1$ receptor antagonists include the "-osins" (prazosin, terazosin, doxazosin) and antagonize peripheral vasoconstriction stimulated by the sympathetic nervous system (which is mediated by alpha$_1$ receptors).

10. How do the alpha$_1$ receptor antagonists cause orthostatic hypotension?

When a person stands up from a sitting position, gravity makes blood pool in the legs, which reduces the mean arterial pressure. Ordinarily the baroreflex compensates for this effect by increasing heart rate and stimulating vasoconstriction. If the alpha$_1$ receptors are blocked in the peripheral vessels, this reflex is less effective at restoring the blood pressure. Nevertheless, a reflex tachycardia, which is mediated by beta receptors, will be maintained.

CASE 3

A 48-year-old man is newly diagnosed with type 2 diabetes and hypertension. In addition to an oral hypoglycemic agent, his physician prescribed captopril for hypertension. After about 1 month the patient developed an annoying dry cough. The physician switched his prescription from captopril to losartan, and the cough disappeared.

1. Why are ACE inhibitors the preferred antihypertensive therapy in this patient?

In addition to reducing the risk of stroke like other antihypertensives, the ACE inhibitors have been proved to reduce the progression of proteinuria in diabetic patients.

2. Describe the physiologic effects of ACE inhibitors.

These drugs prevent the conversion of angiotensin I to angiotensin II. The results are less renal retention of sodium and water because of the lowered angiotensin II and aldosterone levels as well as less peripheral vasoconstriction. In addition, the ACE inhibitors dilate the efferent arteriole of the glomerulus, which reduces glomerular filtration pressures and reduces the damage to the glomerular membrane that occurs in diabetes.

3. Why may the use of beta blockers not be an ideal choice in this patient?

These drugs mask important signs of hypoglycemia, such as tremor and palpitations, that are mediated through the sympathetic nervous system. Beta blockers also antagonize epinephrine-stimulated hepatic gluconeogenesis and glycogenolysis. This contraindication is more important in type 1 diabetics, since they are at greater risk of hypoglycemia secondary to insulin injections.

Note: Although beta blockers may mask many of the symptoms associated with hypoglycemia (e.g., tremors, palpitations), they do not prevent the diaphoresis commonly seen in severe hypoglycemia because sweat glands are innervated by sympathetic cholinergic nerves rather than sympathetic adrenergic nerves.

4. How can loop and thiazide diuretics exacerbate hyperglycemia in diabetics?

This complication may be related to the high incidence of hypokalemia associated with these drugs. Hypokalemia inhibits insulin secretion and end-organ sensitivity to insulin. Remember that insulin stimulates cellular potassium uptake; thus, it makes sense that low serum potassium levels inhibit insulin secretion and action.

5. What is the mechanism by which ACE inhibitors such as captopril can cause cough?

ACE also degrades bradykinin. Accumulation of bradykinin is believed to be the primary cause of the cough. It is thought that the accumulated bradykinin somehow stimulates nociceptors in the airways, thereby initiating the cough reflex. This undesirable side effect can be avoided by using angiotensin receptor antagonists such as losartan.

6. Cover the right-hand column, and for each antihypertensive drug in the left column name the class of drug to which it belongs, the mechanism by which it lowers blood pressure, and the primary side effects associated with its use.

DRUG	CLASS	MECHANISM OF ACTION	MAIN SIDE EFFECTS
Hydralazine	Arterial vasodilator	Unknown	Lupus-like syndrome Reflex tachycardia
Captopril Lisinopril Quinapril Benazepril	ACE inhibitors	↓ ATII production ↓ Peripheral resistance ↓ Aldosterone secretion	Dry cough Hyperkalemia Angioedema Renal failure
Losartan Valsartan	Angiotensin receptor blockers (ARBs)	Inhibit ATII action in tissues	Good side-effect profile
Methyldopa Clonidine	Alpha$_2$ receptor agonists	Decrease CNS sympathetic outflow	Sedation/depression Hypertensive crisis (on withdrawal of clonidine)
Atenolol Esmolol Metoprolol	Selective beta$_1$ receptor blockers	Negative chronotropic and inotropic effects (reduce cardiac output)	Bronchospasm Bradycardia AV block Sexual dysfunction
Propranolol	Nonselective beta blocker	Negative chronotropic and inotropic effects (reduce cardiac output)	Bronchospasm Bradycardia AV block Sexual dysfunction
Prazosin Terazosin Doxazosin	Alpha$_1$ receptor antagonists	↓ Peripheral resistance	Postural hypotension
Labetolol Carvedilol	Combined alpha-beta receptor blockers	Combined effect of alpha$_1$ blockers and beta blockers	
Diltiazem Verapamil	Calcium channel blockers (nondihydropyridine)	↓ Peripheral resistance ↓ Cardiac output	Bradycardia AV block

(Cont'd.)

DRUG	CLASS	MECHANISM OF ACTION	MAIN SIDE EFFECTS
Amlodipine Nifedipine	Calcium channel blockers (dihydropyridine)	↓ Peripheral resistance (more specific for vascular smooth muscle than heart)	Reflex tachycardia
Hydrochloro- thiazide	Thiazide diuretic	Inhibits sodium and water reabsorption in distal convoluted tubule	Hypokalemia Hyperuricemia Hyperglycemia
Furosemide Bumetamide	Loop diuretic	Inhibits sodium-chloride- potassium pump in thick ascending limb of loop of Henle	Hypokalemia Hyperuricemia Hyperglycemia Ototoxicity in combination with aminoglycosides
Spirono- lactone	Potassium-sparing diuretic	Antagonizes action of aldosterone	Hyperkalemia

CASE 4

On a routine office visit, a 45-year-old man is found to have elevated serum levels of low-density lipoprotein cholesterol (LDL-C) and triglycerides and a low serum level of high-density lipoprotein cholesterol (HDL-C). His meager attempts at diet and exercise do not alter his lipid profile significantly, and he is started on simvastatin. Before he takes the first dose, his liver enzymes are checked, and he is told that this test will be repeated in 3 months.

1. **Describe the mechanism of action of simvastatin (and other statins).**
    Statins inhibit the hepatic synthesis of cholesterol by inhibiting HMG CoA reductase, which is the rate-limiting step in the synthesis of cholesterol. Statins are the most potent pharmacologic agents for lowering LDL-C. They also cause a modest reduction of triglycerides but have only a minor effect on increasing HDL-C.

2. **What are the two main sources of plasma triglycerides? How do they enter the circulation?**
    The two main sources of plasma triglycerides are dietary triglycerides and triglycerides synthesized by the liver. Dietary triglycerides are broken down in the gut and then reformed in intestinal enterocytes, where they are packaged in chylomicrons that enter the lymphatics and eventually drain into the venous circulation via the thoracic duct. Nondietary triglycerides are synthesized primarily in the liver and travel within very-low-density lipoproteins (VLDLs). Elevated triglycerides are an independent risk factor for the development of cardiovascular disease.
    Note: Triglycerides are composed of three fatty acids linked to a glycerol backbone.

3. **What enzymatic mechanism clears triglycerides from the circulation?**
    Lipoprotein lipase, which is present on the luminal surface of capillary endothelial cells in adipose tissue, skeletal muscle, and cardiac muscle. This enzyme releases fatty acids from triglycerides present in chylomicrons and VLDL. The released fatty acids then diffuse into the cells.
    Note: Insulin stimulates synthesis of lipoprotein lipase. If this enzyme concentration is low, as in insulin deficiency associated with diabetes, triglycerides accumulate in the circulation and hasten the development of atherosclerosis.

4. **Describe the mechanism of action of the lipid-lowering fibric acid derivatives (e.g., gemfibrozil, fenofibrate).**
    These agents stimulate lipoprotein lipase, causing a significant reduction in triglycerides, with only a modest reduction in LDL cholesterol.

5. **What are the reservations about using the fibrates and statins in combination?**

Both classes of drugs independently can cause muscle damage (myositis) and liver damage; when they are used together, these risks may be increased.

Note: Potential hepatotoxicity is evaluated by periodically monitoring hepatic enzymes such as alanine aminotransferase (ALT) and aspartate aminotransferase (AST), whereas potential myositis and/or rhabdomyolysis can be evaluated by monitoring levels of creatine phosphokinase (CPK).

6. **How does niacin influence the lipid profile? What is the unique pharmacologic feature of niacin in managing lipid levels?**

Niacin (nicotinic acid) is a water-soluble B vitamin that has multiple beneficial effects on the overall lipid profile. It increases HDL-C by 30–40%, reduces triglycerides by 35–45%, and reduces LDL-C by 20–30%. It is unique among the hypolipidemic agents because it is the most potent agent for increasing HDL levels.

Note: An annoying side effect of niacin is facial and upper body flushing (niacin rush). Taking an aspirin before taking niacin can minimize this flushing by reducing the synthesis of vasodilatory prostaglandins.

7. **How do the bile-sequestering resins (cholestyramine, colestipol) lower LDL cholesterol levels?**

The bile-sequestering resins bind bile acids in the intestine and prevent their reuptake in the distal ileum. This process stimulates increased hepatic synthesis of bile acids. Because these acids are formed from cholesterol, increasing their synthesis increases cholesterol catabolism and decreases serum cholesterol levels.

Note: These drugs impair the bile-mediated emulsification, digestion, and absorption of fats and fat-soluble vitamins (A, D, E, and K). Consequently, adverse effects of these drugs commonly include flatulence, abdominal pain, steatorrhea, and deficiencies of fat-soluble vitamins.

8. **Describe the structure of a lipoprotein. Where are lipoproteins synthesized? What are the major types of lipoproteins?**

Lipoproteins are macromolecular structures composed of an inner core of cholesterol esters and triglycerides (more properly referred to as triacylglycerols) and an outer core of apoproteins, phospholipids, and unesterified free cholesterol. The major types of lipoproteins include chylomicrons, very-low-density lipoproteins (VLDL), intermediate-density lipoproteins (IDL), low-density lipoproteins (LDL), and high-density lipoproteins (HDL). Chylomicrons are synthesized within intestinal enterocytes, whereas VLDL is synthesized within the liver. IDL, HDL, and LDL are formed within the circulation via VLDL catabolism.

9. **What are the functions of the various forms of lipoproteins? How are they removed from the circulation?**

Chylomicrons: delivery of dietary triglycerides to adipose tissue, skeletal muscle, and cardiac muscle; cholesterol-rich chylomicron remnants are then taken up by the liver.

VLDL: delivery of liver-synthesized triglycerides to adipose tissue, skeletal muscle, and cardiac muscle; removed by intravascular conversion to IDL and ultimately to LDL.

LDL: delivery of cholesterol to cells throughout the body; removed by internalization via LDL receptor (principally in the liver).

Note: Defects in LDL receptor or internalization of LDL receptor cause familial **hypercholesterolemia**.

HDL: return of excessive cholesterol from cells to the liver for biliary excretion.

10. **What are the putative mechanisms by which HDL-C protects against coronary artery disease?**

HDL-C is involved in reverse cholesterol transport, in which excessive cholesterol is transported from the cells to the liver for metabolism and excretion in the bile. Recall that biliary excretion is the only major mechanism for cholesterol removal from the body. Growing evidence supports a role for HDL-C in preventing LDL oxidation as well. This role may be important, because only oxidized LDL is atherogenic (e.g., macrophages do not phagocytose normal LDL but only oxidized LDL and are then transformed into foam cells).

Note: It is the ratio of total cholesterol to HDL-C that is important, with an optimal ratio ≤ 3.5. A person with a total cholesterol of 180 but an HDL of only 30 has a ratio of 6, which places him or her at high risk for developing coronary artery disease.

11. What is the etiology of the disorder of lipid metabolism known as abetalipoproteinemia?

Abetalipoproteinemia is a genetic disorder characterized by the absence of betalipoprotein B, which results in the inability of intestinal enterocytes to assimilate triacylglycerols into chylomicrons. Intestinal biopsy reveals large, lipid-vacuolated enterocytes. Such patients have markedly decreased (or even absent) plasma chylomicrons.

CASE 5

A 65-year-old man complains of left-sided chest pain with exertion. The pain always resolves with rest and, if needed, sublingual nitroglycerin. He describes the pain as substernal pressure with a bit of a "burning" sensation. The pain remains localized and does not radiate to the arms, shoulder, or jaw. He denies any associated nausea, vomiting, or diaphoresis during these episodes of chest pain. An EKG stress test reveals cardiac ischemia (shown by ST-segment depression) when both heart rate and blood pressure have increased about 50% above baseline.

1. What is the most likely diagnosis?
Angina pectoris.

2. What produces the symptoms of angina pectoris in coronary artery disease?

Impaired blood flow to the myocardium due to atherosclerotic occlusion of the coronary arteries. Myocardial ischemia results in the release of chemical substances secondary to increased anaerobic metabolism (e.g., lactic acid) with a resultant reduction in pH, causing cardiac pain.

Note: Recall that visceral cardiac pain is sensed by sympathetic fibers. Be alert for "silent" cardiac ischemia in patients with autonomic neuropathy (e.g., diabetics) or patients who have received a heart transplant (in which the autonomic fibers have been severed).

3. What is claudication? Why are patients with angina more likely to have it?

Claudication is ischemic muscle pain, often triggered by exertion (e.g., calf pain with walking). Patients with coronary artery disease giving rise to symptoms of angina often have symptoms of peripheral vascular disease due to atherosclerotic occlusion of peripheral arteries.

4. Which disease of the aorta is generally due to atherosclerosis?
Abdominal aortic aneurysm (AAA).

5. What is the difference between stable and unstable angina? Which is more serious?

In **stable** angina, a constant and predictable level of physical exertion elicits the chest pain. In **unstable** angina, the chest pain develops in a setting in which it previously had not, such as at rest or after only mild exertion. Unstable angina is more serious because it indicates a significant change in the atheromatous plaque in the coronary arteries that is causing ischemia. When unstable angina develops, patients are worked up in the emergency department to rule out a myocardial infarction.

6. How can angina occur in the absence of coronary atherosclerosis?

In Prinzmetal's (variant) angina, cardiac ischemia results from vasospasm of the coronary arteries. Patients suffering from Prinzmetal's angina are more likely to suffer anginal pain at rest or in the morning. In addition, severe anemia theoretically can produce angina because of reduced delivery of oxygen to the heart.

Note: To summarize the types of angina: atheromatous disease may cause stable or unstable angina, whereas vasospasm may cause Prinzmetal's (variant) angina.

7. What are the principal physiologic determinants of myocardial oxygen demand (MVO_2)?

- Heart rate
- Contractility
- Intramyocardial wall tension during systole

8. Why is nitroglycerin effective in eliminating anginal pain?

Nitroglycerin is converted within endothelial cells to nitric oxide, which is also called endothelial-derived relaxation factor (EDRF) because of its vasodilatory effects. Perhaps the most important reason that nitroglycerin eliminates anginal pain is its effect on reducing myocardial oxygen demand secondary to venous dilation. Decreases in preload and afterload reduce cardiac contractility and myocardial wall tension, thus allowing greater myocardial perfusion during systole. Nitroglycerin and other organic nitrates also exert effects directly on the coronary vasculature, including vasodilation of the coronary arteries and relief of coronary artery spasm. The precise mechanism by which nitroglycerin reduces anginal pain, therefore, depends on which pathologic mechanism is responsible for the angina in a given patient (e.g., atherosclerotic occlusion, vasospasm).

Note: High doses of nitrates can produce **reflex tachycardia**, which occurs in response to hypotension and may further exacerbate anginal pain. In addition, because nitrates relax both vascular and nonvascular smooth muscle, they can relieve the pain of both angina and esophageal spasm, making it difficult to distinguish between the two conditions based solely on their response to nitrates.

9. What are the mechanisms by which beta blockers decrease myocardial oxygen demand and therefore the symptoms of angina?

- Decreased heart rate (direct effect on the heart)
- Decreased contractility (direct effect on the heart)
- Decreased afterload (secondary to decreased cardiac output and blood pressure), which reduces intramyocardial wall tension.

Note: The compensatory tachycardia that develops because of nitroglycerin-mediated vasodilation can be prevented with beta blockers.

10. A cardiac stress test is typically performed by monitoring the patient during exercise. Why is dobutamine often used for performing a stress test instead of exercise?

Dobutamine has positive inotropic and chronotropic effects on the heart; thus, its administration is physiologically similar to physical exertion (in terms of myocardial oxygen demand).

11. Is increased myocardial oxygen demand met primarily by increased oxygen extraction or by increased coronary blood flow?

Because oxygen extraction from coronary blood is extremely efficient even at baseline (about 70%), the primary compensatory mechanism available to the heart when oxygen demand increases is to increase coronary blood flow. If coronary blood flow becomes compromised, as in coronary artery disease, the cardiomyocytes, unlike other tissues in the body, are unable to extract significant amounts of additional oxygen from the blood and therefore depend on anaerobic metabolism. The resulting accumulation of indicators of anaerobic metabolism (e.g., lactate, potassium, adenosine, hydrogen ions), in addition to causing angina, causes coronary vasodilation and increases coronary blood flow but not to adequate levels.

Note: The highly efficient oxygen extraction from the blood in the coronary circulation explains why blood in the coronary veins is the darkest blood in the body.

CASE 6

A 48-year-old man who is obese and diaphoretic presents to the emergency department complaining of a crushing substernal pressure sensation for the past hour. The pain radiates to his left arm and his jaw. He is concerned because he usually gets chest pain only after exercising, and the pain is typically relieved by sublingual nitroglycerin. An immediate EKG is performed and reveals ST elevation in two consecutive leads. A chest x-ray does not show mediastinal widening or other abnormalities. The patient is given morphine, oxygen, nitroglycerin, metoprolol, and aspirin. The consulting cardiologist decides that he is a suitable candidate for emergent angioplasty, and he is taken to the cardiac catheterization laboratory.

1. What is the presumptive diagnosis?
Myocardial infarction (MI).

2. List common risk factors for MI and coronary heart disease in general.
Male gender, increasing age, hypertension, diabetes mellitus, tobacco use, hyperlipidemia, elevated homocysteine, and increased C-reactive protein.
Note: A common denominator in most of these risk factors is endothelial damage, which alters the endothelium from a normal antithrombotic surface to a pathologic prothrombotic surface. The damaged endothelium is also less effective at causing endothelium-mediated vasodilation.

3. In addition to analysis of the EKG, what serum tests can be ordered to confirm or rule out an MI?
Both the creatine kinase MB fraction (CK-MB) and cardiac specific troponins (cTnT, cTnI) are more sensitive indicators of MI than the EKG.

4. Which lab test is best for detecting an MI that began 4 days ago?
Cardiac troponin, because it is elevated for approximately 7–10 days after onset of an MI. Elevation of CK-MB lasts only about 72 hours.

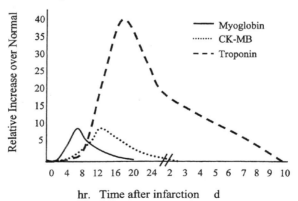

Myoglobin, creatine kinase MB fraction (CK-MB), and cardiac troponin increase after an MI. CK-MB peaks after about 16–24 hours and remains elevated for approximately 72 hours. Troponin peaks around 24 hours after an MI and remains elevated for 7–10 days. (From Henry JB: Clinical Diagnosis and Management by Laboratory Methods, 20th ed. Philadelphia, W.B. Saunders, 2001, p 297, with permission.)

5. What other treatment option is available besides angioplasty to quickly restore coronary blood flow? What are the major contraindications to its use?
Thrombolytic therapy with tissue plasminogen activator (tPA) or streptokinase, which must be performed within a limited timeframe to be effective. Thrombolytic therapy is contraindicated

in patients at high risk for hemorrhage (e.g., recent major surgery, bleeding disorder, severe hypertension, recent hemorrhagic cerebrovascular accident).

Note: Bleeding caused by thrombolytic therapy can be treated with *aminocaproic acid*, which inhibits the activation of plasminogen.

6. How can an MI cause pulmonary edema?

The infarcted myocardium of the left ventricle has reduced contractility, which results in an insufficient ejection fraction, causing backpressure of blood into the left atrium and ultimately into the pulmonary circulation. The resulting increased hydrostatic pressure within the pulmonary veins causes increased transudation of fluid into the pulmonary interstitium. Initially, this interstitial fluid is completely removed by the pulmonary lymphatics. However, when the hydrostatic pressure increases too much (typically > 30 mmHg), the ability of the lymphatics to remove excessive fluid is overcome, and interstitial fluid and intra-alveolar fluid accumulate, resulting in pulmonary edema.

Note: Pulmonary edema reduces oxygen diffusion across the pulmonary membrane, causing hypoxemia, which further exacerbates the failing heart. This is one reason why oxygen therapy is beneficial in patients with MI.

7. What complication of an MI should be suspected if a pericardial effusion develops quite abruptly?

Ventricular rupture, which typically occurs between 3 and 7 days after the infarct.

Note: The inflammatory reaction to necrotic myocardium can also cause pericarditis (usually within 3–5 days after MI). Suspect this condition if you hear a pericardial friction rub.

8. What is Dressler's syndrome?

Pericarditis that develops several weeks after an MI. It is presumed to result from an autoimmune process.

9. What complication of MI can result in a high-pitched holosystolic murmur?

Papillary muscle rupture, which causes severe mitral valve regurgitation.

10. What is sudden cardiac death? Why are patients who have had MIs predisposed to it?

Sudden cardiac death is defined as death within 1 hour of onset of symptoms (usually due to a lethal arrhythmia). People with previous MIs commonly develop arrhythmias, some of which may prove lethal.

11. What is the physiologic rationale for giving beta blockers to patients who have had myocardial infarctions?

As in angina, these drugs lower myocardial oxygen demand, making the heart less susceptible to infarction. In addition, by antagonizing catecholamines, these drugs also may prevent catecholamine-mediated arrhythmias. Regardless of their mechanism, they have been shown to reduce mortality when given after an MI.

12. What is the difference between pale infarcts and hemorrhagic (red) infarcts? Which type is typically found in myocardial infarction?

In hemorrhagic infarcts there is a dual/collateral blood supply to the infarcted region, which, although not sufficient to prevent infarction, does allow blood to seep into the infarct and color it red. This process occurs in the intestines and the lung. In contrast, in pale infarcts there is no dual circulation. Pale infarcts occur in the brain, spleen, kidneys, and heart.

CASE 7

A 72-year-old man with a long history of poorly controlled hypertension presents with fatigue, lethargy, and increasing difficulty with breathing (dyspnea) over the past year. Initially, he experienced difficulty with breathing only with exertion, but recently he has experienced the problem even at rest and admits to supporting himself with two pillows at night to help with breathing (two-pillow orthopnea). Physical examination reveals jugular venous distention, pulmonary rales, hepatomegaly, and bilateral pitting edema of the ankles. A chest x-ray shows cardiomegaly and pulmonary congestion, and an EKG reveals left axis deviation secondary to left ventricular hypertrophy. An echocardiogram does not reveal any valvular abnormalities.

1. What is the diagnosis?

Congestive heart failure, although it is more properly termed heart failure because not all patients have "congestive" symptoms (i.e., pooling of blood in the venous system).

2. Describe the pathophysiology of heart failure.

Heart failure results from either (1) pathologically depressed cardiac output or (2) normal cardiac output that can be maintained only at elevated ventricular filling pressures. Depressed cardiac output causes symptoms such as fatigue, lethargy, and weakness, whereas elevated ventricular filling pressures cause "congestive" symptoms such as pulmonary edema with dyspnea (if left ventricular pressure is elevated) and jugular venous distention, hepatomegaly, and pitting edema (if right ventricular pressure is elevated). This patient has signs of both left-sided and right-sided failure.

Note: The most common cause of right-sided heart failure is left-sided heart failure. Other less common causes of right-sided heart failure include pulmonary hypertension (idiopathic or secondary to pulmonary disease) and pulmonic stenosis.

3. What *causes* heart failure?

Literally, any disease that can impair cardiac function can cause heart failure. Examples include valvular diseases (e.g., aortic stenosis), ischemic disease of the heart (e.g., coronary artery disease), intrinsic myocardial disease (e.g., congenital cardiomyopathy), and longstanding untreated hypertension (as in this patient). This list, however, is not exhaustive. Heart failure can be broadly classified as systolic (pump) failure or diastolic (filling) failure.

Note: The most common cause of heart failure is coronary artery disease, which, when manifesting as heart failure, is referred to as ischemic cardiomyopathy.

4. Discuss the difference between systolic and diastolic heart failure.

Systolic heart failure is characterized by insufficient contractility of the ventricles, with an ejection fraction below 40%. Diastolic heart failure is characterized by poor ventricular compliance, resulting in insufficient filling of ventricles during diastole. It is estimated that approximately two-thirds of patients with heart failure have systolic failure and the remaining one-third have diastolic failure. Unfortunately, the situation becomes messier when one realizes that most patients with systolic dysfunction have components of diastolic dysfunction as well.

Note: The ejection fraction is defined as stroke volume (SV) divided by end-diastolic volume (EDV) and is normally 60–70%.

5. What is the *adaptive value* of the following physiologic responses in heart failure?

Increased sympathetic outflow results in tachycardia and increased contractility of the heart, both of which increase cardiac output (CO). Recall that the determinants of cardiac output are given by the equation:

$$CO = HR \times SV$$

In addition, in the setting of reduced CO (such as heart failure), vasoconstriction caused by elevated sympathetic outflow helps maintain sufficient arterial pressure to provide adequate perfusion to critical organs. Remember, the determinants of mean arterial pressure (MAP) are CO and total peripheral resistance (TPR):

$$MAP = CO \times TPR$$

Note: It is interesting that patients in heart failure secrete 3-4 times more norepinephrine per day than healthy people.

Fluid retention and plasma volume expansion (secondary to activation of the renin-angiotensin-aldosterone system) increases preload. Recall the Frank-Starling relationship, whereby an increased preload has a positive inotropic effect on the heart, which will again increase cardiac output. This inotropic effect is thought to be due to optimal alignment of the actin and myosin filaments in the cardiac sarcomeres that occurs with ventricular stretching.

Note: The reduced CO in heart failure leads to a decrease in renal perfusion and GFR, which activates the renin-angiotensin-aldosterone system and causes fluid retention. In essence, the kidneys sense the reduced CO and decide that they can help by retaining fluid to exploit the Frank-Starling relationship.

The value of **myocardial hypertrophy** depends on the type of overload that occurs in heart failure. In a pressure-overloaded heart (from hypertension or aortic stenosis), concentric hypertrophy (circular thickening of the myocardium) strengthens ventricular contractions to increase ejection fraction in the setting of a significant afterload. In a volume-overloaded heart (aortic regurgitation), the increase in diastolic wall stress from increased end-diastolic volume causes poor alignment of sarcomere fibrils (past the adaptive point of the Frank-Starling relationship); as a result, sarcomeres are added in series to expand the chamber volume and optimize fiber alignment, causing an eccentric hypertrophy. Interestingly, in both the pressure-overloaded ventricle and the volume-overloaded ventricle the homeostatic set point around which the heart remodels is wall stress. In pressure-overloaded ventricles the increased systolic wall stress causes addition of sarcomeres in parallel, which reduces the stress on each sarcomere, and in volume-overloaded ventricles the increased diastolic wall stress stimulates the addition of sarcomeres in series, which normalizes diastolic wall stress.

Note: If an adequate CO is restored by these compensatory mechanisms, the heart failure is said to be compensated. If these physiologic reflexes alone cannot restore adequate CO, the heart failure is said to be decompensated.

6. What are the *pathologic* consequences of fluid retention?

Fluid retention can also cause complications associated with excessive volume expansion, such as pulmonary edema. Because both nitrates and diuretics decrease preload (as well as afterload to some degree), they help alleviate the *symptoms* of congestive heart failure associated with excessive volume expansion.

7. What are the *pathologic* consequences of myocardial hypertrophy?

Oxygen demand of the hypertrophied heart is increased, which may exacerbate an existing ischemic condition. In fact, the vascular supply to the heart often does not increase proportionately to the muscular hypertrophy. In addition, the elevated intramural pressures caused by concentric myocardial hypertrophy further compromise coronary perfusion. Hypertrophy may also result in reduced ventricular compliance, which causes diastolic dysfunction.

8. What are the *pathologic* consequences of increased sympathetic nervous system activation?

The sympathetically mediated chronic vasoconstriction in skeletal muscles that occurs during heart failure is largely responsible for the muscular weakness observed in affected people.

9. How is digitalis, which is used in heart failure, believed to increase cardiac contractility?

Like skeletal muscle fibers, cardiac muscle fibers contract when the intracellular calcium levels rise. Digitalis increases intracellular calcium by an indirect mechanism involving ion exchanges. By inhibiting the sodium-potassium pump, digitalis increases intracellular sodium. However, it is the extracellular-intracellular sodium gradient that drives the sodium-calcium exchanger. Consequently, in the presence of high intracellular sodium less calcium is pumped out of the cell, thus increasing intracellular calcium and contractility.

10. Does digitalis improve mortality rates in patients with congestive heart failure?

No. Digitalis has been shown to improve cardiac performance and quality of life, but it has not been shown to improve mortality rates. In contrast, drugs such as ACE inhibitors and beta blockers have been shown to extend life.

11. Cover the right-hand columns with your hand and attempt to list the mechanism of action for each of the following drugs used in CHF.

DRUG	CLASS OF DRUG	MECHANISM OF ACTION
Digitalis	Cardiac glycoside	Positive inotropic effect, negative chronotropic effect, increased ejection fraction
Metoprolol	Beta blocker	Negative chronotropic and inotropic effects, decreased MVO_2 demand
Captopril	ACE inhibitor	Decreases in aldosterone, plasma volume, and actions of angiotensin II
Losartan	Angiotensin II receptor antagonist	Inhibits actions of angiotensin II

12. Define cardiomyopathy.

Cardiomyopathy is a classification of heart disease in which the myocardium itself is the primary site of disease involvement, and the myocardial dysfunction does not result from coronary atherosclerosis, valvular abnormalities, pericardial disease, or hypertension. The three main types are dilated cardiomyopathy, hypertrophic cardiomyopathy, and restrictive cardiomyopathy.

13. What are the general characteristics of each of these cardiomyopathies?

In dilated cardiomyopathy the ventricular chambers are enlarged, most commonly for unknown reasons, although alcoholism and toxins such as cobalt, lead, and phosphorous, as well as rare infectious diseases (Chagas disease), may be causative. **Hypertrophic** cardiomyopathy is a congenital disorder in which the ventricular septum is abnormally enlarged; hence its synonym, idiopathic hypertrophic subaortic stenosis (IHSS). **Restrictive** cardiomyopathy is characterized by reduced myocardial compliance, which can be due to a host of different factors but often results from infiltration of the myocardium and ensuing fibrosis (as in hemochromatosis, sarcoidosis, and amyloidosis).

14. What is high-output heart failure?

In general, this term refers to the inability of the heart to maintain an elevated cardiac output in pathologic situations that demand it (e.g., thyrotoxicosis, large arteriovenous malformations). A perfectly healthy heart can typically handle the additional circulatory demands of these diseases, but in a heart with some degree of dysfunction these diseases create a load that cannot be met effectively. Nevertheless, if excessive loads are maintained for a long time on a healthy heart, cardiac function may eventually deteriorate, culminating in low-output heart failure.

Note: Bacterial sepsis, in which endotoxemia results in marked systemic vasodilatation and reduction in total peripheral resistance, is another common cause of high-output heart failure.

CASE 8

A 50-year-old man complains of angina that occurs at gradually diminishing levels of physical exertion as well as two recent episodes of syncope while golfing. On physical examination he has a narrow pulse pressure, and his carotid pulse is delayed and weak (pulsus parvus et tardus). Auscultation reveals a systolic ejection murmur heard best in the second right interspace. An EKG reveals left ventricular hypertrophy, and an echocardiogram reveals a bicuspid aortic valve with reduced valvular area.

1. What is the diagnosis?
Aortic stenosis.

2. What predisposed this patient to developing aortic stenosis?
The normal aortic valve is tricuspid, and stenosis generally occurs only in elderly patients secondary to calcification (senile calcific aortic stenosis). However, congenitally bicuspid or even monocuspid valves can calcify and stenose much earlier, usually in the late forties or fifties, as in this man.

3. Why does this patient have left ventricular hypertrophy?
As a compensatory mechanism to overcome the resistance to flow created by the stenotic valve.

4. What are some causes of increased myocardial oxygen demand in aortic stenosis?
Increased left ventricular mass requires more oxygen for normal contractile function. In addition, the increased left ventricular pressures that develop to overcome the outflow resistance increase the workload on the left ventricle, further increasing the MVO_2. Finally, the increased time spent in systole to eject the blood also increases the myocardial oxygen demand.

5. What are some causes of decreased myocardial oxygen supply in aortic stenosis?
Because more time is spent in systole, less time is spent in diastole (when the majority of coronary perfusion occurs). In addition, increased left ventricular pressures during diastole (because of reduced ventricular compliance) further reduce perfusion. Finally, aortic pressure is reduced, which may reduce coronary blood flow.

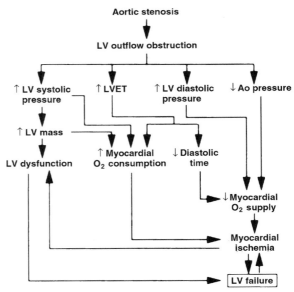

Causes of increased myocardial oxygen demand and decreased myocardial oxygen supply. (From Braunwald E: Heart Disease: A Textbook of Cardiovascular Medicne, 6th ed. Philadelphia, W.B. Saunders, 2001, p 1674, with permission. Derived from Boudoulas H, Gravanis MB: Valvular heart disease. In Gravanis MB: Cardiovascular Disorders: Pathogenesis and Pathophysiology. St. Louis, Mosby, 1993, p 64.)

6. Why is atrial fibrillation a dangerous complication in aortic stenosis (aside from the risk of embolic stroke)?
Because cardiac output is already compromised in this patient, the additional ventricular filling that results from atrial contraction is critical to sustaining cardiac output. Atrial fibrillation will ablate this input and may precipitate severe heart failure.

Note: Reduced cardiac output is most likely responsible for the episodes of syncope in this patient.

7. What causes heart murmurs? Why does this patient have one?

Murmurs are caused by turbulent flow, which occurs at elevated flow velocities. In this case, the stenotic aortic valve forces the heart to contract more forcefully, which generates a significant pressure gradient between the left ventricle and aorta, creating high flow velocities across the aortic valve.

Note: Carotid bruits are due to the same mechanism as murmurs, with the stenotic lumen causing increased flow velocities and a resulting turbulent blood flow that can be auscultated.

8. Explain why this patient has a narrow pulse pressure.

In aortic stenosis, a significant proportion of cardiac energy is devoted to generating sufficient force to overcome the valvular resistance. Consequently, a smaller proportion of cardiac energy is used to eject blood, causing a smaller stroke volume and smaller pulse pressure. In addition, the ventricular hypertrophy can impair diastolic filling, reducing preload and contractility via the Frank-Starling mechanism.

9. Would ventricular myocytes spend more time in isotonic or isometric (isovolemic) contraction as a result of aortic stenosis?

More time is spent in isometric (isovolumic) contraction to overcome the increased afterload forces caused by the stenotic aortic valve. The result is a shortened isotonic ejection phase.

6. FEMALE REPRODUCTIVE SYSTEM

Dave Brown and Thomas Brown

BASIC CONCEPTS

1. What is the normal duration of the menstrual cycle? What are the two ovarian phases? Which occurs first?

Normal cycle time is approximately 28 days, and the ovarian phases consist of the follicular phase and luteal phase, with the follicular phase occurring first. The first day of the cycle is defined as the day on which menses begin, and the follicular phase begins coincident with the beginning of menses.

2. Which phase is generally responsible for a longer or shorter cycle?

Since the luteal phase is fixed at 14 days in the majority of women, differences in the length of the follicular phase account for cycle length differences.

3. What hormonal changes occur in the pituitary during the follicular phase?

Because the corpus luteum, which is the principal source of estrogen during the preceding luteal phase, has involuted before the beginning of the follicular phase, plasma estrogen levels at the beginning of the follicular phase are low. Thus the negative feedback effect of estrogen on pituitary production of follicle-stimulating hormone (FSH) is reduced and FSH secretion begins to rise.

4. What hormonal changes occur in the ovary during the follicular phase?

During the follicular phase, the rising FSH level stimulates the development of several ovarian follicles, eventually causing the emergence of a dominant follicle, which becomes a site of estrogen synthesis. The growing follicle secretes increasing amounts of estrogen, which inhibit pituitary production of FSH, thereby gradually reducing serum FSH levels in the later part of the follicular phase. However, because the dominant follicle becomes increasingly sensitive to circulating FSH, plasma estrogen levels still continue to rise throughout the follicular phase.

Note: Inhibin is also secreted by the ovaries and selectively inhibits FSH secretion with no effect on secretion of luteinizing hormone (LH).

5. What occurs in the uterus during the follicular phase?

After menses, the estrogen secreted by the ovaries stimulates proliferation of the endometrial lining of the uterus throughout the follicular phase.

6. What causes ovulation at the end of the follicular phase?

When plasma estrogen reaches a critical level, it switches from causing negative feedback on the pituitary to causing positive feedback and stimulates the pituitary to release a surge of LH and FSH. The surge of these hormones causes rupture of the follicle and release of the ovum. This is an elegant design feature, because suitably high estrogen levels indicate to the pituitary that the ovarian follicle is sufficiently "mature" to be released .

7. What happens in the ovary and endometrium during the luteal phase?

After ovulation, the cells that lined the follicle (granulosa cells and theca interna cells) form the corpus luteum (yellow body) under the influence of LH. The corpus luteum synthesizes both estrogen and a large amount of progesterone. The progesterone stimulates the endometrium to become more secretory and glandular in preparation for implantation. If fertilization does not occur, the corpus luteum degenerates, the levels of estrogen and progesterone fall, and the endometrium sloughs off as the menstrual flow.

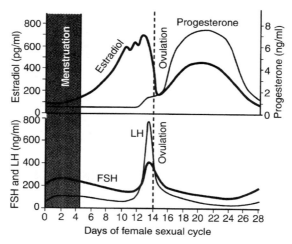

Levels of plasma ovarian hormones and gonadotropins during the female menstrual/ovarian cycles. (From Guyton AC, Hall J: The Textbook of Medical Physiology, 10th ed. Philadelphia, W.B. Saunders, 2000, with permission.)

8. Why does bleeding after the cessation of a brief course of progesterone indicate that the cause of amenorrhea (absence of menses) is lack of ovulation?

If the administration and withdrawal of progesterone cause menses, the endometrium has been sufficiently primed by estrogen and requires only a course of progesterone for menses to occur. However, the only source of endogenous progesterone is the corpus luteum, which forms only after ovulation. If there is no ovulation, there is no progesterone secretion and hence no normal menses.

9. How does fertilization prevent degeneration of the corpus luteum?

If the ovum is fertilized, the developing embryo will synthesize human chorionic gonadotropin (hCG), which acts similarly to LH and maintains the corpus luteum.

10. How does the corpus luteum function in the maintenance of pregnancy?

During the first 6 weeks of pregnancy the corpus luteum is the primary producer of estrogen and progesterone, hormones required for the continuation of pregnancy.

Note: After the sixth week of pregnancy, the placenta begins to take over as the principal site of steroidogenesis. After delivery and removal of the placenta, both estrogen and progesterone levels fall markedly.

CASE 1

A 38-year-old woman who smokes and has hypertension wants to start taking oral contraceptives.

1. Why should estrogen-containing oral contraceptives be used with considerable caution in this patient?

Estrogen-containing oral contraceptives increase the risk of various thrombotic and thromboembolic phenomena, including stroke, myocardial infarction, deep venous thrombosis, and pulmonary embolism. In women who smoke, such contraceptives increase this risk substantially (as does the patient's hypertension) and are therefore relatively contraindicated in such women older than 35 years.

Note: Although estrogens in oral contraceptives have been shown to increase the production of various clotting factors and decrease the production of antithrombin III, no clear relationship between estrogens and bleeding times or clotting times has been shown.

2. **What are the absolute contraindications to using estrogen-containing oral contraceptives?**
   - Thromboembolic phenomena
   - Hepatic tumors (estrogens can make hepatic tumors grow and rupture)
   - Estrogen-dependent cancers, such as endometrial carcinoma or breast carcinoma

3. **What are the typical components of oral contraceptives? Describe their mechanism of action.**

   The two general types of oral contraceptive are the combination pill (estrogen and progesterone) and the progesterone-only pills. In the combination pills, the constant level of estrogen supplied continuously suppresses pituitary gonadotropin secretion, thereby removing the stimulus for ovulation. The progesterone in the combination pills serves two functions: (1) it alters the cervical mucus secretions, essentially making the vaginal/uterine environment less "receptive" to sperm, and (2) it opposes the proliferative effects of estrogen (unopposed estrogen increases the risk for breast and endometrial cancers). The progesterone-only pills are not highly effective at inhibiting ovulation but, as mentioned, they also work by thickening the cervical mucus and altering the motility and secretions of the fallopian tubes.

4. **How can menstrual cycles be made regular by oral contraceptives?**

   For menstruation to occur, there must first be estrogenic stimulation of endometrial proliferation; then progesterone must induce maturation and stimulate secretion by the endometrial glands. Menses then can begin following the decline in progesterone and estrogen levels near the end of the menstrual cycle. In some women, these hormonal events do not occur in such a well-orchestrated manner. Consequently, the estrogen and progesterone stimulation of the endometrium can be provided artificially to mimic the natural menstrual period. Typically, to achieve this type of control, estrogens are given with progesterones for 21 days; then placebo pills are given for 7 days to allow menstruation.

   Note: It is principally the withdrawal of progesterone (not estrogen) that causes normal menses.

5. **How does taking oral contraceptives affect the risk for ovarian cancer? What is supposed to explain this effect?**

   The risk decreases. The proposed explanation is that by inhibiting ovulation, oral contraceptives reduce the inflammatory response and cell proliferation that usually occur on the ovarian surface after each follicle ruptures through the ovarian surface. Presumably, this process predisposes to many ovarian cancers. Consistent with this notion is the fact that the ovarian surface epithelium is the site from which the vast majority of ovarian tumors arise—not the follicular cells.

6. **How do ovarian cysts form? How do oral contraceptives reduce their occurrence?**

   The most common ovarian cysts are "functional cysts" that form when the normal process of follicular maturation and corpus luteum formation becomes somewhat aberrant (follicular cysts and corpus lutein cysts, respectively). Follicular cysts develop after failure of a mature ovarian follicle to rupture and be ovulated. Corpus lutein cysts are formed during the luteal phase and occur when the corpus luteum becomes abnormally large or hemorrhagic (corpus hemorrhagicum). Clearly, the inhibition of follicular maturation and ovulation by oral contraceptives should reduce the chance that such cysts will develop.

7. **Why may the drugs phenytoin, phenobarbital, and rifampin make oral contraceptives less effective at preventing pregnancy?**

   These drugs induce hepatic cytochrome p450 enzymes, which can accelerate the rate of hepatic catabolism of estrogen and progesterone compounds.

CASE 2

A 26-year-old woman has not had a period for approximately 2 months, whereas she was previously regular. She has also had several episodes of nausea and vomiting that she cannot explain. She is absolutely certain that she cannot be pregnant. Physical exam reveals no palpable abdominal or pelvic masses or tenderness. A test for serum β-hCG test is positive.

1. Does an elevated β-hCG test always indicate a developing embryo or fetus?

No. Gestational trophoblastic tumors (hydatiform moles, invasive moles, choriocarcinoma) as well as several germ-cell tumors of the ovary also elaborate beta-hCG. Note, however, that all of these entities are quite rare.

2. What is the normal function of β-hCG, aside from serving as a marker for pregnancy?

Human chorionic gonadotropin is a hormone similar in structure and activity to LH. It is secreted early in pregnancy by the placenta (specifically, the syncytiotrophoblast cells) and functions to maintain the corpus luteum, which is the principal site of ovarian steroidogenesis during the luteal phase. Plasma levels of β-hCG peak in the first trimester (between weeks 9 and 12 of gestation). Then, as the placenta begins to take over as the main site of maternal estrogen and progesterone secretion, the β-hCG levels taper off.

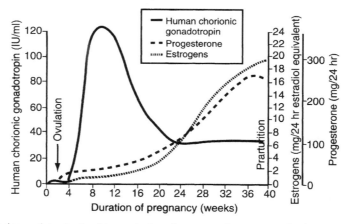

Human chorionic gonadotropin stimulates production of estrogen and progesterone by the corpus luteum. As the levels of this hormone drop, the placenta takes over as the major site of synthesis of ovarian steroids. (From Guyton AC, Hall J: Textbook of Medical Physiology, 10th ed. Philadelphia, W.B. Saunders, 2000, with permission.)

3. Relative to a normal pregnancy, how does the β-hCG level differ for an ectopic pregnancy?

In ectopic pregnancy, since there is poor placentation (with fewer syncytiotrophoblast cells to produce β-hCG), the serum β-hCG is significantly less than would be expected for a normal pregnancy of the same gestational age.

4. Assuming that the positive β-hCG test confirms a pregnancy in this patient, what was the approximate date of conception?

Because ovulation occurs approximately 2 weeks after the onset of menses and her last menses began 8 weeks ago, the approximate date of conception was 6 weeks ago.

5. What is the difference between gestational age and time since conception (also called developmental age)?

The gestational age is the period that has elapsed since the last menstrual period. It is not the time since conception, a mistake that students commonly make. Since conception typically occurs 2 weeks later, the time since conception is 2 weeks shorter than the gestational age.

6. **At what time during development is the embryo/fetus most susceptible to teratogens?**
During the third to eighth week (days 15–56, the "embryonic period"), when organogenesis occurs.

7. **The risk of which fetal developmental abnormalities can be reduced by taking supplemental folic acid early during pregnancy?**
Developmental abnormalities of the central nervous system and spinal cord, which may cause neural tube defects such as spina bifida and/or anencephaly. Ideally, prenatal supplements are taken *before* pregnancy, because significant neural development may already have occurred by the time a woman realizes that she is pregnant.

8. **Is this patient at high or low risk for having a baby with Down syndrome (trisomy 21)?**
The incidence of Down syndrome increases significantly with maternal age, and since she is only 26, the risk is quite low. The risk increases from approximately 1 in 1500 babies of 16-year-old mothers to approximately 1 in 25 babies of 45-year-old mothers.
Note: Maternal serum alpha-fetoprotein (AFP) levels are often checked around the 16th week of pregnancy. High levels may indicate a neural tube defect such as spina bifida, whereas low levels may indicate Down syndrome.   also omphalocel,

9. **Why should ergot alkaloids (e.g., ergonovine), triptans (e.g., sumatriptan), and synthetic prostaglandins (e.g., misoprostol) be stringently avoided during pregnancy?**
All of these agents cause powerful uterine contractions that can result in abortion. The effects of ergot alkaloids and triptans are principally mediated through serotonin receptors. Misoprostol is a synthetic prostaglandin that causes contractions in a fashion analogous to endogenous prostaglandins.

CASE 3

A 26-year-old woman has thought that she was pregnant for the past 2 months because she was amenorrheic and a urine pregnancy test was positive. However, one morning she notices heavy vaginal bleeding and passage of what looks like a cluster of grapes. A pelvic ultrasound reveals a "snowstorm" pattern and no discernible fetus. Serum beta-hCG levels are elevated far above what would be expected in pregnancy.

1. **What is the diagnosis?**
Molar pregnancy.

2. **How can beta-hCG levels differentiate between a normal pregnancy and a molar pregnancy (complete or incomplete mole)?**
Since moles are made exclusively of trophoblastic tissue, the site of beta-hCG synthesis, serum levels of beta-hCG levels are substantially elevated compared with a normal pregnancy of similar "gestational age." Other features that suggest a molar pregnancy include severe vaginal bleeding early in the pregnancy and vaginal passage of molar vesicles.

3. **What is the difference between invasive moles and choriocarcinoma? From what does each generally arise?**
An invasive mole invades the myometrium but does not normally metastasize. The majority arise from benign molar pregnancies. Choriocarcinoma, on the other hand, is often metastatic and spreads hematogenously. Half of these develop from benign molar pregnancies, one-fourth after normal term pregnancy, and one-fourth after miscarriage, abortion, or ectopic pregnancy. A key histologic distinction between invasive mole and choriocarcinoma is that the choriocarcinoma is less differentiated and lacks a villous pattern.

4. Cover the right-hand columns and try to identify the characteristics of the different gestational trophoblastic diseases listed below.

TYPE	BENIGN OR MALIGNANT	KARYOTYPE	FETAL PARTS PRESENT
Complete mole	Benign	Diploid	No
Incomplete mole	Benign	Triploid (69XXY or 69XXX)	Yes
Invasive mole	Malignant	Diploid	No
Choriocarcinoma	Malignant	Diploid	No

CASE 4

A 32-year-old G2P1 woman at 12 weeks' gestation by last known menstrual period complains of occasional palpitations, irritability, and heat intolerance. Except for a gravid abdomen, physical exam is unremarkable. However, because of her symptoms, a thyroid panel is ordered. The results reveal elevated levels of total and free thyroid hormones (triiodothyronine [T_3] and thyroxine [T_4]) as well as reduced levels of thyroid-stimulating hormone (TSH).

1. Does an elevated T_4 necessarily indicate hyperthyroidism? Explain.

No. Elevated *free* T_4 (or free T_3) causes hyperthyroidism. Elevated *total* T_4 can result from increased levels of thyroxine-binding globulin, with no change in free T_4. In fact, during pregnancy the total T_4 is usually elevated because estrogen increases the synthesis of thyroxine-binding globulin by the liver. Notice, however, that this patient also had elevated levels of free T_4.

2. How does the pregnant state predispose to hyperthyroidism?

The presence of hCG in the maternal circulation predisposes to hyperthyroidism. hCG is a glycoprotein synthesized and secreted by the placenta in large amounts. Due to its similarity in structure with TSH, it often hyperstimulates the thyroid gland during pregnancy, resulting in gestational hyperthyroidism. This condition typically resolves spontaneously after delivery of the fetus and placenta.

3. How are maternal levels of FSH and LH likely to be affected in this patient, given that she is pregnant?

They should be low and virtually undetectable because of the significant negative feedback that the high levels of estrogen and progesterone associated with pregnancy produce on the pituitary.

4. Why is the decline in estrogen and progesterone after delivery beneficial for the beginning of lactation?

Both estrogen and progesterone inhibit lactation, and their withdrawal allows the elevated prolactin present at the time of delivery to facilitate milk letdown and lactation. Recall that the placenta is the major site of progesterone and estrogen secretion; thus, its expulsion after delivery reduces the levels of these hormones.

5. How does breast-feeding act as a natural contraceptive?

Nipple suckling by the baby stimulates the release of prolactin by the anterior pituitary gland. Because one of the functions of prolactin is to inhibit the hypothalamic secretion of gonadotropin-releasing hormone (GnRH), the result is reduced secretion of FSH and LH by the pituitary as long as the baby is nursing. Reduced levels of these gonadotropins inhibit ovulation in the nursing mother and act as a natural birth control pill.

Note: This method of contraception has a fairly high failure rate. Do not go crazy trying it at home.

CASE 5

A 28-year-old woman in her thirty-third week of pregnancy is evaluated for proteinuria, an elevated blood pressure of 150/110 mmHg (up from 130/90 mmHg), and +2 pitting edema of both legs. Brisk deep tendon reflexes are also noted on exam. The next week she developed right upper quadrant pain, her proteinuria became worse, and her blood pressure increased to 170/115 mmHg. Lab tests reveal anemia, schistocytes, thrombocytopenia, and elevated serum levels of aspartate aminotransferase (AST) and alanine aminotransferase (ALT).

1. What was the initial diagnosis?

Preeclampsia, which is characterized by hypertension (> 140/90 mmHg), proteinuria (> 300 mg/day), and edema during pregnancy.

Note: The severity of preeclampsia is generally determined by the degree of proteinuria and blood pressure elevation.

2. What syndrome did the patient develop subsequently?

The HELLP syndrome, which can be a complication of severe preeclampsia, consists of hemolysis, elevated liver enzymes, and low platelets. Recall that schistocytes are fragmented red blood cells indicative of a microangiopathic hemolysis.

3. If the patient also develops seizures, how does the diagnosis change?

Assuming that she does not have a preexisting seizure disorder or metabolic abnormality, she has eclampsia, which is defined as seizures in a patient with preeclampsia and no other known causes of seizures.

4. What is the definitive treatment for preeclampsia, eclampsia, and the HELLP syndrome?

Delivery of the fetus is the only definitive treatment. Supportive management includes *magnesium sulfate* ($MgSO_4$) for seizure prophylaxis in eclamptic patients. For preeclamptic patients, $MgSO_4$ is also often given as seizure prophylaxis during labor and delivery.

5. Angiotensin-converting enzyme (ACE) inhibitors and angiotensin receptor blockers (ARBs) should not be used to treat hypertension in women with pre-eclampsia. Explain.

ACE inhibitors and ARBs should not be used to treat *any* pregnant woman, because they carry the risk of causing fetal renal failure and even fetal death.

CASE 6

A 26-year-old woman at 32 weeks' gestation has come to the hospital because she has been having contractions for the past 3 hours, and they are now occurring every 10 minutes. The diameter of her cervical canal is 2 cm. She is told that she may be going into premature labor.

1. What pharmacologic agents can be used to suppress labor?

Agents that inhibit uterine contractions are known as tocolytics. Magnesium sulfate is most widely used. Other classes of drugs include beta-2 receptor agonists (usually *terbutaline* and *ritodrine*) and calcium channel blockers (*nifedipine* is most widely used). These two drug classes are smooth muscle relaxants. Additionally, *indomethacin* and other NSAIDs can decrease uterine contractions by inhibiting prostaglandin synthesis.

Note: After approximately 32 weeks' gestation, there is concern about using nonsteroidal anti-inflammatory drugs (NSAIDs) because of their potential to cause premature constriction of the ductus arteriosus. Remember that prostaglandins are vasodilatory and that NSAIDs inhibit prostaglandin synthesis.

2. What is the main source of risk to the baby of premature delivery?

The principal concern with premature delivery is immature fetal lungs, which can cause neonatal respiratory distress syndrome. Fetal lung maturity is determined by the amount of surfactant present, which can be assessed with amniocentesis and evaluation of the lecithin-to-sphingomyelin ratio, which should be greater than two for mature lungs. Glucocorticoids can be given to a woman in premature labor to increase the production of surfactant. Typically, surfactant production begins by 28 weeks and is complete by 36 weeks.

3. If placenta previa is present at term (or when delivery is necessary), why would a caesarean section be mandatory?

Placenta previa occurs when the placenta covers the internal cervical os. With a vaginal delivery the placenta would have to rupture for the baby to pass through the cervix (a horrifying bloody mess).

4. How can placenta accreta complicate the labor and delivery process?

Placenta accreta occurs when the placenta has invaded and attached firmly to the myometrium. In this situation, the placenta does not separate from the endometrial lining after delivery of the infant.

5. What is oxytocin? How is it used to augment or induce labor?

Oxytocin is a peptide hormone produced naturally by the posterior pituitary and is a stimulant for uterine contractions. Exogenous oxytocin (pitocin) enhances uterine contractions and accelerates the first stage of labor.

Note: During pregnancy the number of oxytocin receptors on the uterus increases, which makes the uterus particularly sensitive to endogenous or exogenous oxytocin at the end of term.

6. What pharmacologic agents may be used if delivery is complicated by postpartum hemorrhage?

Several different pharmacologic agents, including the ergot alkaloids, oxytocin, and certain prostaglandins, cause uterine contractions, which reduce postpartum bleeding by clamping down on bleeding vessels.

Note: Ischemic necrosis of the anterior pituitary gland, known as Sheehan's syndrome, is a potential complication of severe postpartum hemorrhage.

CASE 7

A 28-year-old woman who has never been pregnant and has no history of prior surgeries complains of chronic pelvic pain that is particularly severe during her menstrual period (dysmennorrhea). She also complains of significant pain during sexual intercourse (dyspareunia). Pelvic exam is significant for slight adnexal tenderness. Stains for *Neisseria gonorrhoeae* and *Chlamydia trachomatis* are negative, and a beta-hCG is also negative. A pelvic ultrasound revealed no fibroids or structures suggestive of ovarian neoplasms. Laparoscopy reveals the presence of "chocolate cysts" on both ovaries.

1. What is the most likely diagnosis?

Endometriosis.

2. What causes endometriosis?

Endometriosis is caused by the presence of endometrial tissue in ectopic (extrauterine) locations, such as the ovaries or uterine ligaments. Perhaps the most widely accepted theory to explain the presence of endometrial tissue in extrauterine sites is the phenomenon of retrograde menstruation through the fallopian tubes, a process that is thought to occur in most women. Unfortunately, such retrograde flow does not completely explain the presence of ectopic endometrial tissues in distant anatomic sites such as the pleural cavity.

3. Why is pain worse during the menstrual period in this patient?

Ectopic endometrial tissue undergoes the same cycle of proliferation and breakdown as the normal endometrial lining in response to estrogen and progesterone. The resulting bleeding causes inflammation and pain. Over the long term, this inflammation can lead to tissue damage, fibrosis, adhesions, and compression of adjacent structures, resulting in signs and symptoms such as chronic pelvic pain and infertility. For this reason it is important to diagnose and treat endometriosis early in its development.

Note: Although ectopic endometrial tissue is most frequently found in the pelvis, it can also be found in various other anatomic sites, such as the upper abdomen or thorax. These sites can also become painful during menstrual cycling.

4. What does the presence of ovarian "chocolate cysts" indicate? Why are they black in appearance?

Chocolate cysts are nonfunctional ovarian cysts (endometriomas) that develop from ectopic endometrial tissue present in advanced endometriosis. They are black in appearance because they contain a blood-filled cavity.

5. What is the mechanism of action of leuprolide, a GnRH analog, in treating endometriosis?

The pituitary gland normally releases gonadotropins in response to the *pulsatile* secretion of GnRH from the hypothalamus, but the *continual* presence of leuprolide inhibits the pituitary release of LH and FSH. Suppression of FSH and LH secretion eliminates their stimulation of estrogen and progesterone production, essentially putting the woman in an artificial state of menopause. Without estrogenic stimulation of the endometrial tissue for proliferation and progesterone stimulation for maturation and eventual menses, there is no cycling or bleeding of ectopic endometrial tissue.

Note: Because leuprolide causes an artificial state of menopause, it is used only for brief periods because of the risks of osteoporosis, hot flashes, and other "postmenopausal" problems. Danazol, a derivative of testosterone that nonetheless has some progestational actions, is also used to treat endometriosis. It also decreases pituitary FSH and LH secretion but has some unpleasant side effects (hirsutism, deepening of the voice) due to its androgenic actions.

6. Another option for treating this patient is total abdominal hysterectomy with bilateral salpingo-oophorectory (TAH-BSO). What is the value of excising the ovaries for treatment of endometriosis if they have no endometrial implants?

The estrogens produced by the ovaries are responsible for stimulating the cycling of any ectopic endometrial tissue that is not removed with hysterectomy.

7. Another cause of dysmennorrhea is adenomyosis. What is adenomyosis?

Adenomyosis is ingrowth of the endometrial glands into the myometrium. In addition to dysmennorrhea, it can also cause heavy menstrual bleeding (menorrhagia).

CASE 8

A 37-year-old black woman is evaluated for abnormal uterine bleeding. She has regular periods, but they are heavy. She also has some bleeding between periods. Intercourse has become somewhat painful. Physical exam reveals an enlarged, hardened uterus with nodules. Pelvic ultrasound reveals an enlarged uterus with several tumorous growths within the myometrium.

1. What is the probable diagnosis?

Leiomyomata (leiomyoma for singular), commonly called uterine fibroids. They are benign local proliferations of smooth muscle cells of the uterus.

Note: Uterine fibroids are the most common gynecologic tumor. Black women have a significantly greater risk of developing them.

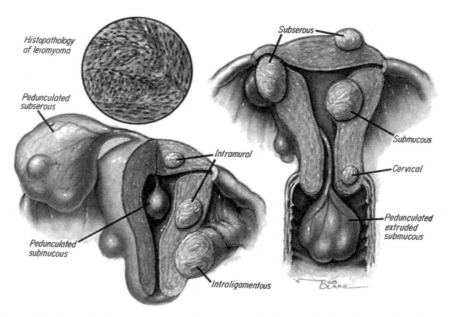

Uterine fibroids are designated subserous, intramual, and submucosal depending on their location. Submucosal fibroids often cause abornmal uterine bleeding. (From Sabiston Textbook of Surgery, 6th ed. Philadelphia, W.B. Saunders, 2000, with permission.)

2. How do oral contraceptives affect uterine fibroids?

Since uterine fibroids are estrogen-sensitive tumors, exogenous estrogens in oral contraceptives may make them grow. Additionally, the substantial increase in estrogen that occurs during pregnancy can make these tumors grow to significant proportions. After menopause, when estrogen levels decline, uterine fibroids often shrink in size and become asymptomatic.

Note: Pharmacologic agents that decrease plasma estrogen, such as leuprolide, danazol, and progesterone, can be used to shrink uterine fibroids.

3. How can uterine fibroids cause urinary urgency and frequency?

By compressing the bladder.

4. What is a leiomyosarcoma?

It is a malignant tumor derived from smooth muscle cells (of the uterus). It is not believed to arise from uterine fibroids.

CASE 9

A 26-year-old woman complains of fever and pelvic pain, neither of which is related to her menstrual cycle. She has multiple sexual partners and rarely uses any form of barrier contraception. Pelvic exam is significant for bilateral adnexal tenderness, a positive chandelier sign, and a purulent cervical discharge. Lab tests reveal a mild leukocytosis and a slightly elevated erythrocyte sedimentation rate (ESR). A quantitative beta-hCG is negative, but a cervical smear is positive for chlamydia.

1. What is the most likely diagnosis?

Pelvic inflammatory disease (PID) secondary to infection with *Chlamydia trachomatis*. *Neisseria gonorrhoeae* is another common cause of PID.

2. What is the chandelier sign? How does it help make a diagnosis of PID?

Severe cervical motion tenderness makes the patient "jump" toward the ceiling. The chandelier sign is provoked by moving tender and inflamed fallopian tubes and pelvic structures.

3. What long-term complications may possibly be prevented by treating this patient?

Tubal strictures can develop from the inflammatory process and may cause infertility or ectopic pregnancy. Adhesions between small bowel and pelvic structures can also develop, causing symptoms of bowel obstruction. Finally, an abscess can form around the tubes and ovaries (tubo-ovarian abscess). Rupture of a tubo-ovarian abscess can be a life-threatening event. Although treatment of PID cannot eliminate these complications, it may reduce their frequency.

4. How should the patient be treated?

With antibiotics. *C. trachomatis*, an obligate intracellular parasite, is typically treated with *doxycycline*. However, endocervical culture often reveals a polymicrobial infection, necessitating the additional use of a broad-spectrum antibiotic such as *ceftriaxone* (a third-generation cephalosporin). Additionally, *N. gonorrhoeae* is generally treated empirically in someone with chlamydial infection (it is susceptible to cephalosporins).

5. If a patient presents with similar signs and symptoms but also has acute onset of right knee pain and swelling without recent trauma to the joint, what infecting organism should you suspect?

N. gonorrhoeae, a gram-negative intracellular diplococcus, which in addition to being a common cause of PID can also cause septic arthritis if it becomes disseminated.

6. Is it sensible to recommend the use of an intrauterine device (IUD) to this patient?

No. IUDs are specifically contraindicated in women who have had previous episodes of PID or multiple sexual partners, because they may increase the risk of subsequent development of PID. Like most implanted devices, IUDs make it easier for bacteria to colonize and cause an infection.

Note: Suspect infection with *Actinomyces israeli* in a woman using an IUD who presents with symptoms of PID. This bacterium can be treated with penicillin.

7. What bacterium is responsible for maintaining the normal acidic pH of the vagina?

Lactobacillus acidophilus ("loves acid"), which maintains the vaginal pH at < 4.5.

8. If a woman complains of a malodorous discharge and a KOH test produces a fishy odor, what is the likely diagnosis? Explain.

Bacterial vaginosis, which results from overgrowth of normal vaginal flora. On microscopy "clue cells" are found, and *Gardnerella vaginalis* is often implicated.

Note: Clue cells are vaginal epithelial cells "studded" with bacteria that adhere to them.

9. What vaginal infection is associated with motile protozoa on microscopy smears?

Trichomoniasis, due to *Trichomonas vaginalis*, which is transmitted sexually. This infection is typically treated with metronidazole.

10. How about a white cheesy exudate with hyphae on microscopy?

Vaginal candidiasis, generally due to *Candida albicans*.

CASE 10

A 30-year-old woman presents to the free health care clinic complaining of postcoital bleeding for several months. She is otherwise healthy and denies any pain with intercourse (dyspareunia) or other gynecologic symptoms. She admits to becoming sexually active at an early age and having multiple male sexual partners. She has a 15-year history of cigarette smoking. A pelvic exam reveals an exophytic growth on the cervix. Colposcopy (light powered magnification of the cervix) and cervical biopsy reveal stage I cervical cancer.

1. **Why was this woman at high risk for developing cervical cancer?**

She has many of the risk factors, including initiation of sexual activity at an early age, multiple male sexual partners, history of smoking, and low socioeconomic status.

Note: In utero exposure of a fetus to diethylstilbestrol (DES) is a risk factor for the development of a rare cancer: cervical or vaginal clear-cell carcinoma.

2. **With what virus has the patient probably been infected?**

Human papilloma virus (HPV), which is believed to cause the vast majority of cervical cancers. Subtypes 16, 18, and 31 are most closely associated with cervical cancer.

Note: HPV types 6 and 11 are associated with condyloma acuminata (genital warts) but curiously do not increase the risk of cervical cancer. The other genital "wart," condylomata lata, is due to secondary syphilis.

3. **What is the mechanism by which the HPV viral proteins E6 and E7 predispose to the development of cervical cancer?**

They interfere with functioning of the tumor suppressor proteins p53 and Rb (retinoblastoma). Specifically, the E6 protein binds p53 and increases its rate of proteolysis, in effect reducing levels of p53. The E7 protein prevents transcription of the Rb gene by binding and displacing bound transcription factors, which are necessary for Rb transcription.

4. **How can cervical cancer cause renal failure?**

The cancer can grow and obstruct the ureters (obstructive nephropathy). This is one of the most common causes of death from cervical cancer.

5. **Why may this patient have benefited from annual Pap smears?**

The Pap smear has been shown to effectively detect preinvasive and early cancerous cervical lesions. Recall that cervical cancers can have a prolonged "latent" period; therefore, early detection via Pap smears and excision of premalignant lesions have drastically reduced mortality from cervical cancer.

Note: Perhaps the major risk factor for developing cervical cancer is simply the failure to have Pap smears on a regular basis.

6. **From what site are cells sampled during a Pap smear?**

Cells are taken from the squamocolumnar junction, the so-called transformation zone, where columnar cervical cells meet stratified squamous vaginal epithelium.

7. **What is cervical intraepithelial neoplasia (CIN)? Differentiate among CINI, CINII, and CINIII.**

CIN is diagnosed only by cervical biopsy (colposcopy with biopsy). CINI corresponds to dysplasia of one-third or less of the depth of the epithelium. CINII corresponds to dysplasia of two-thirds of the epithelium, and CINIII refers to dysplasia of the entire epithelial layer (also known as carcinoma in situ). CIN I, II, and III are also called mild, moderate, and severe dysplasia, respectively. It typically takes about 7 years for CINI to evolve into cervical cancer and 4 years for CINII to evolve into cervical cancer.

CASE 11

A 58-year-old postmenopausal woman presents with abnormal uterine/vaginal bleeding. She has been postmenopausal for 6 years and has not experienced this problem previously.

Physical exam reveals the bleeding to be from the cervical os (i.e., uterine bleeding rather than a vaginal source). No abnormal masses are palpated on bimanual exam, and the uterus is of normal size and shape. Pelvic ultrasound reveals a thickened endometrium, and dilatation and curettage (D&C), which includes scraping and sampling of endometrial tissue, is performed along with hysteroscopy (video visualization of the internal uterus). The pathology report indicates a malignancy.

1. **What is the most likely diagnosis?**
Endometrial carcinoma.

2. **What pathologic uterine abnormality commonly precedes the development of this cancer?**
Endometrial hyperplasia, which also commonly presents as postmenopausal bleeding. Diabetes, obesity, and hypertension also increase the risk of endometrial cancer.

3. **In pathophysiologic terms, why does it make sense that the risk factors for endometrial cancer are similar to those for breast cancer?**
Because estrogen plays an important role in the etiology of both types of cancer. For this reason, obesity (increased peripheral production of estrogen), unopposed estrogens, nulliparity (increased exposure to *cycling* estrogens), and late menopause (increased estrogen exposure) are common risk factors for the development of breast and endometrial cancer.

4. **Why does endometrial cancer, once detected, generally have a much better prognosis than newly diagnosed ovarian cancer?**
Because endometrial cancer is usually detected at a much earlier stage than ovarian cancer, thanks to the fact that abnormal uterine bleeding is an early warning sign. In contrast, there are few warning signs of early ovarian cancer.

5. **If this patient also has atrophic vaginitis, why should vaginal estrogen creams be avoided as a mode of treatment?**
A significant percentage of the cream is absorbed systemically, and since endometrial cancer is an estrogen-dependent cancer, the resulting elevated plasma estrogen can cause the cancer to progress. Remember: estrogen-dependent tumors/cancers are an absolute contraindication to the use of exogenous estrogens.

CASE 12

A 22-year-old woman is evaluated for a breast mass that she detected in the shower. It is round, mobile, rubbery, and nontender. There is no family history of breast or ovarian cancer. An ultrasound reveals the mass to be solid, not cystic, and an excisional biopsy is performed.

1. **What is the most likely diagnosis?**
Fibroadenoma, which is the most common breast tumor in premenopausal women.

2. **What is the difference between fibroadenoma and fibrocystic breast disease?**
Both are benign processes, but fibroadenoma is an encapsulated tumor, whereas fibrocystic breast disease encompasses a wide spectrum of abnormalities, all due to an excessive stromal response to hormones and growth factors. These changes can include cyst formation, nodule formation, and epithelial hyperplasia.

3. **If a woman presents with bloody nipple discharge, what should be done? What are the two diseases that most commonly cause this symptom?**
The discharge should be sent for cytology. A benign process, intraductal papilloma, which is a local proliferation of the epithelial lining of the lactiferous ducts, is one possibility. The other possibility is invasive papillary carcinoma, a malignant process.

4. What differences are detected on physical exam between fibroadenoma and breast carcinoma?

Fibroadenomas tend to be round, soft, and mobile, whereas breast carcinomas tend to be irregular, firm, and immobile. Another clue is that most breast masses in elderly women are carcinomas, whereas most breast tumors in younger women are fibroadenomas.

CASE 13

A 59-year-old woman presents to her family physician because she recently noticed a mass in her right breast while showering. She is concerned about breast cancer because her mother was diagnosed with breast cancer at the age of 72. History is significant for a non-tender mass that does not change in size or shape with her menstrual cycle and a single episode of bloody nipple discharge. Her menstrual cycles began at age 13, and she entered menopause at 55. She has no children and has never been pregnant. On exam, her breasts are asymmetric. There is a firm, nontender, irregular mass on her right breast, with redness and dimpling of the skin, and her right nipple appears slightly retracted. All previous mammograms have been normal. A diagnostic mammogram is ordered, and she is referred to a surgeon.

1. Based solely on the family history and the known genetics of breast cancer, was this patient at high risk for developing breast cancer?

No. The vast majority of breast cancers (~90%) are sporadic. Because her mother was elderly when she developed breast cancer, it is highly unlikely that the patient had a familial predisposition (e.g., BRCA1 or BRCA2 mutations) to develop breast cancer.

2. Based on the physical exam findings, does this woman probably have breast cancer?

Yes. She has many of the classic signs: an irregular, firm breast mass causing retraction or dimpling of the skin or nipple (peau d'orange) and a bloody discharge.

Note: Intraductal papilloma, a benign process, is actually the most common cause of a bloody nipple discharge. Invasive papillary carcinoma is next.

3. Which type of breast cancer is this patient most likely to have?

Infiltrating (invasive) ductal carcinoma is the most common type of breast cancer and should be the presumed diagnosis pending a definitive pathology report.

4. What is the significance of the age at menarche and age at menopause for the risk of developing breast cancer?

The younger the age at menarche and the older the age at menopause, the higher the risk of breast cancer. These relationships are explained by increased cumulative exposure to estrogen.

5. If biopsy reveals estrogen receptor-positive (ER+) and progesterone receptor-positive (PR+) cells, why may treatment with tamoxifen be useful?

Tamoxifen is a selective estrogen receptor modulator (SERM). It acts as an estrogen receptor agonist at certain tissues (e.g., bone, uterus) but as an estrogen antagonist at other tissues (e.g., breast). Because growth of ER+ and PR+ tumor cells is somewhat hormonal-dependent, these cancers can be treated with agents such as tamoxifen. *Raloxifen* is another selective estrogen receptor modulator under evaluation for use in treatment and prevention of breast cancer.

6. If an elderly woman presents with eczematous nipple changes, what should you suspect? What should you do? Why?

Paget's disease of the nipple produces this finding, and a breast biopsy should be done, since an underlying malignancy is found in the vast majority of patients with Paget's disease of the nipple.

7. If a woman has a unilateral inflamed breast with an orange peel (dimpled) appearance to the skin, what disease process should you suspect? Explain the pathophysiology.

She probably has inflammatory breast carcinoma, which is due to embolization of tumor into the dermal lymphatics, which in turn causes redness, swelling, and warmth. Since the tumor has embolized, it is not surprising that axillary lymph node involvement and distant metastases are common.

7. BEHAVIORAL SCIENCES

Thomas Brown, Benjamin Lafferty, and Dave Brown

CASE 1

A 20-year-old college student has been doing poorly for the past 8 months. He has become socially withdrawn and apathetic, and his grades, previously good, have been suffering. He complains to the campus physician that he has been hearing voices and that the TV news anchor has been giving him secret messages, telling him to infiltrate the Russian KGB, and thwart their assassination attempt of the President. He also wants to go into hiding because he believes that the CIA is after him. An extensive work-up to identify organic causes of his symptoms (thyroid function tests, drug screening, CT and MRI) is negative.

1. What is the most likely diagnosis?

Schizophrenia, a thought disorder that occurs in approximately 1% of the population.

Note: The typical age of onset of schizophrenia is 18–24 years in men and 26–45 years in women.

2. According to the DSM-IVTR,[1] what criteria must be met to make the diagnosis of schizophrenia?

Two or more of the following active-phase symptoms must be present for a 1-month period (or less, if successfully treated):

1. Delusions (substantially irrational beliefs, e.g. believe that you're the reincarnation of Fred Astaire)
2. Hallucinations (e.g., hearing voices that only you can hear)
3. Disorganized speech (e.g., incoherence)
4. Grossly disorganized or catatonic behavior
5. Negative symptoms (e.g., social withdrawal)

In addition, the above symptoms must cause negative effects in major areas of functioning, such as work, interpersonal relations, or self-care. The disturbance must persist for at least 6 months, including at least 1 month of active-phase symptoms listed above. Schizoaffective disorder and mood disorder with psychotic features must be ruled out. Finally, psychosis secondary to a general medical condition or psychosis precipitated by substance abuse must be ruled out.

3. What would be the diagnosis if the man had suffered these symptoms for only the past 3 months (with a negative work-up for other causes)?

Schizophreniform disorder, which is diagnosed in a patient displaying symptoms of schizophrenia for longer than 1 month but no longer than 6 months.

4. What would be the likely diagnosis if the man presented with these symptoms and later developed depressive or manic features?

Schizoaffective disorder, because the "affect" is involved. We won't torment you with the usual laundry list of DSM-IV criteria required for this diagnosis.

5. What would be your diagnosis if the man had symptoms of schizophrenia that followed a severe stressor and resolved within 2 weeks?

He would be suffering from a brief psychotic disorder—in this case, a reactive psychosis, because it is associated with marked stressors. A brief psychotic disorder lasts for a short period—less than 1 month but at least one day. It cannot be due to a general medical condition or associated with mood disorder or substance use. Brief psychotic disorder does not require the presence of severe stressors. It also may have postpartum onset (within 4 weeks of delivery), in which case it is called postpartum psychosis. If the disorder had followed or been attributed to a medical illness, it would be diagnosed as psychosis secondary to a general medical condition.

6. What are the four primary types of schizophrenia? Which does the present patient probably have?

Catatonic schizophrenia has two or more of the following: cataplexy (abrupt attacks of muscular weakness or hypotonia, often associated with narcolepsy) or stupor, excessive motor activity, resistance to instructions or attempts at movement, peculiar movements or posturing, peculiar mannerisms or grimacing, or echolalia or echopraxia (mimicking of others' speech or movements).

Disorganized schizophrenia includes disorganized speech and behavior and flat or inappropriate affect and does not meet criteria for catatonic schizophrenia.

Paranoid schizophrenia is characterized by delusions of persecution and absence of disorganized speech, catatonic behavior, and flat or inappropriate affect. This patient's symptoms are most consistent with paranoid schizophrenia.

Residual schizophrenia is characterized by absence of prominent delusions, hallucinations, or catatonia with continuing evidence of disease, such as negative symptoms and odd beliefs.

7. What are the differences between the positive and negative symptoms experienced by schizophrenics?

Positive symptoms are symptoms whose *presence* is abnormal. Examples include thought disturbances, delusions, and auditory and visual hallucinations. Negative symptoms indicate an *absence* of something considered normal. Examples include social withdrawal and isolation, anhedonia, and apathy.

8. What is the relationship between schizophrenia and suicide?

Unfortunately, people with schizophrenia are at increased risk of attempting suicide; 10–15% of schizophrenics successfully commit suicide.

9. What neurotransmitter abnormality is thought to play the primary role in schizophrenia? What evidence suggests this role?

The current theory is that excessive dopamine activity in the brain is the cause of schizophrenia. Several pieces of evidence support this theory. Some researchers have shown that positron emission tomography (PET) scans of the basal ganglia of schizophrenic patients show an increased number of D_2 receptors compared with unaffected controls. In addition, patients with schizophrenia who are treated with dopamine receptor antagonists show a beneficial response. Finally, drugs with dopaminergic effects aggravate existing psychosis and, in some patients, can result in new-onset psychosis.

10. Why should this patient be educated about the symptoms of acute dystonia, tardive dyskinesia, and even neuroleptic malignant syndrome if he will be treated with long-term antipsychotics?

These symptoms are potential side effects of neuroleptic (antipsychotic) administration. **Acute dystonia** is typically caused by extrapyramidal motor dysfunction that results in excessive muscle tone and muscle spasms (e.g., torticollis) after only short-term exposure to antipsychotics. **Tardive dyskinesia** is defined as extrapyramidal motor dysfunction resulting in involuntary tics and movements of the limbs after prolonged exposure (months to years) to high-dose antipsychotics. Finally, **neuroleptic malignant** syndrome is characterized by excessive muscle rigidity and elevated body temperature. It can be treated with dantrolene and/or a dopamine agonist such as bromocriptine.

Note: Akasthesia is a subjective sensation of inner restlessness or desire to move. Individuals with this may appear anxious or agitated, and may move about and pace, unable to sit still.

11. How might this man develop urinary retention and orthostatic hypotension if he is treated with antipsychotics such as the phenothiazines?

Urinary retention. The phenothiazines, in addition to blocking D_2 receptors, also block histaminic, **a**lpha-adrenergic, and **m**uscarinic receptors (in shorthand, the **HAM** receptors). Blockade of the muscarinic cholinergic receptors on the detrusor muscle of the bladder results in urinary retention.

Note: The muscarinic antagonism also causes the common anticholinergic side effects of dry mouth, loss of visual accommodation, and constipation.

Orthostatic hypotension results from alpha blockade, which usually occurs with phenothiazines that are not highly potent D_2 blockers. As a result, higher doses are used, leading to increased antagonism of the alpha receptor.

12. How do typical and atypical antipsychotics differ with respect to mode of action and effect on positive and negative symptoms?

Atypical antipsychotics (e.g., clozapine) are "atypical" in that they are more effective against the negative symptoms of schizophrenia and are much less likely to cause extrapyramidal side effects (e.g., acute dystonia, tardive dyskinesia) than the typical antipsychotics (e.g., chlorpromazine). This more benign side-effect profile of the atypical agents is thought to be due to their more selective affinity for dopamine receptor subtypes.

13. Why is clozapine recommended for use only in schizophrenics who are refractory to other antipsychotics?

Clozapine is an atypical antipsychotic that often works in cases that have been refractory to other antipsychotics. The major drawback of clozapine is that it can precipitate fatal agranulocytosis and therefore requires weekly monitoring of blood levels.

14. How might Parkinsonism develop as a consequence of antipsychotic therapy?

Symptoms of Parkinson's disease (bradykinesia, rigidity, masked facies, resting tremor, shuffling gait) can develop as a consequence of antipsychotic therapy. This phenomenon makes intuitive sense because antipsychotics are dopamine antagonists and essentially deplete (antagonize) central dopaminergic activity. Fortunately, these symptoms are reversible with discontinuation of the antipsychotics.

CASE 2

A 22-year-old college man nicknamed "Roller-coaster" by his friends complains of problems with mood and is referred to a psychiatrist by the campus physician for further evaluation. He states that for the past week he has been incredibly productive because he has required very little sleep. During the interview, the physician notes pressured speech, distractibility, euphoric mood, and psychomotor hyperactivity. The patient denies any history of auditory or visual hallucinations or use of alcohol or other drugs. Just prior to this period, however, he experienced a 2-month period characterized by hypersomnia, anhedonia, decreased appetite, and psychomotor retardation. Physical exam is noncontributory, and lab tests indicate normal thyroid activity.

1. What is the diagnosis?

Bipolar disorder (specifically, bipolar I).

Note: Bipolar I disorder is characterized by manic episodes lasting at least 1 week, whereas the milder bipolar II requires only a hypomanic episode lasting at least 4 days for diagnosis.

2. Was the previous depressive episode required to make the diagnosis of bipolar disorder in "Roller-coaster"?

No. Only a single manic episode is required. All patients who have experienced a manic episode are considered bipolar, regardless of whether or not they have suffered a depressive episode. This point can be confusing, because the term "bipolar" implies manic and depressive features. However, most patients with a history of manic episodes ultimately develop a depressive disorder as well.

3. The physician prescribes lithium and informs "Roller-coaster" that he needs to have blood levels of lithium monitored regularly. Why?

There is only a small difference between the therapeutic and toxic concentrations of lithium (i.e., its therapeutic index is low, which makes it a dangerous drug).

4. After taking lithium for an extended period, "Roller-coaster" develops polyuria and polydypsia. The urine has a low osmolarity, and administration of antidiuretic hormone (vasopressin) does not have a significant effect on either the polyuria or the low urine osmolarity. What is happening?

A distinctive, but rare side effect of lithium is nephrogenic diabetes insipidus. The kidneys do not respond effectively to antidiuretic hormone (ADH) and so do not conserve water or concentrate the urine effectively; hence the polyuria and polydypsia.

5. True or false: Treatment of lithium-induced nephrogenic diabetes insipidus with loop diuretics may be effective in decreasing symptoms of polyuria.

True. Although counterintuitive, loop diuretics and thiazide diuretics actually decrease polyuria in nephrogenic diabetes insipidus.

6. After taking the lithium for a while, "Roller-coaster" also mentions that he has become rather depressed, is having memory problems, and seems to be cold all of the time. Rather than simply prescribing an antidepressant, the physician first orders an assessment of thyroid-stimulating hormone (TSH) and thyroxine (T$_4$) levels. Why?

Another side effect of lithium is hypothyroidism, which can cause the above-mentioned symptoms.

7. Because "Roller-coaster" is not tolerating lithium well, his physician decides to prescribe a drug that is effective not only for bipolar disorder but also for several seizure disorders. What is this drug? What regular monitoring should be done?

Valproic acid, which is also effective for absence seizures, partial seizures, and generalized seizures. Rare but potentially fatal side effects of valproic acid therapy include necrotizing hepatitis (children are at increased risk) and agranulocytosis. Periodic monitoring of liver enzymes and blood cells, therefore, is indicated in patients on long-term valproic acid therapy.

8. At his next visit, "Roller-coaster's" symptoms seem to be well controlled with valproic acid, but his liver enzymes are markedly elevated. The valproic acid is discontinued, and he is prescribed another anticonvulsant that may also cause leukopenia or agranulocytosis but is not hepatotoxic. What drug was he probably given?

Carbamazepine, which is really effective only in acute manic episodes, is known to produce a persistent leukopenia. Therefore, regular monitoring of lab values is required.

9. Why should valproic acid be used with extreme caution in patients also taking phenobarbital?

Valproic acid inhibits the hepatic metabolism of phenobarbital and displaces phenobarbital from plasma proteins. Both effects result in elevated levels of free plasma phenobarbital and put the patient at risk for a barbiturate-induced coma.

10. In patients with a seizure disorder that is well controlled by phenytoin, why may the addition of carbamazepine cause seizures to recur?

Carbamazepine induces hepatic enzymes, which increases the metabolism of phenytoin and can reduce its plasma level to subtherapeutic levels.

CASE 3

A 48-year-old man complains of a poor appetite, insomnia, decreased interest in activities that he used to enjoy, difficulty with concentrating, and loss of energy for much of the past year. He has lost 20 pounds in the past 6 months. On questioning, he denies any illicit drug or alcohol abuse and is not taking any prescription medications. His medical history is significant for closed-angle glaucoma and premature ejaculation. Physical exam is unremarkable. Lab tests show normal T_4 and TSH.

1. **What is the most likely diagnosis?**
   Major depressive disorder.

2. **According to the DSM-IVTR,[1] what criteria must be met to make the diagnosis of major depressive disorder?**
   Major depressive disorder can be diagnosed when at least five of the following symptoms are present on an almost daily basis for at least the past 2 weeks and when at least one of the symptoms is either depressed mood or loss of interest or pleasure in activities that were previously enjoyable (anhedonia):
   1. Depressed mood most of the day
   2. Anhedonia
   3. Significant change in weight or appetite
   4. Insomnia or hypersomnia nearly every day
   5. Psychomotor agitation or retardation nearly every day
   6. Fatigue or loss of energy nearly every day
   7. Feelings of worthlessness or excessive or inappropriate guilt
   8. Diminished ability to think or concentrate
   9. Recurrent thoughts of death, suicidal ideation with or without a plan, or a suicide attempt
   In addition, the above symptoms must cause significant impairment in social, occupational, or other important areas of functioning. These symptoms cannot be better explained by a general medical condition (e.g., hypothyroidism), substance abuse, or loss of a loved one (bereavement).

3. **What does the monoamine deficiency theory propose about the cause of depression?**
   According to the monoamine deficiency theory, a deficiency in one of the neurotransmitters—norepinephrine, dopamine, or serotonin—can result in depression. Accumulating pharmacologic evidence supports this theory because increasing central activity of serotonin, norepinephrine, and dopamine, either individually or in combination, has been shown to be beneficial in the treatment of depression.

4. **Why does hypothyroidism have to be ruled out in this patient?**
   Hypothyroidism can produce symptoms similar to those of depression.

5. **Why may a selective serotonin reuptake inhibitor (SSRI) be particularly suitable as an antidepressant in this patient?**
   SSRIs commonly produce sexual dysfunction and delayed ejaculation in men. In a patient with premature ejaculation, however, the effects of delaying ejaculation would be desirable.

6. **Why have the SSRIs become first-line treatments for depression in preference to tricyclic antidepressants (TCAs)?**
   SSRIs have become a first-line treatment because of their lack of side effects relative to the TCAs, which in excess can cause cardiac arrhythmias, convulsions, and even coma or death. Although SSRIs can cause sexual dysfunction (delayed orgasm or even anorgasmia), this side effect is relatively benign compared with the side-effect profile of TCAs. When treating severe depression with TCAs, one must also consider that they are quite lethal in overdose. A patient

with a suicide plan may save their medication and subsequently overdose on it. The toxic potential of TCAs makes this a very real potential, whereas SSRIs are quite safe, even if ingested in large quantities.

7. Why might you want to avoid administering SSRIs and other antidepressants to a patient whose history is also significant for manic episodes?
Such a patient may have bipolar disorder, and antidepressants can precipitate a manic episode. This effect may occur in approximately 3–5% of bipolar patients.

8. Where does the majority of serotonin and norepinephrine originate in the brain?
The raphe nucleus and the locus ceruleus, respectively.

9. What class of antidepressants may produce symptoms of dry mouth, blurred vision, orthostatic (postural) hypotension, urinary retention, and memory impairment?
TCAs, which have strong anticholinergic side effects (e.g., dry mouth, blurry vision, urinary retention) and antiadrenergic side effects (e.g., orthostatic hypotension).
Note: You should be careful about prescribing TCAs to little old ladies because the side effect of orthostatic hypotension (due to alpha-1 blockade) may cause one of them to fall and break a hip—and it would be all your fault. The anticholinergic effects of the tricyclics (urinary retention) make them effective for treating enuresis (bed wetting). Imipramine is usually used for this purpose.

10. What element in this patient's history makes the use of TCAs such as amitriptyline a very bad idea?
TCAs have anticholinergic actions that can precipitate an attack of narrow-angle glaucoma.

11. The patient responds well to some form of antidepressant therapy but then presents to the emergency department 3 weeks later suffering from priapism. What antidepressant was he probably given?
Trazodone. Priapism is a rare but rather serious complication of trazodone in men.

12. If the patient is addicted to red wine with cheese, what class of antidepressants should be avoided? Why?
Monoamine oxidase inhibitors (MAOIs), such as phenelzine and tranylcypromine. The tyramine present in wine and cheese is ordinarily degraded by monoamine oxidase. If tyramine accumulates, it can cause a hypertensive crisis because it is a potent vasoconstrictor.

13. How do MAOIs work? What are the two classes of MAOIs?
MAOIs inhibit the degradation of monoamines (dopamine, norepinephrine, and serotonin) in presynaptic neurons. Monoamine oxidase A inhibitors primarily reduce the breakdown of norepinephrine and serotonin and are therefore useful in treating depression. Monoamine oxidase B inhibitors (e.g., selegeline) primarily reduce the breakdown of dopamine and are therefore useful in treating Parkinson disease.

14. What is the main danger of prescribing both an SSRI and an MAOI?
The combination of a MAOI and serotonergic drugs, such as SSRIs or TCAs can result in the **serotonin syndrome**. The initial symptoms of myoclonus, tremor, increased muscle tone, and autonomic instability can progress to hallucinations, hyperthermia, and even death.

15. If the patient is suffering from depression and also trying to quit smoking, which drug may be effective?
Buproprion, which has been shown to be effective in smoking cessation, especially when used with nicotine replacement therapy. Although its exact mechanism of action is not completely

understood, it has been shown to inhibit the reuptake of both dopamine and norepinephrine, thereby enhancing both dopaminergic and noradrenergic transmission. Buproprion is a nice alternative to the SSRIs because it lacks their adverse sexual side effects.

Note: One major concern with buproprion is that it lowers the threshold for seizure development, particularly in women with an underlying eating disorder such as anorexia nervosa.

16. If the patient experienced much milder symptoms of depression for more than 2 years, what would be his probable diagnosis?

Dysthymic disorder.

17. How might your diagnosis change if the man was divorced 2 months ago and his symptoms of depression were milder?

Probably he would be suffering from an adjustment disorder with depressed mood. The appearance of emotional or behavorial symptoms in response to an identifiable stressor within the past 3 months is the hallmark of adjustment disorder. To be considered an adjustment disorder, these symptoms must cause either significant distress beyond what would be expected or significant social or occupational dysfunction. On removal of the stressor, the symptoms should resolve within 6 months. If the patient were experiencing loss of a loved one, the disorder would be more appropriately classified as bereavement. The adjustment disorder should be classified as chronic or acute and may be further classified by other modifiers: with depressed mood, with anxiety, with mixed anxiety and depressed mood, with disturbance of conduct, with mixed disturbance of emotions and conduct, or unspecified.

18. If the man's wife died 1 year ago and he is still experiencing these symptoms, what would be the probable diagnosis?

Major depressive disorder. Normal grieving, which can mimic depression, is largely resolved within 6 months.

CASE 4

A 12-year-old boy's twin brother is killed in a car accident. The surviving twin suffers from depressed mood, feelings of guilt, and frequent emotional outbursts. He has begun to wear only his twin's clothing. He has been writing his thoughts in a diary since the accident. He also begins to treat his younger brother badly, talking to him harshly and even physically abusing him.

1. Instead of speaking to his deceased brother, which he believes would be unacceptable, he begins to keep a diary, which he believes is a more acceptable outlet for his emotions. What defense mechanism is being employed?

Sublimation involves altering a socially objectionable aim or object into an acceptable one. By channeling the desire to communicate with his brother into writing his thoughts in a diary, the patient uses sublimation to express his inner thoughts and feelings.

2. Why does the boy begin to wear his brother's clothing? What term is used to describe this type of activity?

Identification involves seeing oneself as like the other person. By wearing his deceased brother's clothing, he feels that part of his brother is still with him and does not have to face the loss.

3. What term is used to describe him taking out his frustrations on his younger brother?

Acting out involves the expression of an impulse through action to avoid dealing with what the feelings mean. By abusing and showing anger toward his little brother, he does not have to be conscious of the anger he feels at having lost his twin.

4. What are the two basic categories of defense mechanisms? Give examples of each.

Immature defenses include acting out, regression, blame, somatization, dissociation, denial, projection, reaction formation, and repression.

Mature defenses include altruism, intellectualization, identification, rationalization, humor, sublimation, and suppression.

CASE 5

A 42-year-old married businessman with six children is diagnosed with Huntington's disease after being seen by a specialist in movement disorders. He is told that there is no cure for his disease and that he will progressively decline both physically and mentally prior to death within 10 years. To make matters worse, he is told that several of his six children may have the disease. He comes home and for the first time in his life is physically abusive to his wife.

1. What are the five stages of grief that this man is likely to experience?

Denial, anger, bargaining, acceptance, and sadness. The grieving person may not experience all of these stages and may pass through a stage quite rapidly, appearing not to pass through it at all.

2. What term is used to describe alleviating his frustration by abusing his wife?

Acting out allows him to express anger without having to deal with the newfound knowledge of his diagnosis. This is obviously an immature defense mechanism.

3. What defense mechanism would he be employing if he ignored the doctor's visit and went on with his life without acknowledging his diagnosis?

Denial involves unconsciously refusing to acknowledge that there is a problem. The patient maintains cognitive and emotional unawareness of the truth and does not believe what he has been told; it does not register emotionally

4. What term would be used to describe his behavior if, while hospitalized, he begins crying for his mother and demanding that other people feed him and take care of matters he is fully capable of tending?

Regression, or attempting to return to an earlier phase of functioning to avoid conflict, is quite common in the medical setting and is a normal phenomenon.

5. Cover the left-hand column and attempt to describe the additional defense mechanisms listed below.

DEFENSE MECHANISM	DESCRIPTION	EXAMPLE
Splitting	Categorization of things into good or bad; everything is black or white, with no gray.	A patient describes you as "the best doctor," whereas her last physician is a "quack."
Altruism	The act of giving or serving, not for feeling of obligation or recognition, but merely for the sake of doing good.	A wealthy widow donates half of her husband's estate to benefit the local children's hospital.
Reaction formation	Turning a strong impulse that is unacceptable into the opposite in order to "undo" the feeling.	A boy is angry with his mother for grounding him and wishes that she would die. Feeling guilty, he runs downstairs, hugs her, and tells her how much he loves her.

(Cont'd.)

DEFENSE MECHANISM	DESCRIPTION	EXAMPLE
Suppression	Consciously or semiconsciously postponing attention to a conscious impulse; discomfort is minimized, but still acknowledged.	A woman tries to avoid thinking about her husband who recently committed suicide by removing his clothing from their shared closet.
Repression	Withholding an idea or feeling from consciousness; impulses are consciously inhibited to the point of losing, not just postponing, goals.	A woman tries to avoid thinking about her husband who recently committed suicide by burning all his clothing and removing all his photos from the wall.

CASE 6

An 8-year-old boy is brought to the physician by his mother for behavioral problems. The mother says that for as long as she can remember he has been much more "difficult" than his brothers and sisters. She is also concerned because he has been doing poorly in the first grade and his teacher has complained to her several times about his disruptive behaviors in class, which include excessive talking and leaving his seat inappropriately. In the physician's office, he appears distracted and fidgety. When asked by the doctor to respond to five questions on a questionnaire, the boy answers only two of them. When addressed by the physician, he seems distracted and does not appear to be listening.

1. What is this patient's likely diagnosis?

Attention deficit hyperactivity disorder (ADHD), a disorder characterized by a pattern of hyperactivity, impulsiveness, inattention, and distractibility. The diagnosis requires that the symptoms be present in at least two settings (e.g., school and at home) and that the onset of the symptoms must occur before 7 years of age.

2. What other diagnoses should be considered before ADHD is diagnosed?

Oppositional defiant disorder, a pattern of negative, hostile, and deviant behavior lasting at least 6 months. Patients must show at least four of the following behaviors: arguing with adults, losing their temper, defying or refusing to comply with requests, deliberately annoying people, blaming others for their mistakes, becoming angry and resentful, spiteful and vindictive.

Conduct disorder is a pattern of behavior in which other peoples' basic rights are violated or societal rules or norms are broken, as demonstrated by at least three of the following behaviors in the past 12 months and at least one in the past 6 months: aggression toward people and animals, destruction of property, deceitfulness and theft, or a serious violation of rules.

3. Using the DSM-IVTR[1] criteria, under what axis would ADHD be listed?

ADHD is listed under axis I. By way of review, the five axes of diagnosis used in psychiatry are as follows:

Axis I: psychiatric conditions (e.g., schizophrenia)

Axis II: personality disorders, mental retardation (e.g., borderline personality disorder)

Axis III: medical conditions (e.g., diabetes mellitus)

Axis IV: social stressors (e.g., bad marriage)

Axis V: global assessment of functioning (a numerical score from 0 to 100 that assesses the patient's emotional, social, and everyday functioning)

4. What class of drugs is the primary treatment for ADHD?

The first-line treatment of ADHD includes the use of amphetamine derivatives (e.g., methylphenidate, dextroamphetamine), which result in increased attention, decreased motor activity, and improvement in learning tasks.

5. What psychiatric symptoms may be evident after an overdose of amphetamines?

Psychotic features, presumably related to increased dopamine, which may explain why a shot of haloperidol (an antipsychotic) usually calms patients who have overdosed on amphetamines. This point also illustrates the importance of ruling out substance abuse before making a diagnosis of schizophrenia.

Note: Ammonium chloride is used to treat amphetamine overdose because it increases the acidity of the urine, which increases the excretion of amphetamines.

CASE 7

A 4-year-old boy is brought to see a psychiatrist by his parents. The mother reports three different episodes of walking in his room while he was masturbating and she is worried that he has some kind of a "problem."

1. If the psychiatrist explains the boy's developmental maturation in terms of psychosexual development, to which psychologist is he referring? What are the stages of psychosexual development?

Sigmund Freud developed five stages of psychosexual development:

Oral stage: birth to 18 months
Anal stage: 1 to 3 years
Phallic stage: 3 to 5 years
Latency stage: 6 years to puberty
Genital stage: puberty to young adulthood

2. Freud also discusses the id, ego, and superego. How do they relate to the boy's behavior?

The **id** represents the instinctual drives with which people are born. The id operates in the subconscious and lacks the ability to delay or change the drives with which one is born.

The **ego** spans both the conscious and the unconscious. Consciously, logical and abstract thinking and verbal expression are handled by the ego. Unconsciously, defense mechanisms are used by the ego. The ego uses external reality to harness instinctual drive of the id and substitutes realities for pleasure.

The **superego** serves to monitor a person's behavior, thoughts, and feelings according to a strict set of morals and values internalized from the parents; it makes comparison with these standards and offers approval or disapproval.

For example, the superego deems it inappropriate for the boy to keep masturbating and causes him to feel guilty about it. The id represents the pleasure that he receives from masturbation. The ego processes the inputs from the id, superego, and external reality. The ego compromises by giving in sometimes and masturbating, but at other times it substitutes other pleasurable activity, such as playing a board game.

3. If the psychiatrist discusses the boy's development in terms of stages of cognitive stages, to which psychologist is he referring? What are the stages of cognitive development?

Piaget developed four stages of cognitive development:

Sensory-motor: Between the time of birth and about 2 years of age, babies begin to develop an understanding of object permanence. No longer do they fear that "mommy is gone" when she covers her face with her hands. Peek-a-boo begins to lose its charm. They develop the ability to control movement and observe their surroundings via their developing senses.

Preoperational: As the child ages from about 2 to 7 years, he or she begins to associate events with external happenings, leading to a belief in phenomenalistic causality. For example, a negative thought directed toward someone who falls and breaks his or her leg causes the child to believe that the fall was caused by the inappropriate thought. Children at this stage also tend to operate in an egocentric fashion. They are unable to process how their behavior or outside events affects other people.

Concrete operations: From ages 7 to 11, children begin to understand conservation of objects. They develop the ability to understand that a small cup full of juice is "less" than a big cup that is half full but still may have trouble understanding that a nickel is less money than a dime ("it's bigger"), because they have not mastered abstract thought. Children in these stages may become strict rule followers; obsessive traits may begin to emerge.

Formal operations: From age 11 until the end of adolescence, teens begin to develop the ability to understand abstract thought and reason. They begin to be able to process ideas and concepts lacking a concrete basis.

4. If the psychiatrist explains the boy's development in terms of development of the ego, to which psychologist is he referring? What are the stages of ego development?

Erikson theorized that a person must overcome certain basic conflicts in eight stages of life in the process of development:

1. **Trust vs. mistrust** (birth to 1 year): the child learns whether basic needs will be met and care providers can be relied upon.
2. **Autonomy vs. shame** (1 to 3 years): toddlers begin to show mastery over excretory functions, such as urination and defecation.
3. **Initiative vs. guilt** (3 to 5 years): children are allowed to initiate behavior and interests, their conscience is established.
4. **Industry vs. inferiority** (6 to11 years): children learn that they are able to master and complete tasks; inadequacy may develop if the social environment is unsupportive.
5. **Identity vs. role confusion** (11 to 21 years): young people develop a sense of who they are and where they are going.
6. **Intimacy vs. isolation** (21 to 40 years): people establish sexual relationships, deep friendships, and deep associations, as long as there is no underlying identity confusion.
7. **Generativity vs. stagnation** (40 to 65 years): people's main interest is in guiding and establishing future generations or improving society.
8. **Integrity vs. despair** (over 65 years): satisfaction is sensed if a person feels that his or her life has been productively lived.

Failure to meet each of these conflicts results in stagnation of development, whereas successful resolution of each conflict allows progression to the next stage of development.

CASE 8

A 37-year-old man presents to a psychiatrist for evaluation of symptoms that he believes may be depression. He reports difficulty with sleeping for the past 6 months, stating that he never feels rested after 7–8 hours of sleep. He also notices decreased concentration at work. He has had relationship troubles with his wife and is recently divorced. He reports that her primary reason for leaving him was that he no longer seemed to care about her; he never wants to go out or do the things that they used to do. She even went so far as to accuse him of having an affair. They stopped sleeping in the same room 2 years ago because his excessive snoring and intermittent bursts of awakening with shortness of breath kept her awake at night. He says that he just does not have the energy to do things anymore. He also relates having been recently reprimanded at work for falling asleep. On exam, he is moderately obese, healthy-appearing, and middle-aged. His mental status exam is unremarkable. He denies any thoughts of suicide, appetite disturbances, or feelings of guilt or hopelessness. He does feel that he has had a depressed mood since his wife left.

1. In addition to a diagnosis of adjustment disorder with depressed mood, what sleep-related disorder probably explains most of the patient's problems?

The patient is suffering from sleep apnea and is appropriately diagnosed with a breathing-related sleep disorder. Such patients are often obese, and a collar size greater than 17 should be a red flag. Presumably the weight of the fat collapses the airway. Sleep is often interrupted at nights because of airway becomes occluded, leading to excessive sleepiness and fatigue. The chronic poor sleep can lead to irritability, poor concentration, and the need to "nap" during the day.

2. What treatment may allow the man to sleep at night?

Therapy involves pressurizing the airway to keep it patent. The patient wears a mask that provides positive airway pressure to keep the airway from becoming obstructed. Positive airway pressure is a treatment option only for patients who suffer from obstructive sleep apnea, like this man. As always, lifestyle modifications are important as well. The patient should be encouraged to lose weight, which should reduce the compressive forces on the airways and thereby decrease the airway obstruction.

CASE 9

A 29-year-old woman presents after an automobile accident in which she fell asleep at the wheel. She notes that she frequently falls asleep during the day and feels rested after these episodes. In addition, she states that sometimes she awakens but is utterly "unable to move a muscle." She adds that she has always been able to fall asleep quickly. She denies any use of drugs or medications. You excuse yourself to answer a page and find her asleep when you return to your office. She is startled at first but then seems to regain her orientation and wishes to know, "What is wrong with me?"

1. What is the likely diagnosis? What are the expected findings of electroencephalography (EEG)?

The patient has narcolepsy. The EEG in a sleep study is likely to show a decreased rapid-eye-movement (REM) latency, meaning that she rapidly progresses into REM sleep. This phenomenon accounts for the restfulness that such patients feel on falling asleep.

2. What treatment is available for narcolepsy?

A regimen of a regular schedule of forced naps during the day can be a successful treatment for some patients. In severe cases of narcolepsy, amphetamines such as methylphenidate (Ritalin) are also used in the treatment of narcolepsy. These agents cause the release of norepinepherine, dopamine, and serotonin.

3. What are the stages of sleep? Describe what happens physiologically in each stage.

Sleep is divided into non-REM (NREM) and REM patterns. NREM sleep is divided into four stages, each involving a deeper level of sleep. The stages are further divided into fast-wave and slow-wave sleep. The earliest two stages are fast-wave sleep, and stages 3 and 4 are termed slow-wave sleep based on the EEG appearance of brain waves. As people fall asleep, they pass through stages 1–4 and then enter REM sleep—usually for the first time after approximately 90 minutes. The first REM episode lasts typically less than 10 minutes, and then the person cycles through the stages again, with further REM episodes of about 15–40 minutes.

During **NREM sleep**, pulse, respiration rate, and blood pressure are decreased and show less minute-to-minute variation. Resting muscle tone is relaxed somewhat, and body movements occur on an episodic basis. Males do not experience erection, and blood flow, including cerebral circulation, is somewhat lower.

REM sleep is characterized by higher pulse rate, higher respiratory rate, and higher blood pressure; EEG patterns are similar to those of the waking state (hence, REM sleep is also termed paradoxical sleep). Men experience partial or full erection. In addition, a person in REM sleep experiences nearly total skeletal muscle paralysis, and movement is quite rare. Abstract and surreal dreams occur during this phase of sleep. Most REM sleep occurs in the last third of the night

4. Name the EEG appearance of each stage of sleep and describe the frequency and voltage of the waves.

STAGE	EEG APPEARANCE	FREQUENCY	VOLTAGE	
Awake	β waves	Random fast waves	Low	$\mathcal{B}$
Eyes closed	α waves	8–12 cycles/sec	Low	A
Stage 1	θ waves	3–7 cycles/sec	Low	T
Stage 2	Sleep spindles K complexes	12–14 cycles/sec slow, triphasic waves	Low	S
Stages 3 and 4	δ waves	0.5–2.5 cycles/sec	High	Drink
REM sleep	β waves	Random fast waves	Low	Blood

5. How do nightmares differ from night terrors?

Nightmares occur almost exclusively in REM sleep. Patients who experience nightmares are able to recall these frightening events, which usually involve threat to life, security, or self-esteem. On awakening, the person rapidly becomes oriented. **Night terrors** occur in deep NREM sleep (stages 3 and 4). Often the person awakes with a panicky scream. They are often unresponsive on awakening, have amnesia for the episode, and show signs of autonomic arousal, such as tachycardia, tachypnea, and diaphoresis.

6. An 82-year-old woman complains that her sleep patterns have changed as she has aged. What changes in sleep are typical as people age?

As people age, they experience a decrease in the amount of time spent in slow-wave sleep (stages 3 and 4) and REM sleep. The typical result is a reduced need for time spent sleeping. Insomnia is common in the elderly population.

7. This woman had been given a benzodiazepine to assist her sleep, which improved for a while. But now she complains of poor sleep once more. Why have her sleep problems returned?

She is experiencing tolerance to the effects of her medication. Benzodiazepines should be used only for short-term management of insomnia and not long-term management, because tolerance and dependence may result. Re-evaluation should follow a 7- to 10-day trial of a benzodiazepine, and other agents should be considered.

8. How do benzodiazepines manifest their pharmacologic effect?

Benzodiazepines are agonists of gamma-aminobutyric acid (GABA) receptors, which are bound to chloride channels. GABA is the primary inhibitory neurotransmitter in the central nervous system (CNS). This CNS inhibition leads to decreased alertness, drowsiness, and less agitation.

9. Why would this pharmacologic effect be another reason to avoid benzodiazepines in the elderly population?

The aged population has a markedly increased (about 25%) incidence of falls when given benzodiazepines due to drowsiness and impaired balance. This effect is especially concerning in elderly postmenopausal women, who may have underlying osteopenia or frank osteoporosis. In addition, the geriatric population is more sensitive to this effect and should be started on a lower dose initially. Again, if a little old lady breaks her hip, it is all your fault.

CASE 10

A 75-year-old man presents to the emergency department. He is diagnosed with chronic pancreatitis and promptly admitted to the medicine service. The patient denies a history of alcohol use until an attractive nurse who seems interested in partying gets him to confess that his wild and crazy days are still alive and kicking. In fact, he had a fifth of vodka this morning with breakfast to put him in the mood for watching Jerry Springer.

1. What concern does this man's alcohol abuse pose to the medicine team?
The pancreatitis is probably due to his alcohol problem. If the underlying disease is not found and treated, the pancreatitis cannot be successfully managed, and all that can be expected is symptomatic control of periodic exacerbations. In addition, patients who consume large quantities of alcohol (or smaller quantities on a regular basis) are at risk for symptoms of withdrawal.

2. What are the expected symptoms of withdrawal? How are they managed?
Withdrawal is displayed in two stages. Early symptoms of withdrawal may include tachycardia, tremors, nausea, vomiting, or hypertension. These initial symptoms are usually controlled with lorazepam (Ativan), a benzodiazapine. The later, more life-threatening concern is the appearance of delirium tremens (DTs). Usually presenting after about 48 hours of abstinence, these severe tremors may be accompanied by hallucinations, delirium, and mild fever. Often DTs are preceded by seizures, which on rare occasions lead to status epilepticus. Seizures can be managed by intravenous benzodiazepines; in patients with a history of withdrawal seizures, prophylactic phenytoin may be started. The DT's can be managed with benzodiazepines and supportive care. This management strategy may require intensive care, especially in the case of autonomic instability. Symptoms typically last for around 3 days but may persist for weeks.

3. What is the mechanism by which benzodiazepines are able to control DTs?
Management of a patient who ceases alcohol intake involves a taper, using benzodiazepines. Alcohol potentiates the GABA receptor, as do the benzodiazepines. Gradual tapering, rather than abrupt termination, of this agonistic effect allows the CNS to acclimate to the increased stimulation experienced as alcohol is removed.

4. What other class of drugs exerts their effect by agonism of the GABA receptor? How do their pharmakokinetic effects differ from those of benzodiazepines?
Barbiturates also agonize the GABA receptor at a site distinct from that of the benzodiazepines. The benzodiazepines eventually reach a maximal effect, whereas barbiturates continue to increase their effect as dosage is increased. The result is that barbiturates are much more likely to cause fatal respiratory depression than benzodiazepines (even though this is still a concern).

5. How are substance *abuse* and *dependence* differentiated?
A person meets the criteria for substance **abuse** when he or she experiences legal problems due to substance use, uses the substance in a hazardous situation, continues to use the substance despite recurrent social problems, and fails to fulfill major obligations at home, school, or work.
The person is diagnosed with **dependence** when three of the following criteria are present: tolerance; withdrawal symptoms; repetitive, unintended excessive use; failure at cutting down use of the substance, reduction in social, recreational, or occupational functioning; spending an excessive amount of time in pursuit of the substance; and continued use despite the knowledge that the substance is causing psychological difficulties.

CASE 11

Law enforcement officials bring a 27-year-old man to the emergency department. He is combative and disoriented and screams that bugs are crawling on his skin. His blood pressure, pulse rate, and respiratory rate are elevated. He appears to be sweating profusely. On exam of the head, you notice dried blood around one of his nostrils and see that his pupils are dilated. Once he settles down and begins talking with you, he complains that he feels light-headed and that his chest hurts.

1. What class of drug abuse should be expected in this patient?
The patient is suffering from intoxication of a stimulant—in this case, cocaine. Tactile hallucinations, impaired judgment, transient psychosis, and agitation are commonly seen in stimulant
intoxication. Other characteristic symptoms include tachycardia or bradycardia, dilated pupils,
hyper- or hypotension, chills or fever, nausea and emesis, and confusion. Amphetamine intoxication may present in a similar fashion.

**2. Should you be surprised if the patient's electrocardiogram revealed myocardial is-
chemia?**
No. Cocaine can cause vasospasm, which can reduce cardiac perfusion and thus lead to
ischemia.

3. Why does the patient have blood around his nostril?
The effect of cocaine on the nasal epithelium is vasoconstriction, which can lead to infarction of the nasal septum and subsequent perforation. This problem is exacerbated by the sympathomimetic effects of cocaine, which lead to increased blood pressure that increases the epistaxis.

4. What symptoms are typical of cocaine withdrawal?
Patients experience extreme fatigue, hunger, headaches, cramps, and perspiration. These
symptoms peak in 48–96 hours. Most patients do not require inpatient management, and symptoms are self-limited. Antipsychotics can be used to control agitation and psychotic symptoms.

CASE 12

A 72-year-old woman with early-stage Alzheimer's disease is admitted to the hospital for
extreme dyspnea and diagnosed with pneumonia. Intravenous fluids and antibiotics are
started. On admission she is alert and oriented to person and time but not to place. She is
able to score 26/30 on a mini-mental status examination administered shortly after her admission. The following morning she is found to be febrile. The attending physician believes that
she is not responding as expected and changes her antibiotic. A few hours later she has
become confused and aggressive and believes that the hospital staff has been trying to kill her.

1. Is the patient's current state best described as dementia or delirium?
The woman is suffering from delirium. Although she may have an underlying dementia, she
has clearly become acutely delirious. This important distinction must be made in all patients with
acute changes in mental status.

2. What is the most likely cause of her delirium?
The two most common causes of a delirious state, especially in the elderly, are prescribed
drugs and acute infections. Pneumonia or the antibiotics used to treat it are most likely the cause
of her delirious state. Other causes that should be investigated include drug or alcohol withdrawal, metabolic derangement, head trauma, epilepsy, and cerebral hypoperfusion.

**3. Distinguish dementia from delirium in terms of onset, course, level of consciousness,
and presence of delusions and hallucinations.**
Dementia typically has a gradual, insidious onset. It often goes unnoticed by family members who see the person everyday. The course tends to be a gradually progressive decline in cognitive function, especially in short-term memory. In early stages, patients can be quite oriented
with a normal level of consciousness. Delusions or hallucinations may or may not be seen in patients with dementia.
Delirium often has an abrupt onset, typically within hours to days. Short-term memory and
poor attention span are common cognitive defects. Delirium involves a sudden impairment in
level of consciousness, and patients can fluctuate rapidly. Delusions are typically fleeting, often

persecutory, and may be related to the disorientation. Hallucinations are common; visual hallucinations strongly suggest delirium.

CASE 13

A 32-year-old previously healthy businesswoman presents to the emergency department (ED) with recent onset of chest pain, shortness of breath, dizziness, and an intense fear that she is dying. Her symptoms appeared "out of the blue" while she was working in her office on a presentation that she is scheduled to give in a few days. She has a strong family history of cardiovascular disease and is convinced she is having a heart attack. An extensive work-up, including an electrocardiogram, chest x-ray, and serial cardiac enzymes, is negative for a myocardial infarction. After a short while in the emergency department, her symptoms appear to resolve.

1. What is the most likely diagnosis?
Panic attack, which patients frequently misinterpret as a heart attack.

2. Distinguish between panic attack and panic disorder.
Panic attacks are a discrete period of intense fear or discomfort during which symptoms develop abruptly and usually peak within 10 minutes. Symptoms may include perspiration, palpitations, chest pain, shaking, sensation of choking, nausea, dizziness, chills, fear of dying, fear of losing control, or a feeling of derealization.

Panic disorder is characterized by recurrent, unexpected panic attacks. Such people have concern about further attacks, fear the consequences of these attacks, and/or significantly alter their behaviors because of the panic attacks.

3. If the woman subsequently develops a fear of leaving the house, what term should be used to describe her "phobia"?
Agoraphobia is intense anxiety felt about being in situations from which escape is difficult (or embarrassing) or in which help may not be available in the event that a panic attack occurs. If the avoidance is limited to specific situations, specific phobias, social phobia, or obsessive-compulsive disorder should be considered. Patients who suffer from panic disorder may or may not experience agoraphobia.

4. Why might the ED intern wish to check blood levels of thyroid hormone and urinary levels of vanillylmandelic acid (VMA) and 5-hydroxyindoleacetic acid (5-HIAA)?
Multiple organic conditions can mimic a panic attack, including hyperthyroidism (or "thyroid storm"), pheochromocytoma (elevated VMA), and carcinoid syndrome (elevated 5-HIAA). These conditions can be ruled out by a laboratory work-up.

5. How can panic disorder be treated?
Selective serotonin reuptake inhibitors (SSRIs) can be used in the treatment of panic disorder. In addition, benzodiazepines can be used to decrease the anxiety associated with panic attacks. Beta blockers can also be used to limit the physiologic effects of anxiety experienced in specific phobias, such as performance anxiety, when a person is certain to be exposed to the triggering situation.

CASE 14

A 16-year-old girl is admitted to a tertiary psychiatric referral center. For several months she has had severe emotional outbursts and fits of anger. She has difficulty with falling asleep and recurrent nightmares when she does sleep. She has a history of sexual and physical abuse by her father at the age of 10 before he left the family. Her nightmares often revolve around these episodes of abuse.

1. What is the most likely diagnosis in this girl?

Posttraumatic stress disorder (PTSD) with delayed onset, because the symptoms appeared more than 6 months after the stressor.

2. What are the requirements for this diagnosis?

The patient has to have been exposed to, witnessed, or subjected to a traumatic event characterized by actual or threatened death or injury or threat to the physical integrity of self or others. In addition, the patient must re-experience the event through distressing dreams, acting out, or intrusive recollections. The person also avoids thoughts, feelings, and activities associated with the event; they may avoid activities, feel detached, and stop expressing their feelings. Arousal is heightened. The person may have difficulty with falling asleep, become irritable or have angry outbursts, have trouble with concentrating, or show an exaggerated startle response. These symptoms must persist longer than 1 month.

3. Is this condition disabling to patients? How is it best managed?

PTSD can be highly disabling and can constitute a life-long impairment. Group therapy has been used successfully in the treatment of PTSD. Patients are encouraged to talk about their trauma with other patients who have suffered from similar experiences. Pharmacologic therapy for PTSD involves the SSRIs. Typically, a combination of group therapy and SSRI is implemented for patients suffering from PTSD.

PERSONALITY DISORDERS

1. A 35-year-old surgeon is 2-hours late for an appointment with his physician and is told by the secretary that he needs to reschedule his appointment. In a loud and argumentative voice he demands to be seen immediately by the physician and states that his time is just as important as the physician's, saying he is entitled be seen that day because he was delayed by an urgent procedure. While waiting to be worked into the schedule, he paces across the room, muttering about how this university-affiliated clinic is not good enough for the leading surgeon in his field. Finally, when seen by the physician, he challenges the doctor's understanding of his condition and argues against the recommended therapy. From what type of personality disorder is the surgeon probably suffering?

Narcissistic personality disorder, often a consequence of being more intelligent than most people (or having a greater *perceived* intelligence).

2. A 22-year-old woman has a long history of unstable relationships. Her history is also remarkable for multiple suicide attempts and episodes of self-mutilation. After being seen by a particular physician for the first time, she says that he is the most amazing doctor she has ever seen. At the next appointment, he begins to discuss lifestyle changes to help with her irregular sleep patterns. At this point she becomes enraged, yelling "You are such a quack! I am going to see Dr. Jones. He knows how to treat insomnia!," and storms out of the office. From what type of personality disorder is the woman probably suffering? What defense mechanism do such patients commonly employ?

The woman probably suffers from borderline personality disorder. Such patients often use splitting (see table in question 5 of Case 5) as a defense mechanism.

3. A 42-year-old woman often appears preoccupied with herself as well as inconsiderate and demanding of others. When seen by a male physician, she is flirtatious and makes inappropriate sexual comments. When the nurse enters the room, she feigns fainting so that the physician has to catch her. She has threatened suicide many times in the past, but her physician is convinced that these threats are not genuine and that the patient is manipulating him. From what type of personality disorder is this woman probably suffering?

Histrionic personality disorder.

4. A 28-year-old man has spent the past 5 years in prison after being convicted for assault and robbery. His behavior has always been characterized by utter disregard for the feelings of others. As a child, he was sexually abused by his father, and he frequently tortured animals for entertainment. He appears to have no conscience and lies whenever it is convenient. His father and grandfather are alcoholics, and he has a long history of alcohol abuse. From what type of personality disorder is this man probably suffering? What type of psychiatric disorder did he probably have as a child?

The man probably suffers from antisocial personality disorder, which can be diagnosed only in a person 18 years of age or older. As a boy he probably suffered from conduct disorder, which can be diagnosed only in children.

5. A physician frequently has calls from a 38-year-old female patient about minor health concerns, such as common colds and minor cuts and scratches. When soliciting the physician's advice about health care at regularly scheduled appointments, she invariably responds that she will do whatever he thinks is best and that her opinion does not matter in the slightest. At home she defers almost all decision making to her husband, on whom she is highly reliant. What type of personality disorder is this woman likely suffering from?

Dependent personality disorder.

6. A 52-year-old man has worked in the same position in a large factory for 30 years. He is an excellent worker but has always turned down offers of promotion. He explains this behavior by saying that he loves his current job, but secretly he fears criticism of his job performance. He does not go out for dinner with his colleagues or attend the annual Christmas party because he becomes anxious in such situations. From what type of personality disorder is this man probably suffering?

Avoidant personality disorder.

7. A 19-year-old female college student normally receives excellent grades in school, but sometimes her grades suffer because of handing in a "perfect" paper past the deadline. She is seen by the campus physician for peeling skin on her hands, which has been caused by constant hand-washing. She is wonderfully reliable to her friends but causes them some frustration due to her insistence on maintaining a fixed rigid schedule and her moralistic and sometimes judgmental views. She pays excruciatingly close attention to minor details and is highly sensitive to any criticism. From what type of personality disorder is this patient probably suffering?

Obsessive-compulsive personality disorder.

8. A 32-year-old accountant is given new responsibilities at his job with which he is not pleased. Instead of discussing with his boss other ways to distribute the additional workload, he expresses his anger by sabotaging assignments, coming to work late, leaving early, and not achieving his usual quality of work. From what type of personality disorder is this man probably suffering?

Passive-aggressive personality disorder.

9. A 38-year-old woman has no close friends and "prefers to do things on my own." She has never had a boyfriend and is unperturbed by the frequent criticism of her parents regarding her unmarried status. Although she is a highly successful professional, she is indifferent to the praise of coworkers and peers. She appears cold and unemotional but is not confrontational. From what type of personality disorder is this woman probably suffering?

Schizoid personality disorder is demonstrated by a detachment from social relationships and restricted affect. Common symptoms include lack of desire to socialize or be part of groups or family, little interest in sexual relations or other pleasurable activities, detachment and emotional coldness, and indifference to the praise or criticism of others.

10. In addition to the above personality characteristics, the woman states that she often sees her soul float away from her body and feels that after this experience she is able to predict the future. She also adds that other people know of her abilities and feels that they are "out to get her." What personality disorder might you diagnose in this woman?

Schizotypal personality disorder, a pattern of social and emotional deficits in addition to some cognitive or perceptual eccentricities. Persons with schizotypal personalities often have odd beliefs, superstitions, or magical thinking. They may have inappropriate affect, odd speech patterns, and a paucity of close friends or confidants.

11. What personality disorder would you diagnose if the woman were reclusive but yearned for social contact?

Avoidant personality disorder is seen in people who are afraid of being ridiculed, and view themselves as inept and inadequate. They desire social interaction, but the anxiety over being placed in social situations keeps them in the shadows. They are reluctant to take personal risks or engage in new activities for fear of being embarrassed.

REFERENCE

1. American Psychiatric Association: Diagnostic and Statistical Manual of Mental Disorders, 4th ed, text revision. Washington, DC, American Psychiatric Association, 2000.

8. MUSCULOSKELETAL SYSTEM

Thomas Brown and Dave Brown

BASIC CONCEPTS

1. What are the components of a diarthrodial joint? Which sites within a diarthrodial joint are vulnerable to disease?

Diarthrodial joints are composed of articulating bones covered by cartilage (usually hyaline cartilage). Additional components include a joint cavity filled with synovial fluid, a synovial membrane, and a fibrous joint capsule. Ligamentous connections provide support and typically allow a large amount of movement. The sites vulnerable to disease are depicted in the figure below.

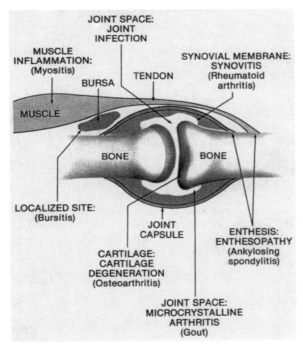

Sites and types of musculoskeletal disease processes. (From Bennett, Goldman (eds): Cecil Textbook of Medicine, 21st ed. Philadelphia, W.B. Saunders, 2000, p 1473, with permission.)

2. What are the vasculitides? How do they typically present clinically?

Although not strictly correct, the best way to think of the vasculitides is as a group of poorly understood autoimmune disorders involving the blood vessels. As inflammatory diseases, they typically present with vague constitutional signs such as fever, malaise, and arthralgias or myalgias. A biopsy of affected blood vessels can be helpful in making a definitive diagnosis, although obtaining a segment of affected vasculature can be difficult. Although it appears that the majority of the vasculitis syndromes are caused by an immune-mediated mechanism, other possible etiologies include drug hypersensitivity reactions and viral infections resulting in immune complex deposition within the vasculature.

131

CASE 1

A 30-year-old woman complains of joint pain for the past several months. The history is also significant for fatigue, pleurisy (pain with breathing), and a facial rash that worsens with sun exposure. Exam reveals a "butterfly" facial rash over the bridge of the nose and malar eminences (cheeks). Blood work reveals positive antinuclear antibodies (ANAs), antibodies against double-stranded DNA (anti-dsDNA), antibodies against RNA (anti-Smith antibodies), and a normochromic normocytic anemia. Urinalysis shows mild proteinuria. The patient is told that she has a chronic autoimmune disease and needs to begin medical treatment immediately.

1. What is the diagnosis? How is it treated?

Systemic lupus erythematosus (SLE). As with many autoimmune diseases, immunosuppression is the mainstay of therapy, typically with steroids such as oral prednisone.

2. What are antinuclear antibodies? Are they sensitive or specific for SLE?

ANAs are a diverse group of autoantibodies, all of which bind antigenic targets within the cellular nucleus. They are sensitive for SLE (> 95% of patients with SLE have them) but not specific, because they are present in many other autoimmune diseases and are often seen in healthy elderly people.

Note: Both anti-dsDNA and anti-Smith antibodies are highly specific to SLE and therefore quite helpful in making the diagnosis.

3. What is the most likely cause of the renal involvement and proteinuria?

Lupus nephritis is associated with immune complex deposition in the glomeruli, a type III hypersensitivity reaction. Several of the extrarenal manifestations of lupus are also due to immune complex deposition, including pericarditis, pleuritis, endocarditis, and malar rash.

4. What is the most likely explanation for the anemia?

Because lupus is a chronic inflammatory disease, the patient most likely has anemia of chronic disease (i.e., anemia of chronic inflammation). This anemia can be either normochromic and normocytic (as in this woman) or hypochromic and microcytic.

5. How does lupus predispose to deep venous thrombosis and a false-positive VDRL test?

A certain percentage of lupus patients produce the lupus anticoagulant, which actually predisposes to coagulation and thrombosis. This substance also causes false-positive results on the Venereal Disease Research Laboratory (VDRL) test for syphilis.

6. Which drugs are well known for causing a lupus-like syndrome?

Procainimide, quinidine, and hydralazine. Procainimide and quinidine are class IA antiarrhythmics, whereas hydralazine is a direct-acting arterial vasodilator used in the treatment of hypertension. Of interest, in drug-associated lupus, anti-dsDNA antibodies are not usually detected, although antibodies against single-stranded DNA (anti-ssDNA) are common.

CASE 2

A 54-year-old woman complains of a puzzling array of symptoms, including a long history of diarrhea, severe heartburn, and weight loss. When specifically questioned, she admits to pain in her fingers and toes in cold weather or when she becomes very emotional. On exam, the skin is fibrotic and thickened on her hands and feet and around her mouth. Several telangiectasias are also observed on her back and chest. Lab tests are negative for scl-70 antibodies but positive for the presence of anticentromere antibodies.

1. What is the likely diagnosis? How is this disease classified?

The likely diagnosis is scleroderma (progressive systemic sclerosis). Scleroderma is generally classified as either diffuse scleroderma, which has more extensive skin involvement, significant visceral involvement, and a poorer prognosis, or localized (limited) scleroderma, which involves primarily the skin and has a more benign prognosis. Localized scleroderma is commonly associated with the CREST syndrome, the symptoms of which this patient displays. **CREST** stands for **c**alcinosis, **R**aynaud's phenomenon, **e**sophageal dysmotility, **s**clerodactyly, and **t**elangiectasia.

Note: Anti-centromere antibodies are specific to limited scleroderma, whereas the scl-70 antibodies are more specific to diffuse scleroderma.

	DIFFUSE SCLERODERMA	LIMITED SCLERODERMA
Organ involvement	Extensive and diffuse skin involvement Significant visceral involvement (lungs, intestines, kidneys)	Limited skin involvement Associated with CREST syndrome Less visceral involvement but can evolve to diffuse scleroderma
Antibodies	+ Scl-70	+ Anticentromere
Prognosis	Poor	Better

2. Describe the pathogenesis of this disorder.

Macrophages in skin and visceral organs stimulate fibroblasts to deposit abnormal amounts of collagen (i.e., fibrosis) in the skin and visceral organs. This process impairs normal organ function, resulting in death secondary to renal failure (from renal arteriole fibrosis), respiratory failure (from pulmonary fibrosis), cardiac insufficiency (from a restrictive cardiomyopathy), and/or intestinal malabsorption (from intestinal fibrosis).

3. How is this condition managed pharmacologically?

Unlike most other rheumatologic diseases, systemic sclerosis does not respond well to immunosuppressant agents such as steroids. However, most patients do respond to therapy with D-penicillamine. Although its precise mechanism of action remains unclear, D-penicillamine appears to inhibit cytokines such as interleukin-1 (IL-1), which stimulates fibroblast proliferation and collagen deposition, and to retard the maturation of newly synthesized collagen. Other drugs used in rheumatoid arthritis include angiotensin-converting enzyme (ACE) inhibitors, which prevent or retard the progression of associated renal dysfunction, and calcium channel blockers such as nifedipine, which alleviate the symptoms of Raynaud's phenomenon.

4. Explain the pathophysiology of the chronic gastroesophageal reflux disease (GERD).

Decreased lower esophageal sphincter (LES) tone due to fibrosis of the LES and decreased esophageal motility.

Note: Malabsorption, diarrhea, and wasting are also frequently seen in scleroderma secondary to fibrosis and decreased motility of the small intestine.

5. What is Raynaud's phenomenon?

Arterial vasoconstriction in the hands and feet, typically triggered by cold or emotional stress and resulting in pain and paresthesias, which can be relieved by heat.

CASE 3

A 55-year-old obese woman complains of bilateral knee pain, right-sided hip pain, and pain in the fingers of both hands for the past 3 months. Her joint pain is relieved by rest and worsened with exertion, and she complains of only brief morning stiffness (about 15–20 minutes). Physical exam is unremarkable except for her hands, which reveal enlarged proximal interphalangeal joints (Bouchard's nodes) and distal interphalangeal joints (Heberden's nodes) of the digits as well as joint pain with movement and severely restricted range of motion. Examination of the knees is significant only for crepitus and slight pain with passive movement. The affected joints are not red, warm, or swollen. Radiographs show joint space narrowing in the knees and right hip (shown below). The patient is prescribed rofecoxib.

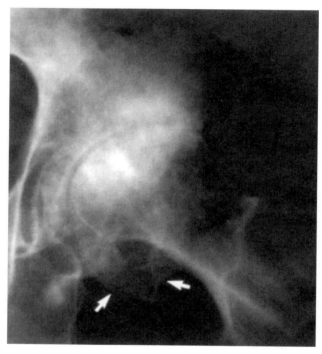

Radiograph showing joint space narrowing in the right hip. Arrows indicate peripheral osteophyte lipping. (From Cotran, Kumar, Collins (eds): Robbins Pathologic Basis of Disease, 6th ed. Philadelphia, W.B. Saunders, 1999, p 1248, with permission.)

1. What is the likely diagnosis?

Osteoarthritis (also known as osteoarthrosis, degenerative joint disease, hypertrophic arthritis), which is a common, slowly progressive disease.

Note: Osteoarthritis can be classified as primary (idiopathic) or secondary (e.g., secondary to trauma, metabolic disorders). The primary form is more common.

2. Is the pathogenesis of this condition primarily related to degeneration of bone, cartilage, or synovial membrane? How is it related to rheumatoid arthritis?

Osteoarthritis is characterized by degeneration of articular cartilage and often associated with overuse or a history of trauma to the joint. However, many other factors play a role (e.g., age, weight, hormones). Women are more commonly affected. In contrast, rheumatoid arthritis is associated with immunologic destruction of the synovial membrane and attendant inflammation, often causing the joints to be red and swollen in this disease.

Note: Recent studies suggest that glucosamine and chondroitin sulfate (a shark cartilage derivative) may be effective both for alleviating symptoms and for slowing disease progression. Joint space narrowing was halted in the treated groups, whereas joint space continued to narrow over time in the placebo groups.

3. What is the anatomic source of the joint pain in osteoarthritis?

Although the joint cartilage is destroyed in osteoarthritis, there is no neural input to cartilage and hence no pain transmission. The pain actually comes from the underlying periosteum/bone. Thus the disease becomes particularly painful when the cartilage has worn away to the point that bone is rubbing on bone.

Note: Joint cartilage is also completely avascular, which explains why injured cartilage does not heal well.

4. What risk factors are associated with osteoarthritis?

Obesity, occupation (repetitive motions), intense physical activity, joint trauma, and muscle weakness (probably via joint instability). Note that all of these factors increase the mechanical forces to which the joint cartilage is exposed.

5. What does an elevated erythrocyte sedimentation rate (ESR) indicate? Would it be elevated in this patient?

An elevated ESR is a nonspecific indicator of a *systemic* inflammatory process. However, because osteoarthritis is a local degenerative disease, it would probably not be elevated in this patient. In addition, although sufficiently severe joint degeneration may have an inflammatory component, it is still *localized* to the joint.

Note: Although osteoarthritis is classically considered a noninflammatory disease, pharmacologic treatment frequently involves the use of nonsteroidal anti-inflammatory drugs (NSAIDs) and intra-articular injections of steroids, which clearly act by reducing inflammation.

6. How do the findings on x-ray generally differ between osteoarthritis and rheumatoid arthritis?

In osteoarthritis the characteristic finding is joint space narrowing, as in this patient; there may also be increased density of the bone abutting the joint. **Rheumatoid arthritis**, on the other hand, is often associated with osteoporotic changes in the adjacent bone, and the joint space is typically normal. However, if the rheumatoid arthritis is severe enough, the inflammatory process may eventually destroy articular cartilage also and narrow the joint space.

7. Both NSAIDs and cyclooxygenase-2 (COX-2) inhibitors are possible treatments for this patient. What is similar about their mechanism of action? What is different?

Both classes of drugs inhibit prostaglandin synthesis by inhibiting cyclooxygenase and thus relieve pain. All of the NSAIDs *reversibly* inhibit COX, except aspirin, which *irreversibly* inhibits COX. The COX-2 inhibitors (rofecoxib, celecoxib) selectively inhibit the form of COX that is induced in inflammatory cells but not the constitutively expressed cyclooxygenase (COX-1) that is produced for various normal body functions.

8. What is the principal therapeutic advantage of the COX-2 inhibitors? What can be given to this patient with an NSAID to prevent their principal side effect?

By not inhibiting gastrointestinal prostaglandin synthesis, COX-2 inhibitors are supposed to cause less gastric ulceration, a common problem with the NSAIDs. Misoprostol, a synthetic prostaglandin analog, can be given orally with NSAIDs to reduce the risk of gastric ulceration and bleeding. Proton pump inhibitors can also be used to reduce the gastrointestinal side effects of NSAIDs.

Note: NSAID use can also precipitate renal dysfunction in a patient with borderline renal function due to reduced synthesis of vasodilatory prostaglandins that help maintain renal perfusion.

9. How does acetaminophen work?

Acetaminophen is a weak inhibitor of prostaglandin synthesis in the peripheral tissues and seems to work more in the central nervous system by raising the pain threshold. Its primary use, therefore, is as an analgesic. Because acetaminophen does not inhibit peripheral prostaglandin synthesis to a significant extent, it does not have the gastrointestinal side effects of NSAIDs.

10. What is the danger of consuming large amounts of acetaminophen?
If ingested in large amounts, acetaminophen is highly hepatotoxic and can even precipitate fulminant hepatic failure. An overdose is treated with n-acetylcysteine. Acetaminophen is especially hepatotoxic in alcoholics.

11. Cover the left side of the chart and specify the class of drug and its mechanism of action.

DRUG	CLASS OF DRUG	MECHANISM OF ACTION	SIDE EFFECTS
Rofecoxib (Vioxx) Celecoxib (Celebrex)	COX-2 inhibitor	Inhibit prostaglandin synthesis by inflammatory cells	Renal toxicity
Indomethacin Naproxen Ibuprofen Etodolac Ketorolac	NSAID	Reversible COX-1/COX-2 inhibition	GI ulcers and bleeding Renal damage
Aspirin	NSAID	Irreversible COX-1/COX-2 inhibition	GI ulcers and bleeding Renal damage
Acetaminophen	No class	Raises pain threshold	Hepatotoxicity

CASE 4

A 45-year-old woman presents with a chief complaint of widespread joint pain for the past 3 months, along with fatigue, depressed mood, and a chronic low-grade fever. She complains of significant morning stiffness, which lasts for well over an hour each morning. Musculoskeletal exam shows symmetrical joint involvement of the metacarpophalangeal (MCP) and proximal interphalangeal joints (PIP) of both hands as well as involvement of both knee joints. Involved joints appear swollen ("boggy"), erythematous, and warm to touch and are slightly painful to palpation. Multiple subcutaneous nodules are also noted on the extensor surfaces of the arms. Lab tests reveal an elevated erythrocyte sedimentation rate (ESR) of 55 mm/hr and are positive for rheumatoid factor. The patient is told that she has a chronic autoimmune arthritic condition and is prescribed methotrexate and celecoxib.

1. What is the probable diagnosis?
Rheumatoid arthritis (RA), which is a progressive systemic inflammatory disorder that primarily affects diarthrodial joints. RA produces a characteristic synovitis (inflammation of the synovial membrane), which causes joint damage and restricted joint mobility.

2. What is rheumatoid factor? Is its presence necessary for a diagnosis of RA in this woman?
Rheumatoid factor (RF) is an autoantibody to the constant (Fc) region of antibodies (usually IgG). The presence of rheumatoid factor is not required to make a diagnosis of RA. Indeed, rheumatoid factor is frequently absent in the first year of symptoms, but approximately 80% of patients eventually convert to a positive status. Because RF may also be present in healthy people and in a variety of other diseases (e.g., Sjögren's syndrome), the test has a low specificity for RA. Nevertheless, RF titers tend to indicate the severity of the disease and help formulate treatment options.
Note: Sjögren's disease (dry eyes, dry mouth) is commonly associated with rheumatoid arthritis. Patients typically present with difficulty in swallowing and multiple dental carries.

3. Which of the major criteria for the diagnosis of RA does this patient have?
At least four of the following seven criteria must be present for the diagnosis of RA:
1. Morning stiffness ≥ 1 hour
2. Arthritis involving ≥ 3 joints

3. Arthritis of hand joints
4. Symmetric arthritis
5. Rheumatoid (subcutaneous) nodules
6. Serum rheumatoid factor
7. Radiographic changes

The patient in this vignette has morning stiffness for greater than 1 hour, symmetrical arthritis, arthritis involving the hand joints, and arthritis involving the knees (i.e., ≥ 3 joints). She also has subcutaneous nodules on exam and tests positive for the presence of rheumatoid factor in her serum. She therefore satisfies six of the seven criteria (radiographic analysis was not performed) and can be definitively diagnosed with RA.

4. Is RA a systemic or localized inflammatory disorder?

Because general indices of systemic inflammation, such as ESR and C-reactive protein, are elevated and because patients frequently complain of systemic constitutional symptoms such as low-grade fever and fatigue, RA is considered a systemic inflammatory disorder. In addition, because of this chronic systemic inflammation many patients with RA suffer simultaneously from normocytic anemia (anemia of chronic disease).

5. What is the likely synovial leukocyte count in this patient?

A mild leukocytosis (≥ 2000 WBCs/mm^3) of the synovial fluid is typically seen in RA; the cells are predominantly polymorphonuclear neutrophils (PMNs). In contrast, septic arthritis (due to joint infection) is associated with a marked leukocytosis (> 50,000 WBCs/mm^3) in the synovial fluid.

6. As the disease progresses, should we expect involvement of the distal interphalangeal joints?

Not usually. Involvement of the distal interphalangeal joints is classically seen in osteoarthritis (Heberden's nodes) but does not typically occur in RA. However, proximal interphalangeal joint involvement in RA can be impressive.

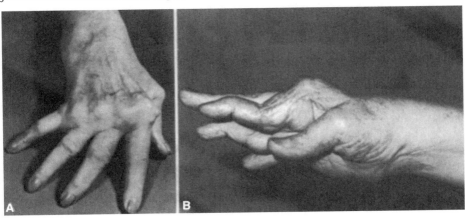

Hand deformities characteristic of chronic RA. **A,** Subluxation of the metacarpophalangeal joints with ulnar deviation of the digits. **B,** Hyperextension ("swan's neck") deformities of the proximal interphalangeal joints. (From Bennett, Goldman (eds): Cecil Textbook of Medicine, 21st ed. Philadelphia, W.B. Saunders, 2000, p 1494, with permission.)

7. In addition to celecoxib to control pain, why was this woman also given methotrexate?

Methotrexate is a disease-modifying antirheumatic drug (DMARD). The DMARDs are used to halt the progression of the disease. Many of these drugs have no direct effect on pain and are used only to slow progression. Other agents in this nonspecific "class" of drugs include gold salts, D-penicillamine, and the immunosuppressants azathioprine and cyclosporine.

8. What disease has the "bamboo spine" appearance on x-ray? What other features are characteristic of this disease?

Ankylosing spondylitis (AS), a spondyloarthropathy that manifests initially as bilateral sacroiliac joint pain and is strongly associated with the HLA-B27 haplotype. More than 90% of patients with ankylosing spondylitis have the HLA-B27 haplotype, although it is present in only 7% of the general population. AS occurs primarily in men.

9. What diagnosis might you suspect in a 30-year-old man who presents with back pain, conjunctivitis, and a recent history of dysuria?

You should suspect Reiter's syndrome, a spondyloarthropathy characterized by the triad of arthritis, urethritis, and conjunctivitis. For the purposes of step 1, you might consider Reiter's as a syndrome in which young men "can't see (conjunctivitis), can't pee (urethritis), and can't climb a tree (arthritis)." As with AS, the HLA-B27 haplotype is commonly associated with Reiter's syndrome.

CASE 5

The parents of a 3-year-old boy are concerned that he is not walking as well as other boys of his age. Both parents are healthy, and there is no family history of neuromuscular disease. Three older brothers are healthy. Physical exam reveals large calf muscles and proximal muscle weakness, as demonstrated by a positive Gower's sign when the boy stands from a sitting position. Examination is otherwise unremarkable. Lab tests are significant only for a markedly elevated creatine kinase (CK). A muscle biopsy shows complete absence of dystrophin staining in skeletal muscle cells.

1. What is the most likely diagnosis?

Duchenne's muscular dystrophy (DMD).

2. Is this condition more commonly acquired or inherited?

About two-thirds of cases of DMD are inherited in an X-linked recessive manner. However, approximately one-third of the cases are acquired secondary to spontaneous mutations within the dystrophin gene. The dystrophin gene is subject to a high rate of spontaneous mutations due to its enormous size ($> 2 \times 10^6$ bases). Because there is no family history of DMD, his condition was probably acquired after a spontaneous mutation in the dystrophin gene.

3. What is the function of dystrophin?

Dystrophin is a cytoskeletal membrane protein that plays an important structural role in skeletal muscle cells. It is absent in DMD.

4. How do the manifestations of Becker's muscular dystrophy (BMD) differ?

BMD is also due to mutations in the dystrophin gene, but some level of protein is present. Thus, the clinical manifestations are not as severe as those of DMD.

5. Why does the boy have such large calf muscle? What term is used to describe this finding in patients with DMD?

Patients with DMD ironically have the appearance of enlarged calf muscles, referred to as *pseudohypertrophy* of the calf muscles. This hypertrophy occurs initially in response to hypertrophy of muscle fibers but secondarily in response to fatty infiltration of the muscle and abnormal proliferation of connective tissue within the muscle.

6. **How is a positive Gower's sign elicited on exam? What does it indicate?**

Gower's sign can be elicited by asking the child to stand from a sitting position. Children with muscular dystrophy and other disorders involving muscle wasting do not have the muscle strength simply to stand. They may instead first roll over into a prone position, push themselves onto all fours, and then "walk" their hands up their thighs to a standing position (positive Gower's sign). Gower's sign indicates marked proximal muscle weakness.

7. **A patient complains of a long history of generalized muscle weakness. On exam, his facial muscles show marked atrophy, and when you ask him to shake your hand, he appears *unable to relax his grip* for an extended period. What diagnosis might you suspect?**

Myotonic dystrophy. The term *myotonia* refers to a sustained involuntary contraction of muscles, which this man exhibits by not being able to release his grip.

8. **What is the mechanism of inheritance of myotonic dystrophy?**

Myotonic dystrophy results from impaired expression of the myotonin protein kinase gene. The mechanism causing impaired expression involves expansion of a trinucleotide repeat sequence located in the 3' untranslated region of the myotonin protein kinase gene. This disorder is inherited as an autosomal dominant disease, and because the mechanism involves expansion of trinucleotide repeat sequences, the phenomenon of amplification is seen (i.e., family members develop the disease at earlier and earlier ages throughout the generations).

CASE 6

A 45-year-old man complains of lower back pain over the past several years. He describes "shooting, electric sensations" that run down the posterior aspect of his left thigh, lateral aspect of his left leg, and sometimes onto the plantar aspect of his left foot. He is pain-free today, of course. Exam reveals pain in his lower back with elevation of his left leg above 60° (positive straight leg test). There is no tenderness to palpation of the vertebral, sacroiliac, or acetabulofemoral (hip) joints. An x-ray reveals no obvious pathology, but an MRI is suggestive of mild disk herniation at the L4–L5 level.

1. **Why are the patient's symptoms commonly referred to as sciatica?**

Because the pain is distributed in an area that the sciatic nerve innervates.

2. **From which spinal nerve roots does the sciatic nerve originate? What are the nerve's two major branches? What muscles do these branches supply?**

The sciatic nerve arises from L4–S3. It then splits into the common peroneal nerve, which supplies the muscles of the lateral and anterior compartments of the leg, and the tibial nerve, which supplies the muscles of the posterior compartment of the leg and the plantar aspect of the foot.

3. **If the L4–L5 disk is herniated, why do the symptoms reflect the distribution of the L5 dermatome instead of the L4 dermatome? After all, the L4 nerve root exits in the intervertebral foramen between L4 and L5.**

The L4 nerve root exits superior to the L4–L5 disk; therefore, it is not susceptible to compression by herniation. In contrast, the L5 nerve root descends immediately posterior to the L4–L5 disk and is susceptible to compression when the disk bulges posteriorly. The same concept applies to L5–S1 herniation, which causes symptoms along the S1 dermatome.

4. **How can spasm of the piriformis cause similar symptoms?**

In approximately 12% of the population, the common peroneal division of the sciatic nerve runs through the piriformis muscle instead of below it. Spasm of the piriformis in such people can cause symptoms mimicking sciatica (so-called piriformis syndrome). This condition can often be treated with muscle relaxants.

CASE 7

A 52-year-old medical receptionist complains of sharp shooting pains in her left hand over the past few months. On closer questioning, she clarifies that the pain radiates along the palmar aspect of her hand through the index finger and middle finger. She admits to several hours of computer work each day, as a large part of her job involves typing physicians' muddled dictations. Thenar wasting is noted on her left hand and a left-sided Tinel's sign is elicited on physical examination.

1. What is the probable diagnosis?
Carpal tunnel syndrome.

2. Describe the pathogenesis of this disease.
Carpal tunnel syndrome is a compression (entrapment) neuropathy caused by compression of the median nerve as it enters the wrist through the carpal tunnel. Such compression can occur secondary to inflammation of the carpal tunnel.

3. How does the median nerve enter the hand? Describe the sensory distribution of the median nerve to the hand.
The median nerve enters the hand via the carpal tunnel, deep to the flexor retinaculum (transverse carpal ligament), along with the tendons of the flexor digitorum superficialis, flexor digitorum profundus, and palmaris longus. Paresthesias in the affected hand occur because the median nerve provides cutaneous innervation to the palmar aspect of the lateral palm and the first three digits as well as the dorsal aspect of the tips of the first three and one-half fingers.

Note: Surgical treatment for carpal tunnel involves release (tension reduction) of the flexor retinaculum. Medical treatment involves steroid injections to reduce the nerve compression due to inflammation

4. How is Tinel's sign elicited?
Tinel's sign is positive when tapping over the median nerve (between the thenar and hypothenar eminences) elicits the same shooting pains or paresthesias of which the patient complains.

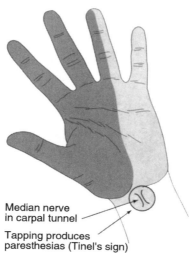

Median nerve
in carpal tunnel

Tapping produces
paresthesias (Tinel's sign)

Tinel's sign in carpal tunnel syndrome. (From Bennett, Goldman (eds): Cecil Textbook of Medicine, 21st ed. Philadelphia, W.B. Saunders, 2000, p 1495, with permission.)

5. Why may the patient develop weakness and incoordination of her left thumb?

The median nerve innervates several muscles of the thenar eminence. These muscles (abductor pollicis brevis, opponens pollicis, and flexor pollicis brevis) coordinate movements of the first digit and therefore may cause weakness and clumsiness of her thumb. Atrophy of these muscles is indicated by thenar wasting on exam.

CASE 8

A 52-year-old man presents with a severe pain in his right big toe. Last night he hosted his daughter's wedding celebration and enjoyed good food and wine until late in the evening. The joint is red, swollen, warm, and painful to the touch. No subcutaneous or tendinous nodules are appreciated. Aspiration of synovial fluid reveals needle-shaped, negatively birefringent crystals under light microscopy.

1. What is the most likely diagnosis?

Gout, caused by precipitation of uric acid crystals within the synovial fluid.

2. How does uric acid deposition within the synovial fluid lead to disease?

Uric acid is deposited within joints in the form of monosodium urate crystals. These crystals are phagocytosed by neutrophils and macrophages. Because these cells are unable to degrade the urate crytals, an inflammatory immune response is activated within the joint (see below).

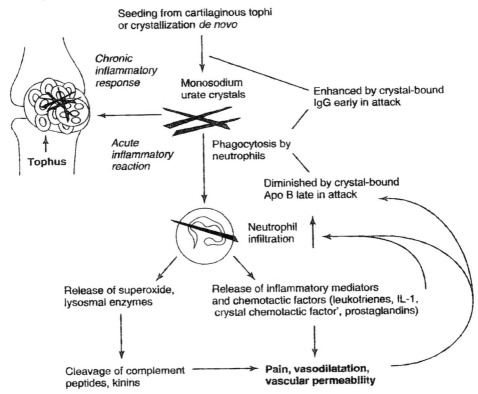

Pathophysiologic processes involved in gout. (From Bennett, Goldman (eds): Cecil Textbook of Medicine, 21st ed. Philadelphia, W.B. Saunders, 2000, p 1544, with permission.)

3. What is the likely diagnosis if crystals found within the synovial fluid revealed positively birefringent crystals?

Pseudogout, which results from deposition of calcium pyrophosphate crystals and more commonly affects the knees. Radiographs often reveal calcific densities that result from calcium pyrophosphate deposition within the cartilage (chondrocalcinosis).

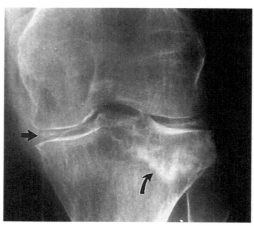

Calcification is seen at the medial (arrow) and lateral joint spaces, representing chondrocalcinosis of the fibrocartilage (menisci). Curved arrow shows stress fracture. (From Katz DS, Math KR, Groskin SA (eds): Radiology Secrets. Philadelphia, Hanley & Belfus, 1998, p 278, with permission.)

4. What is the relationship of gout to elevated serum uric acid levels?

Gout is often associated with hyperuricemia, but hyperuricemia is neither sensitive nor specific for gout. The gold standard for the diagnosis of gout is synovial fluid analysis, which, if positive, will show the presence of needle-shaped, negatively birefringent crystals.

5. If the patient has recurrent attacks of gout, he will likely be put on chronic therapy. What tests can be performed to determine the most suitable type of pharmacologic treatment?

Gout can be caused by the overproduction or the underexcretion of uric acid. Depending on the specific etiology, different treatment strategies may be necessary. The test to discriminate between the two is a 24-hour urinary uric acid excretion, which will be normal in undersecretors and elevated in overproducers.

6. What is the pharmacologic basis for using probenecid in underexcreters of uric acid?

Renal underexcretion of uric acid is due to either impaired tubular secretion or increased tubular reabsorption. Probenecid selectively inhibits renal tubular reabsorption of uric acid, thereby increasing overall excretion.

7. Why should probenecid be avoided in an overproducer of uric acid?

Such patients are at increased risk for uric acid nephrolithiasis, and inhibiting renal tubule reabsorption will increase tubular uric acid levels and the risk of forming a uric acid stone.

8. Why should this patient avoid thiazide diuretics, loop diuretics, and aspirin?

All of these drugs inhibit the organic acid transporter in the distal tubules that secretes uric acid, resulting in increased serum uric acid levels and exacerbations of gout.

9. What is the pharmacologic basis for using allopurinol for overproducers of uric acid?

Uric acid is a product of purine catabolism, and the last step in this pathway is catalyzed by xanthine oxidase, which converts xanthine to uric acid. Allopurinol inhibits this enzyme, resulting in less production of uric acid and greater xanthine levels (which is significantly more soluble).

Note: Recall that the DNA bases adenine and guanine are purines.

10. Why is allopurinol often given to patients undergoing chemotherapy?

By destroying large numbers of replicating cells, chemotherapy causes a significant amount of DNA degradation, and with that significant flux through the purine catabolic pathway, resulting in increased uric acid production. Allopurinol is beneficial because it can attenuate the excess uric acid production and prevent development of *tumor lysis syndrome.*

11. How does hypoglycemia increase uric acid production?

Hypoglycemia reduces cellular adenosine triphosphate (ATP) production, resulting in increased levels of cellular adenosine, a starting substrate for purine catabolism. Interestingly, alcohol is believed to exacerbate gout by causing hypoglycemia.

12. How does Lesch-Nyhan syndrome cause hyperuricemia?

In a normal person, most purines are "scavenged" for reuse by the enzyme hypoxanthine-guanine phosphoribosyl transferase, instead of being degraded to uric acid. The activity of this enzyme is deficient in Lesch-Nyhan, resulting in increased purine catabolism and a resulting increase in uric acid production. Such patients also often have central nervous system symptoms and tend to engage in self-mutilation.

13. If the patient is going to be treated only for an acute attack, what pharmacologic agents are indicated? Describe their mechanism of action.

The two drugs most widely used for acute gouty attacks include colchicine and indomethacin. Colchicine inhibits microtubule polymerization and so prevents phagocytosis of uric acid crystals by macrophages and neutrophils (frustrated phagocytosis of these crystals elicits the inflammatory response in gout). Indomethacin, an NSAID, simply inhibits the inflammatory response.

Note: Colchicine is used cautiously in acute attacks of gout because it can cause pronounced nausea, vomiting, and diarrhea.

14. Why is the absence of subcutaneous or tendinous nodules significant in this patient?

They are findings of tophaceous gout. Tophi are present in chronic gout and consist of a nodular deposit of monosodium urate monohydrate crystals with a foreign body reaction. These tophi can be found in various sites, including cartilage, tendon, bone, and subcutaneous tissue.

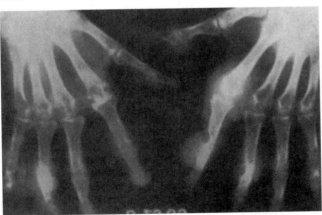

Radiographic evidence of tophi. (From Bennett, Goldman (eds): Cecil Textbook of Medicine, 21st ed. Philadelphia, W.B. Saunders, 2000, p 1546, with permission.)

CASE 9

A 34-year-old obese woman complains of muscle aches "all over" and increasing fatigue for the past 6 months. She says that despite sleeping 8–10 hours each night, she feels more tired in the morning than when she went to bed the previous night. She admits to a long history of anxiety and depression but is adamant that these muscle aches are real. Physical exam is remarkable for muscle tenderness at 14 of 18 trigger points. A thorough laboratory work-up reveals a normal erythrocyte sedimentation rate and normal levels of C-reactive protein and creatine phosphokinase (CPK). Both muscle biopsy and electromyography are normal.

1. **What is the most likely diagnosis?**
   Fibromyalgia, a rheumatologic disorder characterized by fatigue, poor sleep, and musculoskeletal pain, with the presence of specific tender trigger points on exam.
   Note: A diagnosis of chronic fatigue syndrome requires at least 6 months of new-onset, unexplained persistent or relapsing fatigue that is not caused by exertional activity and that is not alleviated by rest.

2. **Who is at greatest risk for developing fibromyalgia?**
   The prevalence of fibromyalgia increases with age and is approximately 7 times more common in women than men. It also appears to be associated with obesity, anxiety and depression, and social stressors (e.g., deadbeat dad and screaming kids). Therefore, the classic patient with fibromyalgia for the purposes of step 1 is an overweight and depressed middle-aged woman who is unhappily married and has to deal with the added stress of raising children. Not terribly flattering, but these associations seem to be real.

CASE 10

A 52-year-old carpenter complains of increasing muscle weakness and muscle pain over the past year or two. He is not taking any cholesterol-lowering drugs. Physical exam is significant only for proximal muscle weakness, as evidenced by marked difficulty in rising from a seated position. Laboratory work-up reveals markedly elevated levels of creatine kinase but a normal ESR, and a muscle biopsy demonstrates lymphocytic infiltration of muscle fibers with perivascular degeneration of fibers.

1. **What is the likely diagnosis?**
   Polymyositis, an autoimmune inflammatory myopathy resulting in muscle destruction, muscle pain, and proximal muscle weakness. Laboratory evaluation typically reveals a markedly elevated creatine kinase but normal ESR.

2. **How would the diagnosis be affected if exam also showed a heliotrope facial rash and the presence of periorbital edema?**
   This presentation is characteristic of dermatomyositis, which involves the skin as well as the muscles.

3. **How is the disease treated? Why?**
   Because polymyositis is an autoimmune inflammatory disorder, immunosuppression with steroids, typically small amounts of oral prednisone, has been effective. However, students should be aware that steroid therapy itself may cause a *glucocorticoid myopathy*, which can present with similar symptoms.

4. **What disease transmitted by pork can cause similar muscular symptoms?**
   Trichinosis, which is caused by eating raw or undercooked meats that contain the viable larvae of the roundworm *Trichinella spiralis*. Although most infections are subclinical, exposure

to a heavy inoculum of larvae can result in trichinosis, which may present clinically with diarrhea, myositis, fever, and periorbital edema. Laboratory evaluation typically reveals hypereosinophilia as well.

CASE 11

Dr. Rheumatoid is a specialist widely known for his interest and skill in treating rare disorders of the musculoskeletal system. His particular expertise is in diagnosing and treating metabolic and developmental disorders of bone. A third-year medical student working with him one afternoon is delighted to encounter one "zebra" after another in clinic and decides that perhaps rheumatology is not as bad as he had originally assumed. Certainly the hours seemed reasonable, and he had not yet heard of any rheumatologic patients dying from painful joints.

1. The first patient encountered by the student was referred to Dr. Rheumatoid with complaints of bone pain and a diagnosis (made by a hematologist) of myelophthisic anemia. A bone scan reveals abnormally thick and dense bones. What is your diagnosis?

Osteopetrosis (also known as marble bone disease).

2. What causes the bones to be dense and thick in this patient?

In osteopetrosis the osteoclasts are less active (or inactive) and therefore do not resorb bone effectively during bone remodeling. In addition, the process whereby woven (immature) bone is converted to compact (mature) bone is disrupted in osteopetrosis. This combination of reduced remodeling of bone and inadequate bone "maturation" results in thick and brittle bones.

3. Why might you see anemia in osteopetrosis? Why is it referred to as a myelophthisic anemia?

The term *myelophthisis* describes the replacement of hematopoietic tissue in the bone marrow with abnormal tissue. Myelophthisic anemia, therefore, is caused by the replacement of bone marrow by abnormal tissue. In the case of osteopetrosis, the failure of osteoclasts to remodel existing bone allows newly formed bone to encroach on the space of the bone marrow, making hematopoiesis less effective and resulting in pancytopenia.

4. A 12-year-old boy with sickle cell anemia is referred for continued right hip pain and intermittent fevers, although he cannot recall any specific trauma to the hip. An x-ray of the hip suggests avascular necrosis of the head of the femur. Infection with what organisms should be suspected?

Although *Staphylococcus aureus* is the most common organism responsible for osteomyelitis, patients with sickle cell anemia are uniquely susceptible to Salmonella bacteremia and osteomyelitis caused by *Salmonella*. This susceptibility stems from the impaired splenic function and impaired mononuclear cell function associated with sickle cell anemia.

5. A 42-year-old woman with end-stage renal failure is referred to Dr. Rheumatoid because recent bone scans revealed marked osteopenia throughout her body. What most likely explains this finding?

The most likely explanation is osteomalacia caused by vitamin D deficiency secondary to renal failure. An important endocrine function of the kidneys is the production of 1,25-dihydroxycholecalciferol, the active form of vitamin D. Because vitamin D is necessary for bone mineralization and because bone is constantly being remodeled, impaired mineralization results in an imbalance between mineralization and degradation, causing marked osteopenia.

Note: Additional causes of renal osteodystrophy include bone buffering of excessive acid and hypocalcemia from calcium phosphate precipitation in hyperphosphatemia.

6. A 6-year-old boy is brought to clinic by his mother because he has suffered multiple bone fractures throughout his short life. All of these fractures were unexpected, because they invariably occurred in response to minor accidents. In addition, the boy has been doing poorly in school recently because he is having trouble hearing the teacher. Exam is remarkable only for slightly blue sclera. What is your diagnosis? What causes this condition?

Osteogenesis imperfecta, which is due to genetic defects that result in structural or quantitative abnormalities of type I collagen, which is the primary component of the extracellular matrix of bones. The wide spectrum of genotypes and phenotypes ranges from very severe to fairly minor.

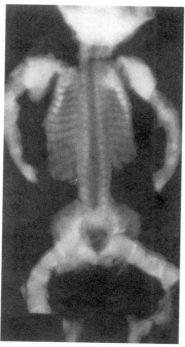

Osteogenesis imperfecta. (From Cotran, Kumar, Collins (eds): Robbins Pathologic Basis of Disease, 6th ed. Philadelphia, W.B. Saunders, 1999, p 1121, with permission.)

7. Cover the right-hand columns and list the pathophysiologic abnormality associated with each of the following disorders.

DISORDER	PATHOPHYSIOLOGY
Osteopetrosis (marble bone disease)	Decreased osteoclast activity, with invasion of bone marrow leading to myelophthisic anemia.
Pseudogout (chondrocalcinosis)	Calcium pyrophosphate deposition.
Achondroplasia	Mutation in fibroblast growth factor receptor prevents endochondral ossification and limits long bone growth.
Paget's disease of the bone	Increased rate of osteoclast activity (perhaps due to viral infection of osteoclasts). Increased rates of bone resorption, formation, and mineralization result in deposition of woven rather than lamellar bone.
Osteogenesis imperfecta	Genetic defects in type I collagen weaken bone.
Gout	Increased uric acid production or decreased uric acid excretion.
Rheumatoid arthritis	Inflammation of synovial membrane.

(Cont'd.)

DISORDER	PATHOPHYSIOLOGY
Osteomalacia	Impaired bone mineralization in adults.
Rickets	Impaired bone and cartilage mineralization in children.
Osteoarthritis	Degeneration of joint cartilage.

CASE 12

Dr. Vasculoid is a rheumatologist widely known for his interest and skill in disorders involving the blood vessels. Like his brother Dr. Rheumatoid, he does not get out much. In any event, because he is employed at a well-known academic medical center, he receives interesting referrals on an almost daily basis, which keeps his medical students quite happy. A fourth-year medical student, who thought that he had seen it all with Dr. Rheumatoid during his third-year clerkship, is surprised to encounter yet another series of interesting patients in clinic.

1. **The first patient is a 75-year-old woman who complains of fever, fatigue, weight loss, and a severe right-sided headache. She denies any recent visual problems or diplopia. Physical exam is significant for palpation causing tenderness along the course of the temporal artery. Lab tests reveal a markedly elevated erythrocyte sedimentation rate (ESR). What is the most likely diagnosis?**
   Temporal (giant-cell) arteritis. The definitive diagnosis is obtained by temporal artery biopsy, which shows granulomatous infiltration of the artery.

2. **If a biopsy of the temporal artery was performed and returned negative, why might it still make sense to treat this woman with prednisone?**
   Because temporal arteritis affects the temporal artery in a segmental fashion, which may explain a negative biopsy result even in the presence of the disease. For this reason, if the clinician has a strong index of suspicion for temporal arteritis, the patient should be treated with prednisone regardless of whether a biopsy is performed or even what the results of the biopsy are.

3. **What does an elevated ESR indicate? How does it relate to treatment with prednisone?**
   An elevated ESR indicates an ongoing systemic inflammatory process, which may be responsive to immunosuppressive agents such as prednisone.

4. **What severe complication of this disorder may be avoided by initiating immunosuppressive therapy as soon as possible?**
   Blindness, which can occur suddenly and without warning (by occlusion of the ophthalmic artery).

5. **The second patient is a 40-year-old man who complains of a 6-month history of sinus problems. More recently he has been coughing up small amounts of blood-tinged sputum (hemoptysis) and admits to occasional blood in his urine (hematuria). A chest x-ray reveals the presence of bilateral nodular and cavitary infiltrates. Testing for plasma anti-neutrophil cytoplasmic antibodies (c-ANCA) is positive. What is the most likely diagnosis?**
   Wegener granulomatosis, a vasculitis that affects both the lungs and the kidneys; c-ANCA antibodies are specific for this disease.
   Note: p-ANCA antibodies are specific for polyarteritis nodosa.

6. **The third patient is a 4-year-old girl who was brought to the emergency department because of a 5-day history of high fever (about 1030 F). Physical exam reveals a wealth of findings, including cervical lymphadenopathy, conjunctival erythema, a desquamating**

maculopapular rash involving the palms and soles, and edema of the hands and feet. Lab tests reveal elevated ESR and C-reactive protein and increased numbers of platelets. A work-up excludes diagnoses of staphylococcal scalded skin syndrome, toxic shock syndrome, and Stevens-Johnson syndrome. What is the likely diagnosis?

Kawasaki's syndrome (also known as mucocutaneous lymph node syndrome).

7. What are the classic presenting symptoms of Kawasaki syndrome?

It may help to recall Kawasaki syndrome by its other name, mucocutaneous lymph node syndrome. The typical signs and symptoms include mucosal inflammation, cutaneous maculopapular rash, lymph node enlargement, and unexplained high fever.

8. How does Kawasaki's disease cause cardiac complications?

The coronary arteries are often inflamed in Kawasaki's disease, resulting in cardiovascular sequelae in about 20% of patients, including coronary artery aneurysms and coronary thrombosis with myocardial infarction.

Note: This is a serious disease. About 1% of children who develop it will die because of rupture of a coronary artery aneurysm or because of coronary thrombosis and infarction.

9. The next patient is a 35-year-old man who complains of fever, muscle aches (myalgias), fatigue, and weakness for the past several weeks. Although he cannot recall being sick with hepatitis, a laboratory evaluation reveals that he is HbsAg-positive. The laboratory work-up also reveals an elevated C-reactive protein and the presence of p-ANCA antibodies. An arterial biopsy reveals inflammation of the tunica media. What is the most likely diagnosis?

Polyarteritis nodosa.

10. What is the significance of the positive HBsAg?

About 20–30% of cases of polyarteritis nodosa are associated with hepatitis B virus antigenemia. In fact, it is believed that immune complex depositions with these antigens may be a cause of polyarteritis nodosa.

11. The next patient is an 8-year-old boy who presents with a maculopapular petechial rash on his buttocks and lower extremities and hematuria, which on microscopic examination reveals red blood cell casts. What is the most likely diagnosis?

Henoch-Schönlein purpura

12. What causes the hematuria in this patient?

Henoch-Schönlein purpura is a cause of glomerulonephritis. A microscopic urinalysis may have shown red cell casts and facilitated the diagnosis.

13. The next patient is a 35-year-old male smoker who complains of pain in his hands and feet with cold weather as well as recurring ulcers on his feet. Oddly, he mentions that when he quit smoking for 6 months, these symptoms disappeared completely. What is the most likely diagnosis?

Buerger's disease (also known as thromboangiitis obliterans), an inflammatory occlusive disease of the arteries of the distal extremities. It is typically seen in male smokers under the age of 40.

14. The next patient is a 35-year-old Asian woman who complains of numbness and tingling in her fingers, which she has experienced for years. On exam, her blood pressure is 90/55 mmHg, and the radial pulse on both wrists is difficult to detect, although her femoral and dorsalis pedis pulses are strong. An aortic arteriography is ordered and reveals stenosis of the branches of the aortic arch but is negative for coarctation of the aorta. What is the likely diagnosis in this woman?

Takayasu arteritis, also known as "pulseless disease."

15. Are small- or large-diameter vessels primarily affected in this disease?

Large-diameter arteries are primarily affected. The most common finding is significant narrowing (caused by intimal thickening) of the great vessels as they come off the aortic arch. Sometimes these arteries can be occluded to varying degrees, resulting in markedly different blood pressures in the upper extremities.

16. What are the three large arteries that branch off from the aortic arch?

Brachiocephalic (which splits into the right subclavian and right carotid arteries), left carotid, and left subclavian arteries.

17. In physiologic terms, why might we expect hypertension if arterial narrowing were to occur in the aorta distal to the ductus arteriosus?

For essentially the same reasons as hypertension secondary to postductal coarctation of the aorta. Decreased renal perfusion results in increased renin secretion, which increases the production of aldosterone and angiotensin II, resulting in hypertension.

18. Cover the right-hand column and describe the classic presentation for each of the following vasculitides.

VASCULITIS	CLASSIC PRESENTATION
Temporal (giant-cell) arteritis	Fever, unilateral headache, markedly elevated ESR.
Wegener's granulomatosis	Hemoptysis, hematuria, presence of c-ANCA antibodies.
Kawasaki syndrome	Unexplained fever, maculopapular rash that starts on hands and feet, bilateral conjunctival injection, cervical lymphadenopathy, and edema of extremities.
Polyarteritis nodosa	Hepatitis B antigenemia, presence of p-ANCA antibodies. Arterial biopsy reveals inflammation of the tunica media.
Churg-Strauss syndrome	History of asthma, labs show eosinophilia.
Takayasu arteritis ("pulseless disease")	Different blood pressures in the arms, diminished radial pulses.
Henoch-Schönlein purpura	Abdominal pain, hematuria, maculopapular rash on lower extremities.
Thromboangiitis obliterans (Buerger's disease)	Young male smoker with distal extremity cold intolerance.

9. ANEMIAS

Thomas Brown and Dave Brown

BASIC CONCEPTS

1. What are reticulocytes?

Reticulocytes are immature red blood cells (RBCs) newly produced by the bone marrow and released into the blood. The number of reticulocytes in the peripheral blood provides an indication of how effectively the bone marrow is producing RBCs.

2. What information can be provided about the cause of anemias by the absolute reticulocyte count?

In anemias caused by inadequate marrow production (ineffective erythropoiesis), the reticulocyte count is lower than would be expected for the degree of anemia. In other words, in the setting of the anemia, the compensatory increase in reticulocyte count is significantly less than would be expected if there were no defect in erythropoiesis. In contrast, in anemias caused by hemolysis, the bone marrow is unaffected and compensates, to a significant extent at least, by substantially increasing reticulocyte production. In either situation, hemolytic anemia or anemia due to ineffective erythropoiesis, the plasma levels of erythropoietin can be similarly elevated, but the bone marrow responds better to the elevated erythropoietin in the hemolytic anemias.

Note: Deficient secretion of erythropoietin also causes anemia, and this is distinct from a defect in the bone marrow or a hemolytic anemia.

3. What are the microcytic anemias? What does their pathogenesis have in common?

The microcytic anemias consist of iron deficiency anemia, anemia of chronic disease, alpha-thalassemia, beta-thalassemia, and lead poisoning. All of these diseases involve a defect in hemoglobin synthesis. They cause microcytic anemias because cell proliferation occurs at a more rapid rate than the defective hemoglobin synthesis; thus, cell division occurs with a less than full or "mature" cytoplasm. Hemoglobin synthesis is impaired in iron deficiency anemia because of iron's crucial role in heme synthesis, and in anemia of chronic disease because of inadequate iron utilization. Lead poisoning inhibits two key enzymes in heme synthesis, alanine dehydratase and ferrochelatase. The thalassemias involve defects in synthesis of the alpha chains and beta chains of hemoglobin.

Note: Anemias due to vitamin B12 and folate deficiency are often macrocytic because hemoglobin synthesis outpaces DNA synthesis and cell division, creating larger cells prior to division. Recall that both vitamin B12 and folate are involved in DNA synthesis.

4. In the hemolytic anemias, what is the difference between intravascular and extravascular hemolysis?

Intravascular hemolysis occurs when red blood cells are directly lysed within the blood vessels—for example, by complement in paroxysmal nocturnal hemoglobinuria, by mechanical prosthetic valves, or by microangiopathic hemolytic anemias that cause mechanical fragmentation of RBCs (as in disseminated intravascular coagulation). In extravascular hemolysis, splenic macrophages or Kuppfer cells in the liver destroy red blood cells (e.g., hereditary spherocytosis, hypersplenism).

5. Why is there a greater degree of hemoglobinemia and hemoglobinuria in intravascular hemolysis than in extravascular hemolysis?

In intravascular hemolysis, lysed red blood cells spill their hemoglobin directly into the bloodstream (hemoglobinemia), which may also leak out into the urine (hemoglobinuria). In contrast, in **extravascular** hemolysis, the hemoglobin in the phagocytosed red blood cells is metabolized intracellularly to bilirubin, reducing the amount of hemoglobin that ends up in the blood or urine.

Note: Haptoglobin, a serum protein that binds free hemoglobin, binds more hemoglobin in intravascular hemolysis, causing a greater decrease in its plasma levels.

	INTRAVASCULAR HEMOLYSIS	EXTRAVASCULAR HEMOLYSIS
Hemoglobinemia	Yes	None or slight
Hemoglobinuria	Yes	None or slight
Plasma haptoglobin	Large decrease	Normal or slight decrease
Anemia	Yes	Yes
Jaundice	Yes	Yes
Hepatosplenomegaly	No	Often
Examples	Microangiopathic hemolytic anemias Disseminated intravascular coagulation Thrombotic thrombocytopenic purpura Paroxysmal nocturnal hemoglobinuria	Hereditary spherocytosis Hypersplenism

6. What is the usual cause of anemia in end stage renal failure?

The anemia in this setting is principally due to reduced production of erythropoietin by the diseased kidneys. However, uremia from renal failure may also make the bone marrow less responsive to erythropoietin. Anemia caused by renal failure typically responds well to exogenously administered erythropoietin.

CASE 1

A 25-year-old African-American man presents with a history of general fatigue and intermittent episodes of sharp abdominal pain. He has had two previous hospital admissions for sepsis caused by encapsulated bacteria. Physical exam is unremarkable except for mild scleral icterus. Complete blood count reveals hemoglobin of 9.0 gm/dl, hematocrit of 27%, and a mean corpuscular volume of 87 fl. A peripheral blood smear, which reveals a marked reticulocytosis, is shown below.

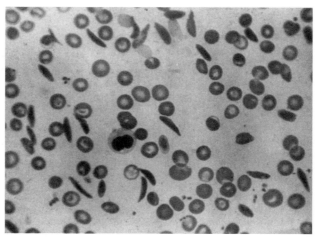

Peripheral blood smear of patient described above. (From Bennett, Goldman (eds): Cecil's Textbook of Medicine, 21st ed. Philadelphia, W.B. Saunders, 2000, p 894, with permission.)

1. What is the expected diagnosis? What is the confirmatory test?

Sickle cell anemia, a hereditary hemoglobinopathy caused by expression of an abnormal beta-globin gene. Note the presence of "sickled" cells on the peripheral smear. The results of hemoglobin solubility testing and hemoglobin electrophoresis can provide definitive evidence to make a diagnosis of sickle cell anemia.

Note: The sickle cell mutation is believed to be more common in African Americans because in its heterozygous form it provides protection from infection with *Plasmodium falciparum*. In fact, in regions of Africa where malaria is common, up to 25–30% of the population is heterozygous for this mutation.

2. What are the three primary types of hemoglobin found within normal adult RBCs? How do they differ in sickle cell anemia?

The three primary types of hemoglobin in adult RBCs include hemoglobin A ($\alpha2\beta2$), hemoglobin A_2 ($\alpha2\delta2$), and fetal hemoglobin F ($\alpha2\gamma2$). The vast majority (> 95%) of hemoglobin in adult RBCs is normally of the hemoglobin A type. Because sickle cell anemia is caused by a mutation in the β-globin gene (a point mutation resulting in a substitution of the hydrophobic valine for the hydrophilic glutamic acid in the β-globin protein), there is deficient production of hemoglobin A (HbA) and increased expression of abnormal hemoglobin S (HbS).

3. What causes "sickling" of RBCs in this disease?

In the deoxygenated form, HbS is significantly less soluble than HbA and is therefore predisposed to precipitate from the cytoplasm under conditions that cause higher concentrations of deoxyhemoglobin (e.g., hypoxemia, acidosis, hyperosmolarity/dehydration). Although the effects of hemoglobin precipitation are initially reversible, repeated bouts of hemoglobin precipitation lead to irreversible defects in structure and function of the RBC membrane, resulting in a chronically sickled cell.

4. What are the vaso-occlusive crises? What factors are thought to increase the risk of these crises?

Vaso-occlusive crises are associated with increased RBC sickling, which occludes blood vessels, resulting in a local lactic acidosis and pain arising from the occluded vascular beds. The same factors that increase deoxyhemoglobin concentrations, such as dehydration, hypoxemia, and acidosis, may also trigger these "crises."

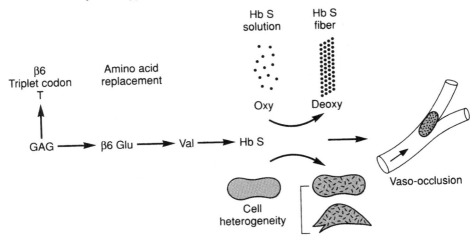

Mechanism of vaso-occlusive crises. (From Hoffman et al (eds): Hematology: Basic Principles and Practice, 3rd ed. New York, Churchill Livingstone, 2000, p 511, with permission.)

5. Describe the mechanism by which dehydration, acidosis, and hyperosmolarity increase sickling. Why might this patient be susceptible to papillary necrosis of the kidneys?

Dehydration, acidosis, and hyperosmolarity increase the *mean corpuscular deoxyhemoglobin concentration (MCHC)*, which causes increased HbS aggregation in RBCs. The conditions of hypoxemia, acidosis, and hyperosmolarity specifically present in the renal medulla cause increased sickling of RBCs, resulting in vaso-occlusion of the vasa recta in the renal papilla and eventually papillary necrosis.

6. How do clinical symptoms differ in patients with sickle cell trait (Hb AS) rather than sickle cell disease (BH SS)?

The heterozygous carrier of the sickle cell mutation is said to have the sickle cell trait, genotypically referred to as Hb AS. Such patients are relatively asymptomatic, with minimal symptoms of anemia, and typically do not experience episodes of pain from vaso-occlusive crises. As previously mentioned, the heterozygous carrier may be less susceptible to infection with Plasmodium falciparum, but approximately 25% of the offspring of two such carriers will have full-blown sickle cell disease.

7. What is the rationale for treating this patient with the chemotherapeutic drug hydroxyurea?

Hydroxyurea increases the production of fetal hemoglobin (HbF), which presumably decreases the amount of HbS expression, and therefore decreases HbS polymerization and RBC sickling. However, the precise mechanism of action of hydroxyurea remains poorly understood. Nonetheless, students should know that it is an important therapeutic agent for sickle cell disease.

8. To what bone "diseases" are patients with sickle cell anemia predisposed? Why?

Vaso-occlusive phenomena in sickle cell anemia can cause avascular necrosis of bones. These avascular areas of bone then become susceptible to the development of infection (osteomyelitis). *Salmonella* osteomyelitis is seen more frequently in sickle cell disease.

9. If the patient presents with complaints of a recent significant increase in fatigue and has developed a facial rash that has a "slapped cheek" appearance, what serious complication should be considered?

The slapped cheek appearance is characteristic of parvovirus infection. Parvovirus is known to infect erythrocyte progenitor cells and cause aplastic crisis in sickle cell anemia. The combination of increased RBC hemolysis (sickled RBCs have a severely reduced life span) and impaired erythropoiesis in sickle cell anemia can precipitate a severe state of anemia.

10. Why should this patient receive vaccinations against encapsulated bacteria (e.g., *Streptococcus pneumoniae* and *Hemophilus influenzae*)?

Recurrent vaso-occlusive crises in the spleen typically lead to fibrotic scarring of the spleen (referred to as *autosplenectomy*), which significantly increases susceptibility to infection by encapsulated bacteria such as *S. pneumoniae* and *H. influenzae*.

11. What are Howell-Jolly bodies? Why may they be seen on a peripheral smear of this patient's blood?

Howell-Jolly bodies are RBCs with inclusions of nuclear chromatin remnants. They are seen in patients with hypoactive splenic function, either secondary to splenic fibrosis and the "autosplectectomy" which occurs in sickle cell anemia or following a surgical splenectomy in patients with sickle cell anemia.

12. Why are parents of children with sickle cell disease taught how to palpate the spleen whenever they develop a febrile illness?

Various viral infections predispose to splenic sequestration crises, in which the spleen enlarges acutely due to massive RBC sequestration and hemolysis. Such splenic sequestration causes a rapid drop in the hematocrit and may cause symptoms of intravascular depletion and hypovolemic shock. If access to medical care (e.g., RBC transfusions) is not available, the mortality rate for sequestration crises can be significant, approaching approximately 15%.

13. Why may the patient's physician suggest that he have a prophylactic cholecystectomy?

Patients with sickle cell disease are highly susceptible to gallstones; about 70% develop symptomatic cholelithiasis. Of note, these gallstones will usually be pigmented due to the hyperbilirubinemia secondary to chronic hemolysis. Having a prophylactic cholecystectomy can also help avoid difficulty in distinguishing gallbladder pain secondary to cholelithiasis from abdominal pain secondary to vaso-occlusive crises.

CASE 2

A 6-month-old boy of Mediterranean ancestry is evaluated because over the past 2 weeks he has seemed abnormally lethargic. Conjuctival pallor, scleral icterus, and hepatosplenomegaly are noted on exam. Complete blood count and peripheral blood smear reveal a markedly hypochromic microcytic anemia. Serum iron, ferritin, and total iron-binding capacity are normal, but a peripheral smear is markedly abnormal, showing the presence of numerous nucleated RBCs and target cells. Gel electrophoresis reveals a complete absence of the beta-globin subunit of hemoglobin. The mother is told that her baby is probably going to require frequent blood transfusions for the rest of his life and that he is likely to have a shortened lifespan.

1. What is the diagnosis?

Based on the severity of signs and symptoms and the electrophoretic pattern of hemoglobin showing a complete absence of beta-globin synthesis, the boy has β-thalassemia major (also known as homozygous β-thalassemia or Cooley's anemia). If the electrophoresis pattern revealed partial expression of beta-globin, a diagnosis of β-thalassemia minor (also known as β-thalassemia trait or heterozygous β-thalassemia) would have been more likely.

2. Why was a normal serum iron profile important in narrowing the differential diagnosis?

The two most common causes of a hypochromic, microcytic anemia are iron deficiency anemia and anemia of chronic disease, in both of which serum iron is decreased.

3. Describe the pathogenesis of the boy's disease.

Beta-thalassemia is caused by impaired synthesis of the beta subunit of hemoglobin. Recall that the normal adult hemoglobin, HbA, is a tetramer formed by two alpha chains and two beta chains. Impaired production of the beta subunit leads to the polymerization and precipitation of excessive alpha chains within RBCs. The *precipitation of alpha subunits* within RBCs results in both premature hemolysis of RBCs within the spleen and ineffective erythropoiesis in the bone marrow. This combination of accelerated destruction and impaired production of RBCs explains the severe anemia seen in the thalassemia major.

4. Since this anemia is inherited, why did it not manifest when the baby was born?

For approximately the first 6 months of life, patients do well because they still have large amounts of fetal hemoglobin. The gradual transition to the adult form of hemoglobin causes the symptoms to manifest.

5. Since in β-thalassemia major there may be no production of hemoglobin beta chains, how can patients have any functional hemoglobin at all?

Because of characteristic increases in the two other types of hemoglobin, HbA_2 and HbF, neither of which has a beta-chain component.

6. What causes the scleral icterus in this patient?

An unconjugated (indirect) hyperbilirubinemia secondary to RBC hemolysis. Recall that the heme component of hemoglobin is degraded into bilirubin (via biliverdin), and elevated levels of unconjugated bilirubin deposit in the sclera, causing icterus.

7. Why might this patient be more susceptible to bone fractures?

Ineffective erythropoiesis in the bone marrow results in markedly hyperplastic bone marrow and bone marrow expansion (see below). This bone marrow expansion erodes away the cancellous and cortical bone, resulting in significant structural weakness.

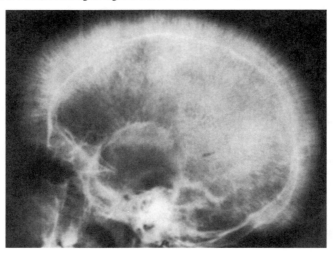

Radiograph showing the "crew-cut" appearance of the skull in beta-thalassemia. (From Cotran, Kumar, Collins (eds): Robbins' Pathologic Basis of Disease, 6th ed. Philadelphia, W.B. Saunders, 1999, p 617, with permission.)

8. Why does hepatosplenomegaly develop?

Hepatosplenomegaly in thalassemia can occur for two reasons. The primary mechanism probably involves increased hemolysis of abnormal RBCs by macrophages in the spleen and liver. However, another contributing factor is the extramedullary erythropoiesis that can occur in the liver and spleen in response to impaired erythropoiesis in the bone marrow. Unfortunately, these organs are no more capable of producing normal RBCs than is the bone marrow, because the defect in thalassemia major is at the level of the beta-globin genes.

9. What long-term (noninfectious) complication can result from the repeated transfusions?

Secondary or acquired hemochromatosis, which is a common complication of repeated transfusions in patients with thalassemia. The excessive iron delivered in the transfused RBC's can lead to iron deposition in such organs as the heart and pancreas, leading to restrictive cardiomyopathy and so-called bronze diabetes, respectively.

Note: Continual treatment with iron-chelating agents such as deferoxamine can reduce the incidence of hemochromatosis. Obviously, phlebotomy to reduce iron stores would be silly for someone receiving transfusions for anemia.

10. How might the clinical presentation differ in a patient with alpha-thalassemia? What would the gel electrophoresis pattern reveal?

Alpha-thalassemia is caused by impaired production of the alpha-subunit of hemoglobin. Whereas there are only two genes for beta-globin (*one on each chromosome*), there are actually four genes for the alpha-globin subunits (*two on each chromosome*). Therefore, unless mutations are present in all four alpha genes, which is unlikely, patients with α-thalassemia still synthesize some amount of alpha hemoglobin. For this reason, patients with α-thalassemia typically present clinically as adults and with much milder symptoms than patients with β-thalassemia major. The gel electrophoresis pattern, in contrast to β-thalassemia major, shows normal expression of beta-globin subunits and decreased expression of alpha-globin subunits.

11. What is hydrops fetalis? Why is it fatal?

Hydrops fetalis is a form of α-thalassemia in which all four alpha chain genes are deleted, resulting in complete absence of the alpha subunit of hemoglobin. Recall that formation of HbA, HbA_2, and HbF requires alpha subunits; in their absence, therefore, none of these hemoglobins can form. Babies with this disease are born with profound edema, which is presumably due to tissue asphyxia as well as congestive heart failure due to the asphyxia.

CASE 3

A 68-year-old man complains of fatigue and shortness of breath. On questioning he admits to seeing some blood in his stool recently and assumed it was from hemorrhoids. However, physical exam does not reveal hemorrhoids or an anal fissure. A fecal occult blood test is positive, and complete blood count reveals a hypochromic microcytic anemia with hemoglobin of 8.1 gm/dl. Both serum iron and ferritin are decreased, and total iron-binding capacity (TIBC) is increased. A colonoscopy is performed, and a biopsy of a necrotic mass is reported as adenocarcinoma.

1. What is the hematologic diagnosis?

Hypochromic microcytic anemia from iron deficiency secondary to chronic GI blood loss.

Note: In any elderly patient who has iron deficiency, always consider a GI bleed as the source, and consider it colon cancer until proved otherwise. In women of reproductive age, iron deficiency is usually due to heavy menstrual flows (menorrhagia).

2. Why is the anemia microcytic and hypochromic?

Iron is required for hemoglobin synthesis. Reduced cytoplasmic hemoglobin results in smaller cells (microcytosis) that have less color (hypochromia). The other anemias that also result from impaired hemoglobin synthesis (e.g., thalassemias, lead poisoning) likewise are often microcytic.

3. Describe the mechanisms whereby dietary iron is absorbed from the GI tract, transported in the blood, and stored in the tissues.

Dietary iron is primarily absorbed in the proximal duodenum, where the acidic pH and presence of ferric reductase enzyme facilitate the conversion of *ferric* iron (Fe^{+3}) to *ferrous* iron (Fe^{+2}), which is more readily absorbed by enterocytes. Dietary iron is then transported in the circulation complexed with the serum protein transferrin, which is primarily secreted by the liver. Transferrin delivers iron to all cells of the body (particularly the liver and bone marrow), where iron is then stored intracellularly complexed to the iron-storage protein ferritin.

Note: Plasma levels of ferritin closely parallel body stores of iron, such that in conditions of iron overload (e.g., hemochromatosis), serum ferritin levels increase, whereas in conditions of iron deficiency (e.g., chronic GI bleeding), serum levels of ferritin decrease.

4. What is the iron-binding capacity? Why is it increased in iron deficiency?

The iron-binding capacity is the amount of serum transferrin that is available to bind iron. When we measure the total iron-binding capacity (TIBC), we are really measuring only the serum transferrin concentration. In iron deficiency, the liver synthesizes more transferrin, and since plasma iron levels are lower also, the iron-binding capacity increases proportionately.

5. How does the temporal course of a GI bleed affect whether the anemia will be normocytic or microcytic?

With a significant GI hemorrhage that rapidly changes the hematocrit (without depressing bodily iron stores), the anemia is initially normochromic and normocytic, but as enough iron is lost, it evolves into a hypochromic and microcytic anemia.

CASE 4

A 42-year-old woman with rheumatoid arthritis complains of lethargy and shortness of breath with exertion. Skin pallor, pale mucous membranes, and slight tachycardia (rate = 105 beats/min) are noted on exam. Complete blood count reveals hemoglobin of 9.5 gm/dl (low), MCV of 75 μl (low), mean corpuscular hemoglobin concentration (MCHC) of 33 (low), and a blunted reticulocyte response. Further studies show low serum iron, reduced total iron-binding capacity (TIBC), elevated serum ferritin, and reduced transferrin saturation.

1. What is the probable diagnosis?

The patient probably has anemia of chronic disease secondary to long-standing rheumatoid arthritis, which typically presents as a mild anemia. This anemia can be either hypochromic and microcytic (as in this case) or normochromic and normocytic.

2. Why does her long-standing inflammatory condition predispose the patient to developing anemia?

Chronic inflammatory disorders with systemic involvement result in elevated plasma levels of various cytokines released by inflammatory cells, such as macrophages. These cytokines increase the phagocytic activity of immune cells, particularly in the spleen, resulting in increased phagocytic destruction of RBCs and a decrease in RBC life span. In addition, the cytokines inhibit the renal secretion of the hormone erythropoietin, which normally stimulates erythropoiesis in the bone marrow. Another contributing factor is that lactoferrin released by inflammatory cells binds serum iron and makes it unavailable for erythropoiesis. Anemia of chronic disease is typically mild; severe cases often respond well to exogenously administered erythropoietin.

3. How is iron normally stored in the body? Why are levels of serum ferritin elevated in this patient?

Ferritin is an intracellular storage form of iron. Plasma levels of ferritin closely parallel body stores of iron; for this reason, levels of ferritin are low in iron deficiency anemia and high in iron-overload states such as hemochromatosis and anemia of chronic disease.

4. Explain the low serum iron, reduced total iron-binding capacity, and reduced transferrin saturation in this patient.

As mentioned previously, chronic activation of immune cells results in release of large amounts of lactoferrin, which sequesters plasma iron. Therefore, reduced levels of plasma iron exist simultaneously with elevated body stores of unavailable iron, as shown by the elevated levels of ferritin in anemia of chronic disease (ACD). The total iron-binding capacity (TIBC) of the blood, which is simply a measurement of plasma transferrin levels, decreases in ACD by an unknown mechanism. Perhaps the same cytokines that stimulate hepatic secretion of ferritin, an acute-phase reactant, inhibit hepatic secretion of transferrin.

5. Iron deficiency anemia can also cause a microcytic anemia. If this woman had heavy menses or a heme-positive guiac stool, how could levels of serum ferritin be used to differentiate between iron deficiency anemia and anemia of chronic disease?

Serum ferritin levels are high in ACD and low in iron deficiency anemia.

6. **Cover the right-hand columns and list the characteristic lab abnormalities expected in anemia of chronic disease and iron deficiency anemia.**

	ANEMIA OF CHRONIC DISEASE	IRON-DEFICIENCY ANEMIA
Iron	Low	Low
TIBC (transferrin)	Low	High
Ferritin	High	Low
% Transferrin saturation	Low	Low
Bone marrow iron stores	High	Absent

CASE 5

A 65-year-old man with a long history of poorly controlled gastritis presents with increasing fatigue as well as tingling sensations in his toes over the past few months. Exam is significant only for slight conjunctival pallor. Lab tests show hemoglobin of 10 gm/dl and MCV of 110 μl (high), and a peripheral blood smear shows hypersegmented neutrophils. An upper GI endoscopy with biopsy of the gastric mucosa reveals chronic inflammation of the mucosal lining of the gastric fundus.

1. **What is the probable diagnosis? What confirmatory tests are available?**
    Pernicious anemia. Serum levels of vitamin B12 (cobalamin) should be low in pernicious anemia. Antibodies to intrinsic factor and/or parietal cells may also be found.

2. **Describe the pathogenesis of vitamin B12 deficiency in this patient.**
    Chronic gastritis, either autoimmune or idiopathic in etiology, results in destruction of gastric parietal cells found primarily in the fundus of the stomach (i.e., atrophic gastritis). Loss of parietal cells results in loss of intrinsic factor, which normally functions to facilitate vitamin B12 absorption in the terminal ileum.
    Note: Vitamin B12 deficiency from inadequate intake can also cause a macrocytic anemia.

3. **What are the normal functions of vitamin B12? How do they relate to the clinical signs and symptoms associated with B12 deficiency?**
    Vitamin B12 is known to be involved in only two enzymatic reactions: one that catalyzes both the conversion of homocysteine to methionine and the conversion of methyltetrahydrofolate to tetrahydrofolate and another that catalyzes the conversion of methylmalonic acid to succinyl CoA. The anemia is believed to be due to reduced levels of tetrahydrofolate, the form of folic acid involved in DNA synthesis. The neuropathy that develops in B12 deficiency is theorized to be due to a deficiency of methionine. Methionine serves as a precursor for S-adenosylmethionine, which is involved in the synthesis of various myelin proteins and phospholipids.

4. **Would we expect the reticulocyte count to be increased, normal, or decreased in this patient?**
    Because B12 is required for nucleic acid synthesis and nucleic acid synthesis is required for erythropoiesis, reticulocyte production in the bone marrow is unable to keep up with normal RBC turnover, resulting in decreased reticulocyte count. The white blood cells (WBCs) and platelets are also often reduced because of a limitation of nucleic acid synthesis.

5. **Other than B12 deficiency, what else can cause macrocytic anemia with hypersegmented neutrophils? How does it do so?**
    Folic acid deficiency. As mentioned, folic acid is also involved in nucleic acid synthesis and affects production of RBCs (as well as platelets and WBCs).

CASE 6

An 8-year-old boy is brought to your office by his mother for evaluation of longstanding fatigue. Both parents are currently healthy, but the mother underwent splenectomy several years ago for "some type of anemia." Physical exam is remarkable for pallor of the skin and mucous membranes, splenomegaly, and mild jaundice. Lab tests show hemoglobin of 7.2 gm/dl and hematocrit of 22%. A peripheral blood smear shows abnormally shaped red blood cells lacking central pallor. A laboratory test using test tubes filled with solutions of increasing salt concentrations reveals an abnormally increased osmotic fragility of RBCs.

1. **What familial anemia might you suspect?**

   Hereditary spherocytosis.

   Note: This condition is most commonly inherited in an autosomal dominant manner, but a more severe form can be inherited in an autosomal recessive manner.

2. **Discuss the etiology of this condition. Why do the RBCs assume a spherical conformation?**

   Hereditary spherocytosis is caused by dysfunction of the protein spectrin, a cytoskeletal protein that provides stability and plasticity to the plasma membrane of RBCs. For spectrin to function appropriately, it must interact with other cytoskeletal proteins, such as ankyrin and protein 4.1. Therefore, mutations in genes other than the spectrin gene can also compromise spectrin function, resulting in spherocytosis. As the name implies, RBCs assume a spherical shape.

3. **Can you explain why splenomegaly is seen in this condition?**

   Dysfunction of spectrin in RBCs results in RBCs with weak and inflexible plasma membranes. During their normal course through the spleen, RBCs must undergo impressive conformational changes to exit the splenic cords (i.e., *cords of Billroth*) and enter the splenic sinusoids. Spherical RBCs are much less able to undergo this conformational change than are normal biconcave RBCs. As a result, spherocytes obstruct the splenic cords and are ultimately phagocytosed by splenic macrophages at an abnormally high rate, resulting in splenomegaly.

   Note: This condition is often effectively treated with splenectomy

CASE 7

A 28-year-old black man who plans a trip to India for a business conference consults his physician about whether he needs to update his vaccines or receive any prophylactic medications before the trip. He is given quinidine for antimalarial prophylaxis. Several days later he returns to the physician with complaints of fatigue and red-tinged urine. Exam is remarkable only for a slight yellowish discoloration of both scleras. Lab tests reveal hemoglobin of 9.6 mg/dl (normal = 12–15 mg/dl) and an elevated total bilirubin of 6.2 mg/dl.

1. **What is the most likely diagnosis?**

   Glucose-6-phosphate dehydrogenase deficiency. This condition is caused by reduced activity of glucose-6-phosphate dehydrogenase (G6PD), the rate-limiting enzyme in the hexose monophosphate pathway.

2. **Is this disease typically acquired or inherited?**

   G6PD deficiency is inherited in an X-linked recessive manner and most commonly affects men (and to a lesser degree woman) of African, Asian, and Mediterranean descent.

   Note: G6PD deficiency is actually the most commonly inherited hemolytic anemia. It is thought that, similar to sickle cell anemia, mutations in the G6PD gene offer a selective advantage to heterozygotes by way of creating a poor habitat in RBCs for the malarial merozoite.

3. **Describe the normal function of the hexose monophosphate shunt in RBCs.**

In RBCs the hexose monophosphate shunt (the pentose phosphate pathway) is used primarily to generate reduced nicotinamide adenine dinucleotide phosphate (NADPH). The NADPH recycles glutathione (via reduction of oxidized glutathione), and the glutathione is involved in combatting various oxidative insults.

Note: Failure of this pathway results in the inability of RBCs to handle increased oxidative stresses (e.g., quinidine, trimethoprim-sulfamethoxazole, infections) and predisposes RBCs to intravascular hemolysis.

4. **Why might a peripheral blood smear reveal the presence of Heinz bodies and so-called "bite cells"?**

Oxidation of the sulfhydryl groups on hemoglobin results in clumping and precipitation of hemoglobin within the cytoplasm of RBCs. These deposits of insoluble hemoglobin are referred to as inclusion bodies or Heinz bodies. These inclusion bodies are then removed by splenic macrophages as the RBCs pass through the splenic cords, producing so-called "bite cells."

5. **Is the hyperbilirubinemia most likely caused by conjugated or unconjugated bilirubin?**

Recall that jaundice or hyperbilirubinemia can have a prehepatic, hepatic, or posthepatic (obstructive) etiology. Hemolytic anemia is clearly a prehepatic cause of elevated bilirubin and therefore is expected to be composed of unconjugated (indirect) bilirubin.

6. **Would haptoglobin levels be high or low in this patient?**

Because haptoglobin is a plasma protein that sequesters free heme, levels of haptoglobin would be reduced.

7. **Why might the mean corpuscular volume (MCV) be slightly elevated? How does this finding reflect the self-limited nature of this hemolytic anemia?**

A compensatory erythrocytosis in response to hemolysis produces increased numbers of circulating reticulocytes, which are premature RBCs that are much larger in size than mature RBCs. This explains the increased MCV. Furthermore, G6PD activity in reticulocytes is much higher than in mature RBCs. A somewhat selective destruction of older RBCs, therefore, occurs in G6PD-deficient patients who are exposed to oxidative stressors. Fortunately, this selectivity limits the nature of the hemolytic crisis, even if exposure to the oxidative stressor continues.

CASE 8

A 1-day-old newborn presents with jaundice that started on his face and spread to his body. Physical exam reveals no hematomas, but in addition to scleral icterus there is some conjunctival pallor. Lab tests show markedly elevated indirect bilirubin, reduced hemoglobin and hematocrit, and an elevated reticulocyte count. A direct Coombs test is positive. Blood typing indicates that the mother is Rh-negative, the father Rh-positive, and the baby Rh-positive. Both phototheraphy and exchange transfusion are used as treatments.

1. **What is the diagnosis?**

Rh-hemolytic disease of the newborn.

2. **What information is provided by the Coombs test?**

It detects the presence of antibodies on the surface of RBCs.

3. **What had to happen previously to the mother for this type of hemolytic disease to occur in the newborn?**

The mother had to be sensitized to the Rh antigen and produce anti-Rh IgG, which can cross the placenta. This process could have happened in a previous pregnancy in which there was mixing of fetal/maternal blood during delivery of an Rh-positive infant. Or it may have been due to a previous spontaneous abortion or miscarriage.

4. What is typically given to the Rh-negative mother before delivery?

Anti-Rh immune globulin can be given. This antibody binds to any fetal Rh antigens that may enter the maternal circulation during delivery and thus prevents the mother from being sensitized to the antigen.

Note: Rh-negative mothers who have had spontaneous abortions, abruptio placentae, or other causes of fetal-maternal blood mixing are also given Rho-gam for the same reason.

5. Why is ABO incompatibility so infrequently a cause of hemolytic disease of the newborn?

Anti-A and Anti-B antibodies are predominantly IgM antibodies, which do not cross the placenta. In addition, multiple other cells express the A and B antigens in the fetus, and these cells "mop up" most of any anti-A or anti-B antibodies that cross the placenta.

6. What is the most serious complication of neonatal jaundice? How does it develop?

Kernicterus, which is deposition of insoluble unconjugated bilirubin in the brain. It can cause brain damage.

7. What is "physiologic" jaundice?

Physiologic jaundice results from the increased destruction of red blood cells with fetal hemoglobin during the newborn period. These cells are replaced by cells with adult hemoglobin (two alpha subunits, two beta subunits). It is believed that infants who develop physiologic jaundice do not have the hepatic capacity to clear the excessive bilirubin that forms during this period.

10. COAGULOPATHIES

Thomas Brown and Dave Brown

BASIC CONCEPTS

1. Differentiate between primary hemostasis and secondary hemostasis.

Primary hemostasis involves the formation of a temporary platelet plug after binding of platelets to exposed collagen, platelet secretion of procoagulant substances (e.g., adenosine diphosphate, calcium), and platelet aggregation. This platelet plug is referred to as *temporary* because it is readily reversible at this stage. **Secondary hemostasis** involves the covalent cross-linking of fibrin between platelets, resulting in the formation of an *irreversible* platelet plug. This process depends on activation of the coagulation cascade.

Note: Disorders affecting platelet function impair primary hemostasis, whereas disorders affecting the coagulation cascades impair secondary hemostasis.

	PRIMARY HEMOSTASIS	SECONDARY HEMOSTASIS
Definition	Temporary platelet plug	Permanent platelet plug
Example diseases	von Willebrand disease	Hemophilia A, hemophilia B
Testing	Bleeding time, platelet aggregation studies	Prothrombin time (PT), partial thromboplastin time (PTT)
Symptoms	Relatively mild (e.g., excessive bleeding after dental work or surgery), mucocutaneous petechiae	Relatively severe (e.g., hemarthrosis)

2. What molecule is responsible for the binding of platelets to collagen?

Von Willebrand factor, which is synthesized by vascular endothelium and attaches to both collagen and platelet receptors (specifically, glycoprotein-Ib [GpIb]).

3. Describe the extrinsic pathway, intrinsic pathway, and common pathway in the coagulation cascade that forms the fibrin clot in secondary hemostasis.

The extrinsic and intrinsic pathways are separate biochemical pathways that activate the coagulation cascade. Both extrinsic and intrinsic pathways lead into the common pathway to cause formation of the fibrin clot.

The **extrinsic pathway** is referred to as "extrinsic" because the factor that activates it (tissue factor) is normally located *outside* the vascular space and is exposed to the vascular space only after damage to the vascular endothelium. The extrinsic pathway includes tissue factor (factor III) and factor VII. All of the constituents of the **intrinsic pathway** are found in blood; hence the term "intrinsic." It is activated by exposure to negatively charged foreign substances. The intrinsic pathway includes factors VIII, IX, XI and XII. As mentioned, the **common pathway** is activated by either the extrinsic or intrinsic pathway and eventuates in the formation of a fibrin clot. This pathway includes factors I II, V, and X. (See figure, next page.)

4. What information can be provided by measuring the prothrombin time (PT) and activated partial thromboplastin time (aPTT)?

To measure the **PT**, a sample of tissue factor is added to the patient's plasma (along with the essential cofactors calcium and phospholipids). This process activates the extrinsic pathway to initiate clot formation. The PT is a measure of how long it takes to form a fibrin clot in this assay system. Since the extrinsic pathway must activate the common pathway to form a fibrin clot, the

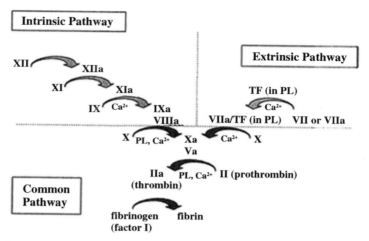

The coagulation cascade. (From Henry JB: Clinical Diagnosis and Management by Laboratory Methods, 20th ed. Philadelphia, W.B. Saunders, 2001, p 643, with permission.)

PT actually reflects the time that it takes for the extrinsic pathway and the common pathway to form the clot.

To measure the **aPTT**, an activator of the intrinsic pathway is added to patient's plasma (along with the essential cofactors) and the time it takes to form a fibrin clot is measured. This time really reflects the time it takes the intrinsic pathway and common pathway to form a clot.

Note: Because the PT measures the time for both the extrinsic and common pathways to form a clot, it can be prolonged by clotting factor deficiencies in either pathway. The aPTT can be prolonged by clotting factor deficiencies in either the intrinsic pathway or common pathway.

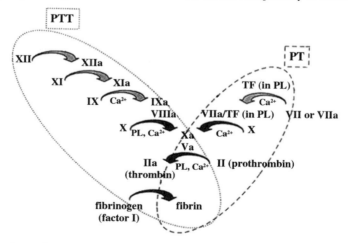

Prothrombin time and activated partial thromboplastin time. (From Henry JB: Clinical Diagnosis and Management by Laboratory Methods, 20th ed. Philadelphia, W.B. Saunders, 2001, p 643, with permission.)

5. What is the bleeding time?

The bleeding time (BT) reflects the time required to form the platelet plug (primary hemostasis) and thus reflects platelet function rather than the coagulation cascade. More commonly, however, in vitro platelet function tests are performed instead of measuring the bleeding time.

6. Describe the mechanism of action of aspirin, heparin, and warfarin. How do they affect the PT, aPTT, and/or BT?

Aspirin inhibits platelet function by irreversibly inhibiting the enzyme cyclooxygenase (COX), which normally functions to synthesize thromboxane A2. Thromboxane A2 normally functions to stimulate platelet aggregation and constriction of blood vessels, both of which act to limit bleeding following vessel trauma. Consequently, inhibition of thromboxane A2 by aspirin results in a prolonged bleeding time.

Note: Because aspirin is an irreversible inhibitor of platelet cyclooxygenase, its effect on platelet function lasts as long as the affected platelets remain in the circulation, about 7 days.

Heparin stimulates the activity of antithrombin III (ATIII), which is a potent inhibitor of thrombin (factor II) as well as several other factors in the intrinsic pathway. Because of this preferential inhibition of the intrinsic pathway, heparin acts rapidly to prolong the aPTT but will prolong the PT only at higher doses. It has no effect on the bleeding time because it does not affect platelet function (except in cases of heparin-induced thrombocytopenia).

Note: Excessive bleeding from heparin toxicity can be rapidly reversed by administering protamine sulfate.

Warfarin inhibits the production of vitamin K-dependent clotting factors in the liver (factors II, VII, IX, and X) by antagonizing the action of vitamin K. It preferentially prolongs the PT more than the aPTT. Because warfarin inhibits the *synthesis* of these clotting factors rather than their activity in the blood, there is a delay between administration and onset of action (typically a few days). For this reason, patients who require long-term anticoagulation are usually started on heparin and warfarin simultaneously, and once the patient is sufficiently well anticoagulated with warfarin, the heparin can be discontinued and the PT maintained within a therapeutic range.

Note: The effects of warfarin can be reversed by administering vitamin K; the process of reversal takes about 1 or 2 days. For emergent surgical procedures, fresh frozen plasma can be given to immediately replace the deficient clotting factors. Warfarin also inhibits the production of protein C and protein S, both vitamin K-dependent proteins secreted by the liver that exert *anti*coagulant effects. Consequently, inhibition of protein C and protein S synthesis by warfarin can initially result in a hypercoagulable state (prone to clotting). For this reason, "loading" doses of warfarin are not recommended.

7. What is the mechanism of action of tissue plasminogen activator (tPA)?

As its name suggests, tPA is an enzyme that activates the plasma enzyme plasminogen by converting it into its active form, plasmin. Plasmin is an enzyme that proteolytically cleaves fibrin strands, thereby degrading fibrin clots that may obstruct vessels. Like streptokinase and urokinase, tPA is sometimes referred to as a "clot buster."

Summary of Agents Related to Hemostasis

	MECHANISM OF ACTION	EFFECT ON CLOTTING PROFILE	ANTIDOTE
Aspirin	Inhibits thromboxane synthesis	Increases BT	
Heparin	Activates antithrombin III	Increases aPTT	Protamine sulfate
Warfarin	Inhibits synthesis of factors II, VII, IX, X	Increases PT	Vitamin K Fresh frozen plasms
tPA	Stimulates production of plasmin, which degrades fibrin		Aminocaproic acid

CASE 1

A 7-year-old boy is brought to your office by his mother because of a swollen right knee. When questioned, she states that the swelling has appeared in the absence of significant trauma several times over the past few years. He does not appear febrile, and a complete

blood count (CBC) is normal. **Both parents are healthy, although the mother says that her father (the boy's maternal grandfather) "had some type of bleeding disorder." She offers no specific information.**

1. What is the most likely diagnosis?

Hemophilia (A or B). Hemophilia typically presents with hemarthrosis or prolonged bleeding after dental procedures or minor surgery.

2. What causes this disorder? How is it inherited?

Hemophilia is caused by a hereditary deficiency of either factor VIII (hemophilia A) or factor IX (hemophilia B) and is inherited as an X-linked recessive disease. The absence or deficiency of factor VIII results in prolonged bleeding. In the above vignette, in which the maternal grandfather was affected, the boy's mother was an asymptomatic female carrier who transmitted the "bad" X chromosome (from her father) to the child.

3. What is the mainstay of medical treatment?

Infusion of the missing factor (factor VIII for hemophilia A or factor IX for hemophilia B) is the mainstay of medical treatment.

Note: Historically, isolation of clotting factors from pooled collections of blood resulted in HIV-contaminated fractions. This problem was most pronounced before the beginning of HIV screening of the blood supply. Currently, factors VIII and IX can also be produced by recombinant DNA methods, which obviate this problem.

CASE 2

A 35-year-old woman with a missed abortion (the fetus dies, but the conceptus is retained in utero for a few months) develops petechiae on her skin and buccal mucosa, begins coughing up some blood (hemoptysis), and also observes blood in her stool. While evacuation of her uterus is being arranged, a complete blood count reveals anemia and thrombocytopenia. A peripheral smear reveals schistocytes, the PT and PTT are elevated (although she is taking no anticoagulants), and the D-dimer level is increased. Fresh frozen plasma and platelets are ordered.

1. What is the most likely diagnosis?

The woman appears to be experiencing disseminated intravascular coagulation (DIC), a disorder that is characterized by thrombocytopenia, elevated PT and PTT, and an elevated D-dimer level.

2. Describe the pathogenesis of DIC.

Procoagulant (thromboplastic) substances are released throughout the circulation and activate the clotting mechanism. This process depletes the clotting factors and platelets (consumption coagulopathy) and thus results in excessive bleeding. DIC, therefore, is characterized by the *simultaneous occurrence* of excessive clotting and bleeding throughout the body. The main disease states in which DIC occurs are obstetric complications (missed abortion, abruptio placentae), gram-negative sepsis, and malignancies.

3. What are schistocytes? Why do they form in DIC?

Schistocytes are fragmented red blood cells (RBCs) that have been "clothes-lined" by fibrin strands that streak across blood vessels, tearing off part of the RBC membrane as the RBCs pass by. The widespread fibrin deposition that occurs in disseminated intravascular coagulation can lead to the formation of schistocytes.

Note: Schistocytes are a hallmark of microangiopathic hemolytic anemia (hemolytic anemia due to intravascular fragmentation of RBCs).

4. How does the pathophysiology of thrombotic thrombocytopenic purpura (TTP) differ from that of DIC?

TTP involves thrombosis, thrombocytopenia, and abnormal bleeding as evidenced by purpura on exam. It is precipitated by widespread damage to the endothelium. Because platelets adhere to the exposed subendothelial collagen of damaged vessels, massive activation of platelet binding and aggregation can cause thrombocytopenia, resulting in bleeding (purpura). However, in marked contrast to DIC, the coagulation factors are not consumed as they are in DIC (so-called *consumption coagulopathy*). In addition, the cause of most cases of TTP is unknown. Both disorders show evidence of a microangiopathic hemolytic anemia.

5. What is the pentad of TTP? How does it differ from hemolytic uremic syndrome?

Actually, TTP and hemolytic uremic syndrome (HUS) are now considered essentially the same entity. The pentad consists of microangiopathic hemolytic anemia, thrombocytopenia, neurologic symptoms, fever, and renal dysfunction. Most of the manifestations are explained on the basis of clot formation, with fibrin strands causing the microangiopathic hemolytic anemia. The neurologic symptoms and renal dysfunction are due to clots and occlusion of the cerebral circulation and glomerular capillaries, respectively.

Note: Enterohemorrhagic *Escherichia coli* O157 and *Shigella* species are well known for producing HUS (or TTP since the two disorders are now considered the same entity).

6. Cover the right-hand columns and try to differentiate TTP and DIC on the basis of pathogenesis, changes in blood elements, bleeding time, and changes in PT, PTT, and D-dimer levels.

	TTP/HUS	DIC
Pathogenesis	Endothelial damage leads to platelet consumption	Release of procoagulants or endothelial damage
Changes in formed blood elements	Thrombocytopenia Schistocytes Microangiopathic hemolytic anemia	Thrombocytopenia Schistocytes Microangiopathic hemolytic anemia
Bleeding time	Increased	Increased
PT	Normal	Increased
PTT	Normal	Increased
D-dimer levels	Normal	Increased

CASE 3

A 27-year-old man presents to the emergency department with a complaint of bleeding gums since the dentist cleaned his teeth earlier in the day. On exam, his gums appear to be bleeding profusely, and his mouth requires packing with gauze pads to limit the bleeding. He denies any history of abnormal bleeding or any family history of bleeding disorders. He is not taking aspirin or other nonsteroidal anti-inflammatory drugs (NSAIDs). The review of systems is significant only for painful swelling of his right knee intermittently over the past 10 years. Suspecting a diagnosis of hemophilia, the intern orders PT and aPTT, both of which are normal. However, bleeding time is prolonged at 15 minutes.

1. Based on the prolonged bleeding time, what is the most likely diagnosis?

Because the prolonged bleeding time indicates platelet dysfunction, the patient probably has von Willebrand disease, which is the most common inherited disorder of platelet dysfunction.

2. What is the normal function of von Willebrand factor? Describe the pathogenesis of the disease.

Von Willebrand disease is caused by a quantitative or qualitative deficiency in von Willebrand factor (vWF), a high-molecular-weight protein primarily produced and secreted by vascular endothelial cells. It normally functions to "anchor" platelets to exposed subendothelial collagen, one of the first steps required for clotting.

3. Why may a patient with von Willebrand disease be mistakenly diagnosed with hemophilia A?

Levels of factor VIII are commonly low in von Willebrand disease because vWF acts as a carrier protein for factor VIII. Although his clinical presentation (bleeding gums and possible hemarthrosis) is suggestive of hemophilia, the normal PT and aPTT rule out hemophilia as a diagnosis.

4. What is the mechanism of action whereby desmopressin acetate (DDAVP) may help the patient's symptoms?

DDAVP is useful in many of the bleeding disorders, because it induces the hepatic production of plasma clotting factors. It is effective in von Willebrand disease because it stimulates the release of vWF from endothelial cells. However, DDAVP may not be effective in variants of von Willebrand disease caused by qualitative defects in vWF function.

5. If levels of functional vWF were normal and specialized platelet function studies revealed a defect in platelet adherence to collagen, what rare disorder of platelet function might you suspect?

Bernard-Soulier syndrome, which is caused by a lack of or abnormal function of the platelet gpIb–IX receptor. The gpIb–IX receptor functions in platelet adherence to subendothelial collagen by binding to vWF (which is bound to subendothelial collagen).

6. If specialized platelet function studies demonstrated that platelets were able to adhere to collagen properly but were unable to aggregate with other platelets, what other rare disorder of platelet function might you suspect?

Glanzmann's thrombasthenia. This rare disease is caused by a lack of the gpIIb-IIIa receptor on platelets, which mediates platelet aggregation via a "fibrinogen bridge."

7. Given the function of the gpIIb–IIIa receptor, why are drugs such as abciximab (ReoPro) and eptifibatide (Integrillin) given to patients with cardiovascular disease?

These drugs prevent platelet aggregation by antagonizing the gpIIb-IIIa receptors on platelets and therefore lower risk for thromboembolic events in high-risk patients.

8. Why might you suspect an abnormal bleeding time if the patient suffered from diabetic nephropathy or osteoarthritis for which he routinely took aspirin?

Uremia and NSAIDs are common causes of acquired platelet dysfunction

9. Cover the right-hand columns and try to describe the mechanism of action of the following antiplatelet drugs.

DRUG	MECHANISM OF ACTION	NOTES
Aspirin	Irreversible inhibition of COX-1 and COX-2 (inhibits thromboxane A2 synthesis)	Most common cause of platelet dysfunction
Clopidogrel, ticlopidine	Inhibits platelet ADP-receptor activation	
Abciximab, eptifibatide, tirofiban	Platelet GpIIb–IIIa Inhibitors	Mimics Glanzmann's thrombasthenia

CASE 4

A previously healthy 35-year-old woman complains of easy bruising and occasional nose-bleeds over the past few months. She does not take any medications. Physical exam reveals multiple petechiae and ecchymoses diffusely located on her body. Lab tests show a platelet count of 12,000/μl, white blood cell count of 7200/μl, red blood cell count of 4.6 × 10⁶/μl, and normal PT and aPTT. A peripheral blood smear is unremarkable. Specialized testing reveals the presence of antiplatelet antibodies.

1. What is the most likely diagnosis?
Immune thrombocytopenic purpura (ITP).

2. What causes ITP?
The precise cause is not known, but ITP is often preceded by an upper respiratory tract infection. In children ITP is usually short-lived, but in adults it is often chronic.

3. Is a bone marrow biopsy likely to reveal increased or decreased numbers of megakaryocytes? Why?
The number of megakaryocytes, the precursors to platelets, is likely to be normal to increased. This finding indicates that the thrombocytopenia is due to increased platelet destruction rather than reduced production.

4. What anticoagulant is well known for causing thrombocytopenia?
Heparin. As many as 1–3% of patients receiving heparin may develop heparin-induced thrombocytopenia, which, oddly enough, can present with either excessive bleeding or excessive thrombosis (these two "syndromes" are sometimes referred to as HITS and HITT for heparin-induced thrombocytopenia syndrome and heparin-induced thrombocytopenic thrombosis, respectively). The mechanism behind this thrombocytopenia is generally due to an autoimmune reaction whereby Ig autoantibodies against platelets cause platelet destruction and thrombocytopenia.

5. Why does the absence of splenomegaly help determine the cause of thrombocytopenia?
Splenomegaly/hypersplenism can result in increased platelet sequestration and thrombocytopenia. Most commonly, splenomegaly results from congestion due to portal hypertension, but it may also result from leukemias, lymphomas, and several other disease processes.

6. Can pregnant women with ITP affect the platelet count of the fetus?
Yes. ITP can cause neonatal thrombocytopenia because the autoantibodies, predominantly IgG, are able to cross the placenta and attack fetal platelets.

7. What is the treatment strategy for ITP?
The usual treatment for ITP is corticosteroids, such as prednisone, to suppress the immunologically mediated destruction of platelets. IV immunoglobulin may also be given if the thrombocytopenia is severe. If medical treatments fail, a splenectomy may be helpful to prevent the abnormal destruction of platelets by the spleen.

CASE 5

A 58-year-old woman complains of a swollen and painful right leg since returning from a trip to Europe two days ago. Past medical history is significant for metastatic breast cancer; she is currently between chemotherapy regimens. On exam, her right calf is warm and tender to palpation and measures 26 cm in diameter; her left calf, which is nontender to palpation, measures 16 cm in diameter. She has a positive Homan's sign on the right (pain in the calf with dorsiflexion of the toes). Compression ultrasonography reveals a clot in the right femoral vein.

1. What is the diagnosis?
Deep venous thrombosis (DVT).

2. From what site do DVTs that lead to pulmonary embolism usually arise?
DVTs that embolize and occlude the pulmonary circulation arise predominantly from the deep veins of the proximal leg (above the popliteal vein) and the pelvis.

3. What is Virchow's triad? How does it relate to this patient?
Virchow's triad includes the three main general causes of increased clotting: (1) abnormalities of the vessel wall (e.g., vasculitis, atherosclerosis), (2) abnormalities of blood flow (e.g., stasis), and (3) abnormalities of blood coagulability (e.g., deficiencies of anticoagulants, presence of procoagulants). This patient had a recent history of immobilization during her long flight, which can cause venous stasis. In addition, she probably has a hypercoagulable state secondary to the malignancy.

4. How do deficiencies of proteins C and S and antithrombin III predispose to DVT?
Protein C, protein S, and antithrombin III are inhibitors of various clotting factors. A deficiency of any of the three, therefore, results in a hypercoagulable state.

Note: Protein C normally functions to degrade factor V (among other actions). Patients with the factor V Leiden mutation synthesize a factor V that is resistant to degradation by activated protein C, resulting in a hypercoagulable state.

11. HEMATOLOGIC MALIGNANCIES

Dave Brown and Thomas Brown

BASIC CONCEPTS

1. What are the two principal lineages along which leukocytes differentiate?

The **lymphoid lineage** gives rise to B and T lymphocytes as well as natural killer (NK) cells.

The **myeloid lineage** gives rise to the granulocytes (eosinophils, basophils, neutrophils), monocytes, platelets, and erythrocytes (i.e., the nonlymphoid cells).

2. What categories of hematologic malignancy arise from the lymphoid lineage?

1. The lymphomas, including Hodgkin's lymphoma and the various types of non-Hodgkin's lymphoma.

2. The lymphocytic leukemias, including acute lymphoblastic leukemia (ALL) and chronic lymphocytic leukemia (CLL).

3. Tumors of plasma cells (antibody-secreting B cells), which include multiple myeloma and lymphoplasmacytic lymphoma.

Note: All lymphoid neoplasms arise from a single transformed cell and are consequently phenotypically monoclonal.

3. What is the general distinction between lymphoma and leukemia?

Leukemia generally indicates significant bone marrow involvement with neoplastic cells, as well as significant peripheral blood involvement. **Lymphoma** indicates a primary mass in the peripheral tissues. However, this line is often blurred because of lymphomas that can evolve to a leukemic picture, and tumors otherwise identical to leukemias may start out as peripheral tissue masses similar to lymphomas. Currently, leukemia or lymphoma refers to the usual pattern of specific tumor types.

4. Distinguish between chronic lymphocytic leukemia and small lymphocytic lymphoma.

They are essentially the same entity with the exact same immunophenotyping and genetic alterations. The "distinction" is that when the peripheral blood lymphocytes reach a certain level, the disorder is considered "leukemic." This is an excellent example of the blur between leukemias and lymphoma.

Note: Smudge cells are a characteristic feature of CLL on a peripheral smear.

5. What categories of hematologic neoplasms arise from the myeloid lineage?

1. Acute myelogenous leukemia

2. Myelodysplastic syndromes

3. Myeloproliferative disorders (polycythemia vera, chronic myelogenous leukemia, and essential thrombocythemia)

4. Histiocytoses (of monocyte/macrophage origin)

Note: All myeloid neoplasms arise from a transformed hematopoietic progenitor cell. Consequently, features of these neoplasms often overlap, confusing medical students and physicians alike. All of the foregoing neoplasms of the myeloid lineage may infiltrate the bone marrow, resulting in anemia, thrombocytopenia, and leukopenia. In addition, both acute and chronic lymphocytic leukemia, as well as many types of lymphoma, can have significant bone marrow involvement.

6. What is the distinctive feature of acute myelogenous leukemia on bone marrow biopsy?

A substantial amount of the bone marrow is replaced by relatively undifferentiated blast cells that resemble one (or more) early steps of myeloid differentiation. Consequently, there are multiple subclassifications of acute myelogenous leukemia, depending on which early cell type predominates (e.g., acute promyelocytic leukemia, acute myelomonocytic leukemia, acute megakaryocytic leukemia).

7. What is the distinctive feature of myelodysplastic syndromes?

A mutant multipotent stem cell that *can give rise to all cell types of the myeloid lineage* replaces the bone marrow (partly or wholly). However, this mutant stem cell produces cells of the myeloid lineage in an ineffective manner. Consequently, anemia, thrombocytopenia, and leukopenia are seen.

Note: The myelodysplastic syndromes can evolve to acute myelogenous leukemia.

8. What is the distinct feature of the myeloproliferative disorders?

In myeloproliferative disorders, a transformed hematopoietic progenitor cell causes a pathologically increased production of one of the final products of the myeloid lineage (granulocytes, erythrocytes, platelets). Examples include polycythemia vera (increased red blood cells), essential thrombocytosis (increased platelets), and chronic myelogenous leukemia (increased granulocytes).

Note: Chronic myelogenous leukemia is unique among the myeloproliferative disorders in that it has a characteristic genetic defect: a chromosomal translocation (t9:22), known as the Philadelphia chromosome.

9. What are histiocytes? What are the histiocytoses?

A histiocyte is a tissue macrophage found within the interstitium. The histiocytoses are disorders involving uncontrolled proliferation of histiocytes. For the Step 1 exam, students need be familiar only with Langerhans cell histiocytosis (also known as histiocytosis X), which, depending on age at presentation and clinical course, is classified as Letterer-Siwe disease, Hand-Schuller-Christian disease, and/or eosinophilic granuloma. A characteristic feature of histiocytosis X is **Birbeck granules** in the cytoplasm, which you can easily recognize on Step 1 because they look like miniature intracellular tennis rackets.

Note: Eosinophilic refers to protein staining—not to the type of cell.

10. Summarize the categories of hematologic malignancies and their associated cell types.

LINEAGE	CELL TYPE/COMMENTS
Lymphoid	
Acute lymphoblastic leukemia	Precursor B or T lymphocytes (lymphoblasts)
Chronic lymphocytic leukemia/ small lymphocytic lymphoma	Smudge cells on peripheral smear
Hodgkin's lymphoma	Reed-Sternberg cells
Non-Hodgkin's lymphoma	Multiple types, which are generally classified according to site in lymph node they resemble (e.g., follicular, mantle zone, marginal zone)
Multiple myeloma	Plasma cells (mature B cells: IgG- and IgA-secreting)
Lymphoplasmacytoma	Plasma cells (mature B cells: IgM-secreting); common cause of Waldenstrom's macroglobulinemia
Myeloid	
Acute myelogenous leukemia	Cells of early myeloid lineage
Myelodysplastic syndromes	Hematopoietic stem cell with ineffective hematopoiesis that replaces bone marrow

(Cont'd.)

LINEAGE	CELL TYPE/COMMENTS
Myeloid (cont'd.)	
Myeloproliferative syndromes	Clonal expansion of a multipotent hematopoietic stem cell, ultimately giving rise to excessive numbers of one or more final products of the myeloid lineage
Histiocytosis	Langerhans cell (of monocyte/macrophage origin)

11. Describe the relationship between myelofibrosis and the myeloproliferative diseases.

Myelofibrosis is simply fibrosis of the bone marrow, which can be due to multiple causes (e.g., radiation, drugs, chemicals) but is most commonly idiopathic. It can also occur as a result of the myeloproliferative disorders. The resulting fibrosis can impair hematopoiesis, resulting in pancytopenia, which unfortunately can be rapidly fatal.

12. How does the leukocyte alkaline phosphatase help differentiate reactive leukocytosis from a true leukemia?

Reactive leukocytosis is an increase in white blood cell (WBC) count that occurs in response to infection and is associated with high levels of leukocyte alkaline phosphatase (LAP). On the other hand, the abnormally large increase in WBCs seen in leukemia is typically associated with low levels of LAP.

13. Cover the right-hand column and define the hematologic terms in the left-hand column.

TERM	DEFINITION
Hemarthrosis	Bleeding into joints
Leukemia	Malignant proliferation of blood cells within the bone marrow and circulatory system
Lymphoma	Proliferating *mass* of B cells (most common), T cells, NK cells, or histiocytes (rare)
Myelofibrosis	Fibrosis of bone marrow, often causing extramedullary hematopoiesis that results in hepatosplenomegaly
Myelophthisic anemia	Anemia that arises from a space-occupying lesion that displaces normal hematopoietic elements
Leukemoid reaction	Abnormally high WBC count, similar to that occurring in various forms of leukemia, but not as the result of leukemia (typically in response to infection)

CASE 1

A 65-year-old man complains of malaise and recurring sinus infections over the past few months and the recent onset of back pain. He cannot recall any recent accidents or trauma that might explain his back pain. Physical exam is significant only for focal tenderness to palpation at the level of the T12 vertebra. An x-ray of the skull for evaluation of his sinus infections reveals multiple "punched-out" lytic lesions (shown below). Serum protein electrophoresis reveals a monoclonal spike (M protein). A 24-hour urinary protein collection tests positive for Bence Jones proteins. Blood work reveals a hematocrit of 29%, hemoglobin of 9.2 gm/dl, albumin of 2.2 gm/dl (normal = 3.1–4.3 gm/dl), total plasma protein of 8.6 gm/dl (normal = 6.3–8.2 g/dl), blood urea nitrogen (BUN) of 22 mg/dl (normal = 7–20 mg/dl), and creatinine of 3.2 mg/dl (normal = 0.7–1.4 mg/dl). A bone marrow aspiration reveals the presence of abnormal plasma cells that account for approximately 30% of all marrow cells.

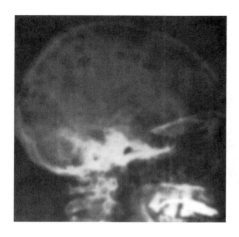

"Punched-out" lytic lesions revealed on skull x-ray. (From Cotran, Kumar, Collins (eds): Robbins Pathologic Basis of Disease, 6th ed. Philadelphia, W.B. Saunders, 1999, p 663, with permission.)

1. What is the expected diagnosis?

This is a classic presentation of multiple myeloma.

2. Describe the pathophysiology of multiple myeloma. How does the patient's blood work support a diagnosis of multiple myeloma?

Multiple myeloma is caused by an abnormal proliferation of plasma cells, which are terminally differentiated antibody-secreting B cells. These malignant cells continuously secrete excessive amounts of a single monoclonal immunoglobulin, explaining the presence of the M (for myeloma or monoclonal) spike seen on serum protein electrophoresis. This secretion of excessive amounts of a single immunoglobulin is referred to as a **monoclonal gammopathy**. The resulting hypergammaglobulinemia explains the elevated total plasma protein levels commonly seen in multiple myeloma. The hypoalbuminemia is also typical of multiple myeloma and is thought to result from elevated cytokine levels (e.g., interleukin-6) that reduce the hepatic synthesis of albumin.

3. What is the association between Bence Jones proteinuria and the above-mentioned monoclonal gammopathy?

Bence Jones proteins are immunoglobulin light-chain subunits (most commonly of the *lambda* isotype) that are filtered by the kidney and excreted in the urine.

Note: The malignant plasma cells also secrete heavy-chain immunoglobulins subunits, but these are of high enough molecular weight that they are not typically excreted in the urine.

4. Why is this patient predisposed to develop amyloidosis?

This monoclonal gammopathy results in elevated levels of free light chains in the blood, which can undergo processing and be pathologically deposited in tissues throughout the body as amyloid. Histologic staining of involved tissues with Congo red reveals the classic apple-green birefringence under polarized light.

5. How does multiple myeloma predispose to carpal tunnel syndrome?

As mentioned, processing of elevated free plasma light chains results in amyloid deposition throughout the body. Among these complications, carpal tunnel syndrome can occur secondary to amyloid deposition in the carpal tunnel, which causes compression of the median nerve. Carpal tunnel syndrome is a common manifestation of multiple myeloma.

6. Explain why this patient is at an increased risk for infection even though plasma levels of immunoglobulins are abnormally elevated.

Although total immunoglobulins are high, this finding is due predominantly to the M protein. The remaining immunoglobulins are low, predisposing to infection.

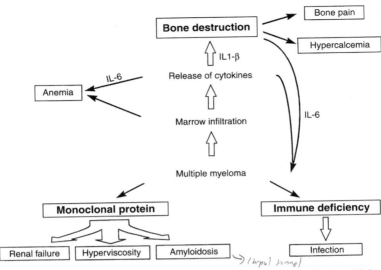

Cycle of bone destruction and immune deficiency, with predominance of M protein, in multiple myeloma. (From Hoffman et al (eds): Hematology: Basic Principles and Practice, 3rd ed. New York, Churchill Livingstone, 2000, p 1402, with permission.)

7. What is the characteristic finding on a peripheral blood smear? Why?

Rouleaux formation, in which red blood cells (RBCs) are stacked on each other like a row of coins. It is due to an antibody causing agglutination of RBCs.

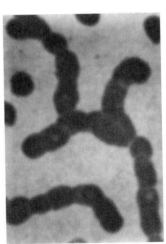

Stacking of red blood cells with rouleaux formation in myeloma. (From Hoffman et al (eds): Hematology: Basic Principles and Practice, 3rd ed. New York, Churchill Livingstone, 2000, p 371, with permission.)

8. How might the presence of elevated serum kappa light chains and amyloidosis affect kidney function in this patient?

Both can seriously impair renal function, making renal failure a major cause of mortality in multiple myeloma. Elevated serum kappa light chains result in renal filtration and excretion of large amounts of light chains. These proteins are toxic to renal tubular epithelial cells and also may combine with the urinary glycoprotein (Tamm-Horsfall protein) and form casts that obstruct the tubules. Renal deposition of amyloid, which may occur in primary amyloidosis, can also seriously compromise renal function.

Note: Primary amyloidosis is due to amyloid deposition from an immunocyte dyscrasia, whereas secondary amyloidosis is a consequence of a chronic inflammatory or process. Other factors associated with multiple myeloma, such as hypercalcemia and hyperuricemia, that predispose to nephrolithiasis can impair renal function.

9. What causes the hypercalcemia that is often seen in multiple myeloma?

Hypercalcemia occurs frequently in multiple myeloma secondary to bony destruction, which may also predispose to pathologic fractures. Lytic lesions in multiple myeloma occur partly in response to secretion of osteoclast-stimulating cytokines by the tumor cells.

Note: Symptoms of hypercalcemia include confusion, weakness, polyuria, polydypsia, and constipation.

10. What is the pharmacologic basis for giving the patient allopurinol before and during chemotherapy?

Allopurinol inhibits the enzyme xanthine oxidase, which catalyzes the conversion of the purine metabolite xanthine to the relatively insoluble uric acid. In patients receiving toxic chemotherapy, DNA catabolism secondary to increased cell death results in the excessive production of purine metabolites and, ultimately, uric acid. Such patients, therefore, are at increased risk for developing painful gout. Allopurinol reduces this risk by decreasing the production of uric acid.

11. If a patient work-up reveals an IgM monoclonal gammopathy, what disease might you suspect?

Waldenstrom's macroglobulinemia (*macro* refers to the large pentameric IgM molecule). It is most commonly due to lymphoplasmacytic lymphoma (a plasma-cell tumor that secretes IgM).

12. Why does Waldenstrom's macroglobulinemia predispose to visual disturbances and neurologic problems?

The increased concentration of IgM increases plasma viscosity, which impairs blood flow and causes sludging in the retinal vessels and cerebral vasculature (as well as elsewhere).

13. Does the finding of an M spike on serum protein electrophoresis necessarily indicate a malignancy?

No. In the phenomenon known as monoclonal gammopathy of undetermined significance (MGOS), no tumor is found. However, approximately 20% of such patients eventually manifest multiple myeloma or lymphoplasmacytic lymphoma.

CASE 2

A 4-year-old girl is evaluated for fatigue, night sweats, poor appetite (anorexia), and a 10-lb weight loss over the past month. She also complains of pain in her lower back that she is unable to localize precisely. Because of this pain, she has started walking with a limp and, whenever possible, tries to avoid walking at all. Physical examination is significant for conjunctival pallor, hepatosplenomegaly, painless lymphadenopathy, and diffuse petechiae. Complete blood count reveals marked lymphocytosis, thrombocytopenia, and anemia. A bone marrow biopsy reveals > 50% lymphoblasts, karyotype analysis of which reveals multiple chromosomal translocations. Immunostaining of the abnormal marrow cells is positive for terminal deoxytransferase.

1. What is the likely diagnosis?

Acute lymphoblastic leukemia/lymphoma (ALL), which is caused by a malignant proliferation of immature precursor B or T lymphocytes (i.e., pre-B or pre-T cells). It is the most common cause of cancer in children.

Note: Terminal deoxytransferase (TdT) is an enzyme involved in the normal gene rearrangement of immature lymphocytes (lymphoblasts) that creates unique antigen specificity. It is present in the majority of patients with ALL.

2. Why are fatigue, petechiae, and fever commonly seen in patients with acute lymphoblastic leukemias and/or myeloproliferative diseases?

The pancytopenia that occurs in these diseases as a consequence of marrow replacement is responsible. The anemia causes fatigue, thrombocytopenia causes petechiae, and leukopenia predisposes to infection and fever.

3. How does lymphadenopathy due to infection differ from lymphadenopathy due to malignancy?

Tender lymph nodes indicate a reactive (infective) process, whereas painless lymphadenopathy may indicate cancer, particularly when associated with constitutional symptoms such as fatigue, anorexia, weight loss, night sweats, and/or fever.

4. How does the presentation classically differ if the ALL is caused by a malignancy of pre-T cells rather than pre-B cells?

ALL caused by **pre-B cells** has a peak incidence at the age of 3–4 years. This type of ALL is primarily a leukemia, with predominant bone marrow and peripheral blood involvement. However, the less frequent ALL, caused by **pre-T cells**, typically occurs in adolescents and presents primarily as lymphomas, with predominant involvement of the lymphatic system. This lymphomatous type of ALL may present with mediastinal masses, marked lymphadenopathy and splenomegaly, and thymic involvement.

Note: Because pre-B and pre-T cells can be difficult to distinguish morphologically, immunophenotyping based on cell surface markers is necessary to make a definitive diagnosis.

5. What is the French-American-British (FAB) classification of ALL? How should this patient be classified if chromosomal analysis shows an 8:14 chromosomal translocation?

The FAB system classifies ALL into three categories (L1, L2, and L3) on the basis of histologic appearance of the "blasts." L1 blasts are small and of uniform size, with a small amount of cytoplasm, few cytoplasmic granules, and absent nucleoli. L2 blasts are larger and variable in size and may have nucleoli. L3 blasts are characterized by a basophilic cytoplasm and typically have very obvious nucleoli.

FAB CLASSIFICATION	ALTERNATIVE NAME	CHROMOSOMAL TRANSLOCATIONS
L1	Acute lymphoid leukemia, childhood variant	Various, including t9:22*, t4:11, and t1:9
L2	Acute lymphoid leukemia, adult variant	—
L3	Burkitt-like acute lymphoid leukemia	t8:14

* The 9:22 translocation in the childhood variant of ALL is a poor prognostic indicator. However, the 9:22 translocation is substantially more common in chronic myelogenous leukemia.

6. If the patient is started on high-dose chemotherapy and suddenly develops marked hyperuricemia, hyperkalemia, hyperphosphatemia, and hypocalcemia, what has happened?

She has developed tumor lysis syndrome, a metabolic emergency that is caused by massive destruction of tumor cells after initiation of high-dose chemotherapy. The death of large numbers of tumor cells results in the metabolism of large amounts of DNA. This process produces excessive amounts of uric acid, which can precipitate in the renal tubules and cause renal damage. Intracellular ions such as potassium, phosphate, and calcium are also released in large amounts by dying tumor cells. The released potassium can cause marked hyperkalemia, resulting potentially in fatal arrhythmias, whereas the hypocalcemia and hyperphosphatemia can cause calcium phosphate precipitation within tubules, further contributing to renal damage. Immediate hydration and correction of electrolyte and uric acid abnormalities are necessary to prevent irreparable renal damage.

CASE 3

A 35-year-old woman complains of fatigue for the past 3 weeks and recurrent spontaneous nose bleeding. Physical exam is significant for nontender lymphadenopathy, hepatosplenomegaly, truncal petechiae, and multiple ecchymoses. A peripheral blood smear shows the presence of numerous myeloblasts, cytogenetic analysis of which shows a translocation between chromosomes 9 and 22 (the Philadelphia chromosome). Complete blood count reveals a hematocrit of 25%, hemoglobin of 7.2 gm/dl, WBC count of 22,000/μl, and platelet count of 30,000/μl.

1. What is the likely diagnosis?

Chronic myelogenous leukemia (CML). The presence of a translocation between chromosomes 9 and 22 (the so-called Philadelphia chromosome) is highly suggestive of CML.

2. Describe the pathogenesis of this disorder.

CML is a myeloproliferative disorder in which a transformed hematopoietic progenitor cell causes increased production of granulocytic cells (the myeloid lineage) in the bone marrow, causing a myeloid leukocytosis (predominantly neutrophils). Bone marrow biopsy in such patients reveals an abnormally increased myeloid-to-erythroid ratio of approximately 15-20:1. The Philadelphia chromosome, present in the majority of patients with CML, is caused by a translocation between the *BCR* gene on chromosome 9 and the *ABL* gene on chromosome 22.

3. Explain the blast crisis that occurs in CML.

A blast crisis is an acute worsening of the disease associated with substantial medullary or extramedullary proliferation of blasts. Marrow blasts often exceed 30% of marrow cells. Blast crisis is an ominous prognostic sign.

4. Compare and contrast chronic lymphocytic leukemia (CLL) and CML.

	CLL/SLL	CML
Immunophenotype and genetics	B-cell tumor that expresses CD5 (unique to T cells) Varied chromosomal abnormalities	9:22 translocation (Philadelphia chromosome) *BCR-ABL* fusion gene product
Peripheral blood smear	Smudge cells	Blasts, myelocytes
Evolution	To prolymphocytic lymphoma or large B-cell lymphoma (both ominous events)	Blast crisis (ominous)
Typical age at onset	Older adult	Young to middle-aged adult

SLL = small lymphocytic lymphoma.

CASE 4

A 28-year-old woman is evaluated for a 2-month history of fatigue, occasional night sweats, and anorexia with a 10-lb weight loss. Her past medical history is unremarkable. On exam, nontender supraclavicular lymphadenopathy is noted as well as a feeling of fullness in the upper left abdominal quadrant. Her primary care physician immediately referred her to an oncologist for further evaluation. CT scan shows a mediastinal mass, which on biopsy reveals the presence of large, binucleated (owl's-eye) cells amid lymphocytes, histiocytes, and granulocytes.

1. What is the diagnosis?
Hodgkin's lymphoma. The owl's-eye cells (Reed-Sternberg cells) are characteristic.

2. What are the main variants of Hodgkin's lymphoma? How do they relate to prognosis?
  1. **Nodular sclerosis:** lacunar variant of Reed-Sternberg cell with fibrotic collagen bands that divide tumor into circumscribed nodules.
  2. **Mixed cellularity type:** heterogeneous (mixed) cellular infiltrate of lymph nodes.
  3. **Lymphocytic predominance:** predominantly lymphocytic infiltrate of lymph nodes.
  Note: The lymphocytic depletion variant is controversial and therefore is not addressed.

3. What is the value of distinguishing Hodgkin's lymphoma from non-Hodgkin's lymphoma?
Unlike other lymphomas, Hodgkin's disease begins as a localized process and spreads in a consistent fashion to adjacent nodes, commonly affecting only a single set of axial nodes. Extranodal involvement is rare. Consequently, the tumor is often susceptible to local cure. Other types of lymphoma frequently involve multiple peripheral nodes and extranodal sites and are less likely to benefit from purely localized therapy.

4. What are the genetic alterations in the following non-Hodgkin's lymphomas?
  Follicular lymphoma: translocation between chromosomes 14 and 18 involving *BCL-2* (antiapoptosis)
  Burkitt lymphoma: translocation between chromosomes 8 and 14, involves *c-myc* on chromosome 8; EBV is common in African Burkitt lymphoma

5. Describe briefly the other non-Hodgkin's lymphomas.
  Diffuse large B-cell lymphoma: highly aggressive lymphoma; follicular lymphoma may evolve into this type.
  Mantle-cell lymphoma: cells resemble mantle zone cells that surround follicular centers.
  Marginal zone lymphoma (MALToma): begins as reactive polyclonal B-cell proliferation and culminates in monoclonal B-cell neoplasm.
  Cutaneous T-cell lymphoma: mycosis fungoides and Sezary syndrome.

6. Cover the right-hand column and list an associated disease.

DESCRIPTION	DISEASE
Massive splenomegaly, B-cell proliferation, and the presence of tartrate resistant acid phosphatase in B cells	Hairy-cell leukemia
8:14 translocation	Burkitt lymphoma
Philadelphia chromosome	Chronic myelogenous leukemia (CML)
Smudge cells on PBS	Chronic lymphocytic leukemia (CLL)
14:18 translocation involving *BCL-2*	Follicular lymphoma
Bence Jones proteinuria	Multiple myeloma
Auer bodies	Acute myelogenous leukemia (AML)
Reed-Sternberg (lacunar) cells	Hodgkin's lymphoma
> 30 % myeloid blasts in bone marrow	Acute myelogenous leukemia (AML)
HTLV-1 infection	Adult T-cell leukemia

12. RESPIRATORY SYSTEM

Thomas Brown and Dave Brown

BASIC CONCEPTS

1. What are the driving forces and source of resistance for inspiratory and expiratory airflow?

Inspiratory airflow. For inspiration, the driving force for airflow into the lung is a negative pressure difference between the alveolar air spaces and the external environment. This gradient is created by descent of the diaphragm and expansion of the chest wall, which create a negative intrapleural pressure that is transmitted to the alveoli. The sources of resistance for inspiratory airflow include airway resistance and the inherent resistance to stretch (elasticity) of the alveolar air spaces. This elasticity is due both to alveolar elastic tissue and alveolar surface tension.

Note: Pulmonary surfactant reduces alveolar surface tension, making it easier to expand the lungs.

Expiratory airflow. For expiration, the driving forces include an increase in intrapleural pressure from elastic recoil of the diaphragm during quiet respiration. During forced expiration, elastic recoil of the diaphragm and chest wall is accompanied by contraction of the abdominal muscles, both of which increase the intrapleural pressure. This increased pressure is transmitted to the alveoli and drives expiration. In addition, the recoil forces from the alveoli that were stretched during inspiration promote expiration. The primary source of resistance to airflow during expiration is the diameter of the airways, which are smallest during expiration because of increased intrathoracic pressures.

Note: Inspiration is normally an active (energy-requiring) process; both contraction of the diaphragm and expansion of the chest wall require energy. Expiration is normally a passive process. With exercise or severe lung disease (e.g., emphysema), however, expiration can become an active process requiring the use of accessory muscles.

2. What is minute ventilation?

Minute ventilation is the total volume of air that enters and exits the lung per minute. The normal (resting) minute ventilation is a function of respiratory rate (RR) and tidal volume (TV).

$$\text{Minute ventilation} = RR \times TV$$

For example, for a person with an RR of 12 breaths/min and a TV of 500 ml/breath, minute ventilation is 6 L/min.

3. What is alveolar minute ventilation?

Alveolar minute ventilation is the volume of air that enters and exits the alveoli per minute. To calculate this value, the anatomic dead space has to be taken into account and subtracted from the tidal volume. The typical anatomic dead space is about 150 ml.

$$\begin{aligned}\text{Alveolar ventilation} &= RR \times (TV - \text{anatomic dead space}) \\ &= 12 \text{ breaths/min} \times (500 \text{ ml/breath} - 150 \text{ ml}) \\ &= 4.2 \text{ L/min}\end{aligned}$$

The alveolar ventilation is a much better representation of functional ventilation, because gas exchange occurs in the alveoli.

4. What is "dead space"? What is the difference between anatomic dead space and physiologic dead space?

Dead space in the lungs refers to volume that is ventilated but not perfused; thus, no gas exchange takes place in this space. **Anatomic dead space** refers to lung volume that receives ventilation but in which no pulmonary capillaries are available for gas exchange. Anatomic dead space includes the trachea, bronchi, and conducting bronchioles. **Physiologic dead space** includes both anatomic dead space and alveoli that are ventilated but in which the capillaries are not open (alveolar dead space).

Note: By impeding blood flow, pulmonary vasoconstriction can increase the physiologic dead space, as can a pulmonary embolus that occludes blood flow to a large segment of alveoli.

5. What does the ventilation/perfusion (V/Q) ratio measure? What is its approximate value? What is an "ideal" value for this ratio?

The V/Q ratio measures how well pulmonary perfusion and pulmonary ventilation are matched and indicates the efficiency of blood oxygenation in the pulmonary capillaries. Normally, the lungs receive close to the entire cardiac output (about 5 L/min), and a 70-kg man has an alveolar ventilation rate of roughly 4 L/min (as shown above). A ventilation rate of 4 L/min and a pulmonary perfusion rate of 5 L/min yield a V/Q ratio of 0.8, which implies a suboptimal matching of pulmonary ventilation and perfusion. A V/Q ratio of 1 is ideal because it represents optimal matching of pulmonary ventilation and perfusion. This situation in fact typically occurs during exercise, when alveolar ventilation increases to a greater extent than cardiac output, thereby increasing the V/Q ratio closer to 1.

Note: The V/Q ratio can be applied to the lungs as a whole or to separate areas of the lungs and is a measure of the efficiency of ventilation in separate areas as well.

6. What conditions cause an increase in the V/Q ratio?

The V/Q ratio increases whenever pulmonary ventilation is proportionately greater than pulmonary perfusion. As discussed above, exercise is a normal situation in which ventilation increases proportionally more than perfusion, and thus optimizes the V/Q ratio. A pathologic condition that increases the V/Q ratio is pulmonary embolus. In this condition, patients are often tachypneic (respiring rapidly), which increases ventilation, but the clot in the lungs reduces pulmonary perfusion. Both of these processes increase the V/Q ratio.

Note: The pathologic consequence of an increased V/Q ratio is that ventilation is "wasted" in lung areas that are not adequately perfused.

7. What is the relationship between the V/Q ratio and physiologic dead space?

An increase in physiologic dead space is an increase in volume of the lung that cannot participate in gas exchange because of lack of pulmonary capillary blood flow, although this volume does get ventilated. Consequently, increasing the physiologic dead space increases the V/Q ratio.

8. What causes a decrease in the V/Q ratio?

Generally, any lung disease in which the process of ventilation is compromised will decrease the amount of oxygen that the pulmonary blood flow receives, predisposing to hypoxia. This effect is deleterious because less oxygen diffuses into the blood that flows through the lungs. Additionally, less carbon dioxide can be blown off, predisposing to hypercapnia. An example is asthma, in which bronchoconstriction impairs ventilation and reduces the V/Q ratio.

9. What effect does chronic obstructive pulmonary disease (COPD) have on the V/Q ratio?

Airway obstruction in COPD can reduce ventilation relative to perfusion, thus decreasing the V/Q ratio. However, pulmonary capillary loss in COPD can increase ventilation relative to perfusion, causing an increased V/Q ratio. In fact, if these two processes occur in the same patient, the patient may have a normal V/Q overall, despite severe V/Q mismatches in different parts of the lung!

10. What influences the diffusion of gases from the alveoli into the pulmonary capillaries and vice versa?

Gas diffusion across a membrane (the pulmonary membrane in this case) is described by Fick's law for diffusion:

$$V_{gas} = \frac{A \times D \times (P1 - P2)}{T}$$

where V_{gas} is the volume of gas that traverses the membrane per unit time, A is the surface area of the membrane, D is the diffusivity of the particular gas in the particular membrane, P1–P2 is the partial pressure difference of the specific gas across the membrane, and T is the thickness of the membrane. All pulmonary diseases that create respiratory dysfunction affect one or more of the parameters in the diffusion equation. For example, in asthma the impaired ventilation reduces the pressure gradient for oxygen across the membrane. In emphysema the surface area of the pulmonary membrane is reduced from loss of alveoli.

Note: The "diffusing capacity" of the pulmonary membrane is defined as the volume of gas (typically measured using carbon monoxide) that can diffuse across the pulmonary membrane per mmHg pressure difference across the membrane. It can be seen from Fick's law that the diffusing capacity depends on the surface area, gas diffusivity, and membrane thickness.

11. What is the alveolar-arterial oxygen gradient? Discuss the clinical significance of its magnitude.

The alveolar-arterial oxygen gradient is a measure of the difference in oxygen tension between the alveoli and arterial blood. In a healthy person, a typical alveolar oxygen tension (PAO_2) might be roughly 110 mmHg, whereas the arterial oxygen tension (PaO_2) might be roughly 100 mmHg. In such a healthy person, this slight 10-mmHg difference in the partial pressure of oxygen between the two "compartments" reflects the highly efficient diffusion of oxygen across the pulmonary membrane. A high alveolar-arterial oxygen gradient implies the presence of pulmonary disease that impairs diffusion of alveolar oxygen across the pulmonary membrane, resulting in hypoxemia.

12. What are the primary controls of the respiratory drive?

Respirations do not occur without input from the nervous system, which comes from the medullary respiratory center (or from conscious drive). The respiratory center responds to changes in peripheral oxygen, carbon dioxide, and pH levels as well as pH changes in the central nervous system (CNS) and attempts to maintain these parameters within specific limits. Hypoxia, hypercapnia, and low arterial pH stimulate peripheral chemoreceptors that then transmit to and stimulate the respiratory center to increase the rate and depth of respirations. Hypercapnia also stimulates central pH-sensing chemoreceptors by way of carbon dioxide (CO_2) diffusing across the blood-brain barrier and dissolving to form carbonic acid, thereby lowering the pH of the CNS.

Note: The predominant mechanism of respiratory suppression of the barbiturates, benzodiazepines, opiods, and general anesthetics is to make the medullary respiratory center less responsive to increases in partial pressure of carbon dioxide (pCO_2).

13. How does increasing or decreasing the arterial pCO2 affect the pH?

When CO_2 dissolves in water, the following reaction occurs:

$$CA$$
$$CO_2 + H_2O \leftrightarrow HCO_3^- + H^+$$

where CA = carbonic anhydrase. Addition of CO_2 pushes the reaction to the right, creating more hydrogen ions and lowering the pH. Conversely, removal of CO_2 pushes the reaction to the left; removal of more H^+ from solution results in an increase in pH. The lungs exploit this reaction to compensate for alterations in arterial pH. By increasing or decreasing ventilation and thereby affecting the arterial pCO_2 levels, the pH can be raised or lowered.

14. What is respiratory acidosis? Respiratory alkalosis?

In **respiratory acidosis**, the lungs are not ventilating well, and the build-up of carbon dioxide shifts the above equation to the right, lowering the pH to an abnormal level. In **respiratory**

alkalosis, the lungs blow off too much CO_2, shifting the above equation to the left and raising the pH to an abnormal level. In both cases, respiratory rate and depth are pathologically mismatched to the physiologic demands/needs.

Note: The kidneys attempt to compensate for respiratory acidosis by retaining bicarbonate and for respiratory alkalosis by increasing bicarbonate excretion, exploiting the other side of the above chemical reaction. However, in contrast to compensation by the lungs, renal compensation is slow and can take several days to be complete.

15. Define FEV_1 and FEV_1/FVC ratio.

FEV_1 is the maximal amount of air that can be expired in one second after a full inspiration. Forced vital capaticy (FVC) is the total amount expired after a full inspiration. The FEV_1/FVC ratio describes the proportional relationship between the two parameters.

16. What is the principal difference between "restrictive" and "obstructive" lung disease?

In restrictive lung disease (e.g., pulmonary fibrosis), decreased compliance of the alveoli limits *inspiratory* volumes and therefore reduces ventilation. Such patients tend to take frequent shallow breaths to compensate for reduced lung expansion. In contrast, in **obstructive** lung disease (e.g., chronic bronchitis, emphysema), *expiratory* airflow is impaired secondary to airway narrowing and possibly also to decreased elastic recoil of damaged alveoli in emphysematous COPD.

Note: Although both FEV_1 and FVC decrease in restrictive airway disease, the $FEV_1/$ FVC ratio may actually be slightly increased because FVC often decreases proportionally more than the FEV_1. In contrast, in obstructive airway disease the impaired expiratory airflow reduces the rate of expiration, which is reflected by a decreased FEV_1 and FEV_1/FVC ratio.

CASE 1

A 23-year-old woman is evaluated for a chronic cough that is worse at night, episodes of shortness of breath, and chest tightness. She denies ever smoking but complains of seasonal allergies when pollen levels are high. Her respiratory symptoms tend to be worse during this time also. On exam no wheezes are auscultated initially, while the patient is asymptomatic, but a methacholine challenge causes pronounced expiratory wheezes and shortness of breath. During this methacholine challenge the FEV_1/FVC ratio is 60%. However, one puff of an albuterol inhaler restores the FEV_1/FVC ratio to 75%.

1. What is the probable diagnosis?
Bronchial asthma.

2. What is the difference between allergic (extrinsic) asthma and idiosyncratic (intrinsic) asthma? Which type does this patient probably have?

Allergic asthma is associated with a personal or family history of allergies such as urticaria, rhinitis or eczema. Serum IgE is usually elevated, and attacks can often be provoked by a known antigenic stimulus. **Idiosyncratic asthma**, on the other hand, does not have any association with allergy and typically develops in the setting of a viral upper respiratory tract infection, cold, exposure to aspirin, or exercise. In both types of asthma, however, inflammatory mediators stimulate bronchoconstriction. Because this patient has pollen sensitivity and seasonal allergies, she is more likely to have extrinsic asthma, a subtype of which is called allergic or atopic asthma.

3. What pathophysiologic process causes respiratory symptoms in allergic asthma?

Antigen from the environment enters the lungs and binds to IgE antibodies that are bound to mast cells and basophils. This process stimulates cross-linking of the membrane-bound antibodies and results in cellular degranulation. Histamine and other proinflammatory mediators that cause bronchoconstriction are released, resulting in *reversible* bronchoconstriction that causes symptoms of dyspnea, wheezing, coughing, and chest tightness.

4. About 5% of asthmatics are sensitive to aspirin, and some may even develop fatal bronchospasm from ingesting aspirin. What is currently believed to be the biochemical basis of this reaction?

Aspirin inhibits cyclooxygenase (COX) and therefore prevents the synthesis of prostaglandins while simultaneously shunting substrates into the synthetic pathway for leukotrienes in certain inflammatory cells. Pulmonary leukotrienes are potent bronchoconstrictors and therefore may exacerbate bronchospasm in asthmatics (and even nonasthmatics).

Note: Asthmatics who also suffer from rhinitis and nasal polyps seem to be particularly sensitive to this effect of aspirin and may need to avoid aspirin altogether.

5. Explain the decreased FEV_1/FVC ratio in this patient.

This ratio is reduced in asthma because bronchoconstriction increases airway resistance and impairs the rate of expiratory airflow.

6. Although this patient probably has allergic asthma, why does methacholine cause the FEV_1/FVC ratio to decrease?

The common denominator in the different types of asthma is *hyperreactivity of the tracheobronchial tree*, especially to inflammatory mediators. Methacholine is a cholinomimetic that causes bronchoconstriction, to which asthmatics of various types (with hyperirritability of the bronchi) have a heightened response.

7. What is the residual volume? How is it affected in an asthma attack?

Residual volume is the volume of air left in the lung after a maximal expiration. The elevated resistance to expiratory airflow that develops during bronchoconstriction does not allow normal expiration of the usual percentage of alveolar gas at typical intrathoracic pressures, resulting in an increase in residual volume. This increase in residual volume is typical of obstructive airway diseases.

8. Why is wheezing generally heard best during expiration in asthmatic patients?

During expiration, positive intrathoracic pressure further decreases the diameter of airways that are already narrowed from bronchoconstriction, making it more difficult for air to flow, creating a "turbulent" and noisy airflow.

9. With respect to the pathophysiology of asthma, what are the two mechanistic targets of pharmacologic intervention?

Because bronchoconstriction and pulmonary inflammation play such an important etiologic role in asthma, pharmacotherapy is primarily aimed at stimulating bronchodilation (or preventing bronchoconstriction) and at inhibiting the pulmonary inflammatory process. Dugs used for these purposes are discussed below.

10. Cover the right-hand column and list the class of drug and mechanism of action of the following antiasthmatic agents.

DRUG	CLASS	MECHANISM OF ACTION
Albuterol	β_2 agonist	Bronchodilation
Cromolyn sodium	Mast cell stabilizer	Prevents release of histamine and other proinflammatory substances
Ipratropium	Anticholinergic	Bronchodilation (or more accurately, inhibition of bronchoconstriction)
Monteleukast	Leukotriene-receptor antagonist	Inhibits activity of proinflammatory leukotrienes
Zileuton	5-lipoxygenase inhibitor	Inhibits synthesis of leukotrienes
Beclamethasone	Steroid	Anti-inflammation via inhibition of synthesis of wide variety of proinflammatory agents

11. Why are albuterol and salmeterol preferable to isoproterenol in treating asthma?

Although all three drugs are beta agonists, only albuterol and salmeterol are selective beta2 agonists. The beta$_2$-adrenergic receptor type is present in the lungs and mediates bronchodilation. Isoproterenol has both beta$_2$ and beta$_1$ agonist activity and can therefore stimulate cardiac beta1 receptors, resulting in tachycardia and palpitations.

Note: The beta blockers should be avoided in asthmatics because they can precipitate or exacerbate bronchospasm. Although the more selective beta$_1$ blockers (e.g., *atenolol, esmolol, metoprolol*) can be expected to have less effect on respiratory function, they still have enough beta$_2$ antagonist activity to warrant their avoidance.

12. This patient was put on a combination inhaler that contained a beta$_2$ agonist and a corticosteroid. A month or so later she noticed a white, cheesy exudate on her soft palate and pharynx. What probably happened?

She probably developed oropharyngeal candidiasis (due to the fungus *Candida albicans*), a well-known side effect of inhaled glucocorticoids. This infection develops because of glucocorticoid-mediated suppression of the local immunologic response.

13. Why are cromolyn sodium and nedocromil useful in the prevention but not treatment of asthmatic attacks?

Cromolyn sodium and *nedocromil* inhibit mast cell degranulation and release of histamines and prostaglandins in an allergic-response asthmatic attack. However, once the mast cells have degranulated, these agents have no significant effects on the activity of the inflammatory mediators that are released. Thus, it is essentially too late to use these drugs once symptoms have developed.

14. What histologic changes would be expected in the bronchial smooth muscle and mucosa if a biopsy were performed in this patient?

Smooth muscle hypertrophy secondary to recurrent bronchoconstriction and mucosal edema (with a relative eosinophilia) secondary to a chronic subacute inflammatory process.

15. What is theophylline? What are some of the disadvantages of its use?

Theophylline is a methylxanthine derivative (i.e., it has a structure similar to caffeine and purine bases) that can be used in the treatment of asthma. Its effectiveness is due to its bronchodilatory and anti-inflammatory actions, although the precise mechanisms by which it mediates these actions are beyond the scope of this book. Because theophylline is so inexpensive, it remains the drug of choice for the treatment of asthma in many nonindustrialized countries and is still used fairly commonly in the United States for cases that have proved refractory to beta agonists, steroids, and other newer agents. Unfortunately, theophylline has a low therapeutic index and can precipitate seizures, cardiac arrhythmias, and even death. Plasma levels, therefore, have to be monitored regularly.

CASE 2

A few weeks ago a 36-year-old man walked into his physician's office and said, "Doc. I don't understand it. I just bought this farm a month ago, and every time I go out there I get short of breath after only a few hours." He is diagnosed with asthma and sent home with an albuterol inhaler to be used every time he goes to the farm. The patient is now in your office and upset that his inhaler "doesn't do a darned thing!" He has been using his inhaler properly.

1. What disease may he have?

Hypersensitivity pneumonitis, which is also known as extrinsic allergic alveolitis.

2. Describe pathophysiology of this disorder. Why is albuterol not helpful?

Hypersensitivity pneumonitis is an acute inflammatory disease of the alveoli, which results from an allergic reaction to a wide variety of allergens, and causes acute shortness of breath.

However, unlike asthma, the bronchioles are not affected. Albuterol works in the bronchioles and therefore is not helpful for this patient. The "allergic" reaction, however, is *not* IgE-mediated.

Note: Hypersensitivity pneumonitis subsumes a wide variety of diseases with the same underlying etiology and pathogenesis but results from exposure to different allergens (e.g., farmer's lung, pigeon handler's lung).

3. Why should this disease be suspected?

The patient has acute attacks of shortness of breath with a classic exposure history, and an albuterol inhaler does not help.

4. How is hypersensitivity pneumonitis treated?

The most crucial aspect of treatment is avoidance of exposure to allergens. Continuous exposure to the offending allergen and continual alveolar inflammation (alveolitis) can result in pulmonary fibrosis.

CASE 3

A man with a known history of allergic asthma presents to the emergency department with severe shortness of breath and a mild fever. He says that his albuterol inhaler has not helped relieve the symptoms to any significant extent. The intern thinks that the patient is in status asthmaticus and starts him on oxygen and a nebulizer with atropine and albuterol. A third-year medical student (of all people) requests a chest radiograph and complete blood count (CBC), which reveal pulmonary infiltrates and marked eosinophilia, respectively. The same student orders a sputum sample that shows the presence of fungal hyphae and additional lab tests that show marked elevations of serum IgE.

1. What is the probable diagnosis?

Allergic bronchopulmonary aspergillosis (ABPA), which is characterized by fever, eosinophilia, and pulmonary infiltrates. It occurs predominantly in patients with asthma.

2. What other tests can be done to establish this diagnosis with greater confidence?

Skin sensitivity tests to the fungus *Aspergillus fumigatus* as well as Aspergillus-specific serum IgE tests.

Note: Several other fungi can also cause identical clinical and laboratory findings but do so less commonly than *Aspergillus* species.

3. What causes the pulmonary infiltrate?

Marked infiltration of the pulmonary parenchyma with eosinophils. Because of this finding, the disease is known as one of the "eosinophilic pneumonias."

Note: The eosinophilic pneumonias encompass a spectrum of diseases of different etiology, all of which have in common eosinophilic infiltration of the lung; peripheral blood eosinophilia is often present, as in this patient. Allergic bronchopulmonary aspergillosis and other eosinophilic pneumonias are treated with corticosteroids.

CASE 4

A 65-year-old woman with a 50 pack-year history of smoking complains of an insidiously developing and progressive dyspnea over the past 10 years. Physical exam is significant for hyperresonance of the chest, decreased breath sounds bilaterally, and a prolonged expiratory phase. Pulse oximetry on room air shows an arterial oxygen saturation of 85%, and her pulse is strong and regular. A chest x-ray shows hyperinflation and hyperlucency of the lungs, an increased anteroposterior chest diameter, and flattening of the diaphragm. Pulmonary function tests (PFTs) yield a FEV_1/FVC ratio of 45%, with only slight improvement

after the administration of bronchodilators. An EKG reveals right ventricular hypertrophy, and CBC shows an elevated hemoglobin and hematocrit.

1. What is the most likely diagnosis?

Emphysema, an obstructive lung disease commonly associated with a long exposure to cigarette smoke.

2. What histopathologic changes would a biopsy of the patient's lung probably reveal?

The destruction of alveolar elastin that occurs in emphysema results in permanent abnormal
enlargement of the airspaces distal to the terminal bronchiole, accompanied by destruction of
their alveolar walls but without obvious fibrosis. This process causes the hyperlucency on chest
x-ray.

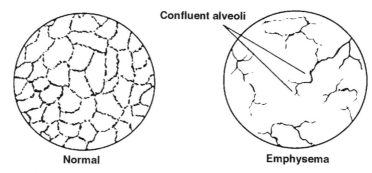

Pulmonary changes in pneumonia and emphysema. (From Guyton AC, Hall JE: Textbook of Medical
Physiology, 10th ed. Philadelphia, W.B. Saunders, 2000, p 487, with permission.)

3. What is the pathophysiologic explanation for the decreased FEV_1/FVC in this patient? In other words, why is emphysema classified as an obstructive lung disease?

The widespread destruction of alveolar septa and alveolar elastin in emphysema causes decreased elastic recoil of the alveoli, which is one of the major forces for expiratory airflow.
Another important contributing factor to airway obstruction in emphysema is luminal narrowing
of the terminal bronchioles, which occurs secondary to chronic infection of the airways and also
excessive mucus secretion.

4. What was the most likely cause of emphysema in this woman?

Chronic cigarette smoking is the most common cause of emphysema. Smoking is thought to
damage the respiratory bronchioles and alveoli, resulting in chronic activation of alveolar
macrophages and neutrophils. These cells release large amounts of elastase and other proteases,
which degrade alveolar elastin and collagen, resulting in alveolar destruction and loss of elastic
recoil during expiration. Cigarette smoke is also thought to directly inhibit alveolar elastin synthesis and to inhibit the activity of alpha1 antitrypsin, a protease inhibitor synthesized and secreted by the liver.

5. How do centriacinar and panacinar emphysema differ in morphology and etiology?

Centriacinar emphysema is much more common than panacinar emphysema and is typically
acquired secondary to a long history of cigarette smoking. In centriacinar emphysema, respiratory bronchioles are abnormally enlarged, whereas the distal alveoli are spared. Panacinar emphysema is associated with alpha1-antitrypsin deficiency and involves abnormal enlargement of
the distal alveoli, alveolar ducts, and respiratory bronchiole. This disease should be suspected in
any younger patient with symptoms of emphysema but minimal exposure to cigarettes.

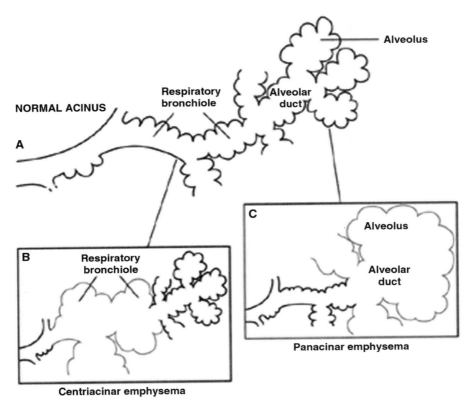

Centriacinar vs. panacinar emphysema. *A*, The normal acinus consists of a respiratory bronchiole, alveolar duct, and alveoli. *B*, In centriacinar emphysema, the respiratory bronchiole is the initial site of dilation. *C*, In panacinar emphysema, the alveoli, alveolar ducts, and eventually repiratory bronchiole are pathologically dilated. (From Cotran: Robbins' Pathological Basis of Disease, 6th ed. Philadelphia, W.B. Saunders, p 708, with permission.)

6. Is the diffusing capacity in this patient's lungs likely to be low, normal, or above normal?
The diffusing capacity is low due to alveolar destruction, which reduces the surface area of the pulmonary membrane available for gas exchange.

7. Why may administration of large volumes of concentrated oxygen to this patient cause hypoventilation?
Patients with COPD may have become adjusted to abnormally high levels of plasma CO_2 (hypercapnia), such that ventilatory drive is maintained only by low plasma oxygen (hypoxemia). Oxygen therapy, therefore, may remove this ventilatory stimulus, resulting in hypoventilation and possibly even respiratory failure.

8. How can emphysema cause the right ventricular hypertrophy seen on this patient's EKG?
First, recall that the pulmonary vessels respond to hypoxia by constricting and diverting blood flow from poorly ventilated to well-ventilated regions of the lung. This widespread pulmonary vasoconstriction in COPD can elevate pulmonary resistance and consequently pulmonary arterial pressures. Second, emphysematous destruction of the alveolar septa and walls reduces the number of pulmonary capillaries, which forces increased blood flow through remaining blood vessels, further increasing pulmonary pressures. These elevated pressures eventually cause right ventricular hypertrophy, which, if severe enough, can lead to cor pulmonale.

Note: Cor pulmonale is much more common in the chronic bronchitis form of COPD than in the emphysematous form of COPD, probably due to a greater degree of hypoxemic pulmonary vasoconstriction in chronic bronchitis.

9. What is the pathophysiologic explanation for this patient's elevated hemoglobin and hematocrit?

Patients with COPD are often hypoxemic, which stimulates erythropoietin production, resulting in an elevated hematocrit and oxygen-carrying capacity of the blood.

10. Why is person with with alpha$_1$ antitrypsin deficiency at increased risk for developing emphysema?

Alpha$_1$ antitrypsin inhibits the activity of various proteolytic enzymes in the serum. Some of these enzymes, such as neutrophil elastase, degrade alveolar elastin. Widespread alveolar elastin degradation in the lungs then produces early-onset emphysema throughout the entire acinus (panacinar emphysema). Generally, this disease should be suspected in a nonsmoker who develops emphysema at an early age.

11. What pharmacologic agents are used to treat COPD?

COPD DRUG	MECHANISM OF ACTION	CLINICAL USE
Albuterol	Dilation of airways	Acute symptoms
Ipratropium	Prevent bronchoconstriction	Prophylaxis
Glucocorticoids	Reduce Inflammation	Prophylaxis, acute exacerbations

CASE 5

A 55-year-old man who has been smoking two packs of cigarettes per day for the past 20 years complains of "a productive cough on most days for at least 3 months during the past 2 years." He is also fat and blue.

1. What is the diagnosis?

Chronic bronchitis, another form of COPD.

2. What is the pathogenesis of chronic bronchitis? How does it differ from emphysema as a cause of obstructive lung disease?

Chronic bronchitis is caused by chronic irritation by inhaled substances (e.g., cigarette smoke) and repeated infections of the airways. Histopathologically, hypertrophy of submucosal glands and goblet cells results in mucus hypersecretion in both large and small airways, which reduces their diameters and makes expiration more difficult. Cigarette smoking also causes paralysis of the mucociliary tract, which predisposes to repeated infection, a necessary step in the development from early, relatively benign, bronchitis to chronic bronchitis, which can be as serious a condition as emphysema.

Note: Clinically, a diagnosis of chronic bronchitis is made in any patient with a productive cough for 3 months in at least 2 consecutive years.

3. What is the physiologic basis of the reduced FEV$_1$/FVC ratio in chronic bronchitis?

In the chronic bronchitis form of COPD, reduction of airway diameter is the principal cause of expiratory airflow limitation, with little effect on elastic recoil of the alveoli.

4. What is an acute exacerbation of COPD? What classes of medications should be avoided or prescribed with great caution in these situations?

An acute exacerbation entails the acute onset of significantly greater dyspnea as well as alterations in blood gases, such as worsening hypoxemia or hypercapnia. These exacerbations are usually due to respiratory infections such as acute bronchitis or pneumonia. Drugs that suppress respiration, such as opiod analgesics, benzodiazepines, and barbiturates, should be used quite cautiously in such patients.

Note: Beta blockers are contraindicated in patients with COPD in general and certainly should not be used in an acute exacerbation of COPD, because they inhibit catecholamine-mediated bronchodilation.

5. What acid-base abnormality is commonly found in patients with COPD? What is its origin?

Because of depressed ventilation, hypercapnia ensues, resulting in respiratory acidosis. As a compensatory response, the kidneys excrete additional hydrogen ions and reabsorb and generate increased amounts of bicarbonate, thereby restoring the pH toward normal.

6. How can artificial ventilation cause respiratory alkalosis in a COPD patient?

If tidal volume and respiratory rate are set too high, the patient may float to the other end of the spectrum, causing them to blow off too much CO_2 and go into respiratory alkalosis. The kidneys attempt to compensate for this condition by excreting more bicarbonate to lower the pH back to normal.

Note: Respiratory acidosis or alkalosis can develop rapidly, over minutes to hours. However, renal compensation occurs more slowly, and can take several days for complete compensation.

7. Why may cigarette smoking predispose to chronic lung infections?

Cigarette smoking impairs the normal protective mechanisms of the airways. Specifically, nicotine and other substances within cigarette smoke cause partial paralysis of the bronchiolar epithelial cilia and excessive mucus secretion. This combination creates an environment suitable for infecting organisms, leading to chronic infections.

CASE 6

A 50-year-old man is evaluated for chronic dyspnea. He indicates that it developed after he had been working in a shipyard for about 12 years and has become progressively worse over time. He denies any history of smoking or any association of the dyspnea with recumbency (orthopnea). Pulmonary function studies show an FVC < 50% of predicted for his age, height, and sex, but his FEV_1/FVC ratio is greater than 80%.

1. What is the probable diagnosis?

Pulmonary fibrosis, possibly secondary to asbestos exposure (asbestosis) while working in the shipyard.

Note: The greatly varied causes of pulmonary fibrosis include silicosis, granulomatous diseases of the lung (e.g., sarcoidosis), connective tissue diseases (e.g., lupus, rheumatoid arthritis), and certain medications (e.g., amiodarone). It is also commonly idiopathic.

2. Does this patient have pneumoconiosis?

Most likely. Pneumoconiosis is defined as lung inflammation generally leading to fibrosis from inhalation of various types of dust particles in different occupational settings.

3. What is the pathophysiologic explanation for the reduction in FVC?

In pulmonary fibrosis, the fibrosis of the alveolar walls and septa makes the alveoli less compliant. The alveoli, therefore, do not expand as well for a given drop in intrathoracic pressure during inspiration, resulting in a reduced inspiratory volume, which, of course, translates into a reduced expiratory volume. However, the process of expiration itself is not compromised in restrictive lung diseases such as pulmonary fibrosis; for this reasons, the FEV_1/FVC ratio is not reduced in restrictive diseases.

4. What lung biopsy finding is unique to asbestosis?

Ferruginous bodies (or asbestos bodies), which are fibers of asbestos lined by hemosiderin deposits.

5. For what tumor types is asbestosis a predisposing factor?

Malignant mesothelioma (tumor of the pleura) and bronchogenic carcinoma.

Note: Smoking markedly increases the risk for developing asbestos-related bronchogenic carcinoma but does *not* increase the risk for developing asbestos-related mesothelioma. Pleural plaques are a characteristic x-ray finding in asbestosis.

CASE 7

A 45-year-old woman complains of chronic fatigue as well as shortness of breath with exertion. Her history is significant for rather heavy menstrual bleeding (menorrhagia). She has never smoked. She has no signs of cyanosis, and the only truly notable finding on physical exam is conjunctival pallor. Lab tests show hemoglobin of 7.5 gm/dl and hematocrit of 25%. Arterial oxygen saturation on room air is 95%. Further testing shows decreased serum iron and ferritin, decreased transferrin saturation, and increased total iron-binding capacity.

1. What is causing the dyspnea?

The patient is suffering from severe iron deficiency anemia, probably secondary to heavy menstrual flows (see Chapter 9 for a detailed description of iron deficiency anemia).

2. What is the difference between PaO_2 and arterial oxygen concentration?

PaO_2 is the partial pressure of oxygen dissolved in arterial blood, also referred to as the oxygen tension. If exposed to the same level of atmospheric oxygen, both water and blood equilibrate with the oxygen and have the same partial pressure. The level of partial pressure depends only on adequate exposure to oxygen. Similarly, in the body the partial pressure of arterial oxygen is principally mediated by adequate respiration and is unrelated to hemoglobin (Hb) concentration. Therefore, even in severe anemia (i.e., water), the PaO_2 can be completely normal as long as respiratory function is normal.

Arterial oxygen concentration is a measure of the total quantity of oxygen in a given volume of blood and is heavily influenced by the concentration of Hb in the blood. Hb does not alter the partial pressure, but it does increase substantially the amount of oxygen that is dissolved in blood at a given partial pressure of oxygen. Because each gram of Hb can bind approximately 1.34 ml of oxygen at normal PaO_2, the average person with Hb of 15 gm/dl has an arterial oxygen concentration of 20% (i.e., 15 gm Hb/dl × 1.34 ml O_2/gm Hb = 20 ml O_2/dl, or 20 ml O_2/100 ml). In anemia, the reduced hemoglobin level clearly reduces the arterial oxygen concentration.

Note: The PAO_2 is the *alveolar* oxygen tension.

3. What is the arterial oxygen saturation?

Arterial oxygen saturation is a measure of the percentage of oxygen-binding sites on hemoglobin to which oxygen is actually bound. It is determined by the PaO_2, with higher values causing greater oxygen saturation. This parameter is also unaffected by anemia. (See figure, next page.)

Summary of Terms

PAO_2 (mmHG)	PaO_2 (mmHG)	ARTERIAL OXYGEN CONCENTRATION (mg/dl)	OXYGEN SATURATION (%)
Partial pressure of alveolar oxygen	Partial pressure of dissolved oxygen in arterial blood	Total quantity of oxygen dissolved in volume of arterial blood	Percentage of oxygen-binding sites on Hb to which oxygen is bound

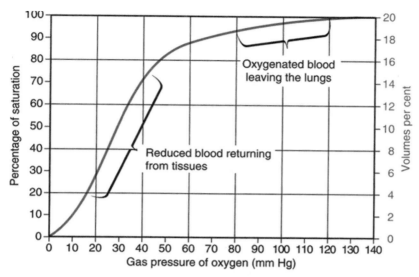

Effect of partial pressure of oxygen in blood on the quantity of oxygen bound with hemoglobin in each 100 ml of blood. (From Guyton AC, Hall JE: Textbook of Medical Physiology, 10th ed. Philadelpha,W.B. Saunders, 2000, p 467, with permission.)

4. Why does the patient's anemia *not* make her cyanotic?

Cyanosis is caused by the presence of at least 5 gm/dl of arterial *deoxy*hemoglobin, which occurs at a low PaO_2 with reduced arterial oxygen saturation. As long as the PaO2 is normal in anemia (as it should be in the absence of respiratory disease), the patient has good oxygen saturation and minimal deoxyhemoglobin. Note that in this patient the oxygen saturation is 95%, indicating good respiratory function. Nevertheless, because the oxygen-carrying capacity of the blood is reduced, she still suffers the symptoms of anemia (e.g., fatigue).

Note: Methemoglobinemia is another potential cause of cyanosis. In this disease heme iron is oxidized to its ferric form (which cannot bind oxygen), thereby increasing the concentration of deoxyhemoglobin.

5. How does anemia contribute to the patient's dyspnea?

The peripheral chemoreceptors cannot "sense" the low arterial oxygen concentration; they can sense only the PaO_2, which is normal because ventilation is unimpaired. However, the low oxygen delivery causes increased tissue lactic acid production, which lowers arterial pH and increases respiratory drive.

6. What are typical values for arterial and venous PaO_2? What do they represent with respect to the hemoglobin dissociation curve?

At a normal arterial PaO_2 of 100 mmHg, hemoglobin is fully saturated, corresponding to the "loading" portion of the hemoglobin dissociation curve. In the capillaries, oxygen diffuses rapidly from the blood to the tissues, so that the PaO_2 in venous blood drops to approximately 40 mmHg, corresponding to hemoglobin that is only ~ 75% saturated (i.e., bound to three molecules of O_2). (See figure, next page.)

7. Would exposure to carbon monoxide be expected to affect the PaO_2? Explain.

Not necessarily. Carbon monoxide exhibits its effect by binding to hemoglobin and preventing oxygen from dissociating from the hemoglobin, but it does not affect the amount of oxygen dissolved in plasma. Therefore, exposure to carbon monoxide usually should not alter the PaO_2, although the oxygen *saturation* will decrease secondary to decreased binding of oxygen to hemoglobin.

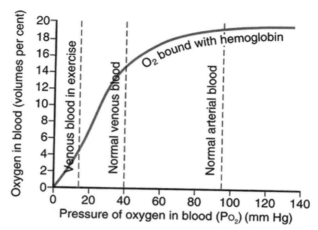

Normal partial pressure of oxygen in venous and arterial blood. (From Guyton AC, Hall JE: Textbook of Medical Physiology, 10th ed. Philadelphia, W.B. Saunders, 2000, p 467, with permission.)

8. Differentiate between external and internal respiration. Which is affected by anemia?

Gas exchange between the alveoli and blood in the pulmonary capillaries is referred to as **external** respiration, whereas the exchange of gases between capillary blood and the interstitial fluid is referred to as **internal** respiration. External respiration may be compromised by low atmospheric oxygen (e.g., high altitude) or poor alveolar ventilation (e.g., pneumonia). In anemia, less oxygen can be transferred from the capillary blood to the interstitial tissues.

Note: Cellular respiration refers to the exchange of gases between the cells and the interstitial fluid.

CASE 8

A 35-year-old male victim of multiple blunt trauma went into hemorrhagic shock because of splenic rupture, underwent surgery, and was sent to the intensive care unit. The next day he became acutely short of breath; the chest x-ray showed diffuse, bilateral pulmonary infiltrates; and arterial blood gas analysis revealed severe hypoxemia. A Swan-Ganz catheter was threaded through the superior vena cava (SVC), right atrium, and right ventricle into the pulmonary artery and shows a normal pulmonary capillary wedge pressure.

1. What is the expected diagnosis?

Acute respiratory distress syndrome (ARDS; formerly known as adult respiratory distress syndrome). It is also referred to as shock lung.

Note: ARDS is diagnosed by the presence of acute onset respiratory failure, bilateral diffuse pulmonary infiltrates, severe hypoxemia, and the coexistence of a disease known to cause it.

2. Summarize the etiology and pathogenesis of ARDS.

ARDS occurs secondary to a wide variety of diseases, including sepsis, shock, severe pancreatitis, gastric aspiration, and near drowning. The common link in all of these conditions is widespread pulmonary capillary endothelial damage. This damage leads to inflammation and fluid extravasation into the alveoli and interstitium, resulting in significant alveolar and interstitial edema (hence the infiltrates on x-ray) and, consequently, severe hypoxemia.

3. How is ARDS managed?

Supportive therapy with a ventilator to maintain oxygenation and treatment of the underlying disease. Unfortunately, this condition can be quite challenging to treat, because delivering a high FiO$_2$ (percent inspired oxygen) via a ventilator can produce damaging free radicals that further exacerbate the condition.

4. Which parameter in the diffusion equation is influenced most by the high concentration of inspired oxygen?

Recall that the diffusion equation relates an increase in diffusion rates to increases in partial pressures of a gas across the membrane, increased solubility of the gas, or an increased surface area available for diffusion. The high inspired oxygen increases the partial pressure of oxygen across the pulmonary membrane, which attenuates the reduction in diffusion that occurs because of the increased membrane thickness (from edema).

5. Both congestive heart failure and ARDS can cause significant pulmonary edema. How does the cause of pulmonary edema differ in these two settings?

In **congestive heart failure**, increased hydrostatic pressures due to back-up of fluid in the pulmonary system causes the edema. In this situation the pulmonary capillary wedge pressure is elevated as a result of fluid back-up. In **ARDS**, increased capillary permeability is the basis for the edema; there is no cause for an increase in pulmonary capillary wedge pressure, which remains normal.

6. Why is it necessary to be particularly cautious in giving fluids to this patient?

Excessive fluids can push the patient into congestive heart failure. The resulting increase in pulmonary edema can seriously compromise an already inadequate respiratory function (the increased edema makes the diffusion barrier even thicker).

7. Using the diffusion equation, explain why each of these conditions is associated with hypoxemia.

Recall the diffusion equation from question 10 of Basic Concepts:

$$V_{gas} = \frac{A \times D \times (P1 - P2)}{T}$$

CONDITION	EXPLANATION FOR HYPOXEMIA
Neuromuscular respiratory insufficiency	Decreased ventilation reduces P
Pulmonary edema	Increased thickness of pulmonary membrane/diffusion barrier
Emphysema	Reduced surface area of pulmonary membrane from alveolar degradation; reduced pressure gradient from impaired ventilation
Pneumonia	Decreased oxygen diffusion due to pulmonary edema (i.e., T increases in diffusion equation) and reduced "available" surface area of pulmonary membrane
Asthma	Reduced P because of ventilatory insufficiency
Neonatal respiratory distress syndrome	Reduced surfactant increases surface tension in alveoli, causing alveoli to collapse, impairing ventilation (P) and reducing surface area of pulmonary membrane.
Acute respiratory distress syndrome (also called diffuse alveolar damage)	Diffuse pulmonary infiltrates increase thickness of pulmonary membrane.

CASE 9

A 75-year-old woman with a 90-pack-year history of cigarette smoking complains of hemoptysis, shortness of breath, fatigue, and an involuntary 30-lb weight loss over the past 6 months. Chest x-ray is characteristic of COPD, with increased anteroposterior diameter

and flattening of the diaphragm, but also reveals a large mass in her right upper lobe. Biopsy establishes that the mass is malignant. Lab tests show a plasma sodium level of 125 mEq/L (normal = 135-145), and the urine osmolarity is > 300 mOsm.

1. What type of lung cancer does this patient probably have?

Small-cell (oat-cell) carcinoma of the lung. Various paraneoplastic syndromes, including the syndrome of inappropriate secretion of antidiuretic hormone (SIADH), are commonly observed in small-cell lung carcinoma. Hyponatremia and increased urine osmolarity make small-cell carcinoma more probable.

2. If a patient with small-cell carcinoma develops bilateral ptosis (droopy eyelids) as well as neuromuscular weakness, what paraneoplastic syndrome should be suspected?

Lambert-Eaton syndrome, which occurs quite frequently (~ 60% of cases) in small-cell carcinoma. It results from antibodies that attack the voltage-gated calcium channels on the terminal bouton of presynaptic motor neurons.

3. If a lung tumor is growing in the apex of the lung and compressing the cervical sympathetic chain on that side, what manifestations might you see?

Since the cervical sympathetic chain supplies the superior tarsal muscle (which elevates the eyelid), the dilator pupillae, and the sweat glands of the face, cutting off this nerve supply can result in ipsilateral ptosis, miosis, and anhydrosis (i.e., Horner's syndrome). This syndrome differs from Lambert-Eaton syndrome, in which the ptosis is bilateral.

Note: Tumors in the apex of the lung are known as Pancoast's tumors.

4. Although there are several different histologic types of lung cancer, what are the two principal classes? What is their significance?

Small-cell lung cancer (SCLC) and non-small-cell lung cancer (NSCLC). The therapeutic and prognostic considerations do not differ for subtypes of non-small cell cancers, and all are generally treated with surgery. Small-cell carcinomas, however, readily metastasize and are highly susceptible to radiation therapy. Radiation therapy, therefore, is generally the first line of treatment.

5. Why are radon levels routinely measured before homes are purchased?

Because excessive exposure to radon is another cause of lung cancer.

6. How can squamous-cell carcinoma cause hypercalcemia without bony metastases?

This type of lung cancer is known to release parathyroid hormone-related peptide (PTHrP), which stimulates bone resorption in much the same fashion as parathyroid hormone.

7. If a patient with small-cell carcinoma has hypertension, hypernatremia, hypokalemia, abdominal striae, and a buffalo hump, what should be suspected?

Cushing's syndrome due to ectopic production of adrenocorticotropic hormone, which is another common paraneoplastic syndrome in small-cell carcinoma.

CASE 10

A 38-year-old black woman presents with a nonproductive cough and shortness of breath with exertion. She also complains of generalized fatigue, night sweats, and a recent 15-lb weight loss. Physical exam reveals erythema nodosum (erythematous cutaneous nodules that do not ulcerate, scar, or exfoliate) and mild hepatosplenomegaly. A chest x-ray shows bilateral hilar lymphadenopathy. Lab tests show hypercalcemia. These findings prompt the physician to request a mediastinal lymph node biopsy, which reveals noncaseating granulomas.

1. What is the most likely diagnosis?

Sarcoidosis, a systemic granulomatous disease of unknown etiology.

2. Why was the lymph node biopsy performed?

Bilateral hilar lymphadenopathy is quite characteristic of sarcoidosis, suggesting the diagnosis. A lymph node biopsy confirms the diagnosis by showing noncaseating granulomas, another characteristic feature of the disease.

3. How can sarcoidosis cause cor pulmonale (right ventricular failure)?

As an inflammatory pulmonary disease, sarcoidosis can cause widespread pulmonary fibrosis, with obliteration of the pulmonary vascular bed, resulting in significant pulmonary hypertension. The pulmonary vasoconstriction that occurs in hypoxemia due to pulmonary fibrosis may also contribute to this process.

4. How can sarcoidosis cause a restrictive cardiomyopathy?

Granulomatous infiltration of the myocardium can cause fibrosis and consequently reduced ventricular compliance. This process is fairly similar to the pathogenesis of restrictive cardiomyopathy that develops from infiltration in amyloidosis and hemochromatosis.

Note: Because elevated levels of angiotensin-converting enzyme (ACE) are frequently associated with sarcoidosis, the diagnostic work-up often includes a measurement of serum ACE. The hypercalcemia that develops in sarcoidosis is due to increased production of 1,25 dihydroxyvitamin D3 by the macrophages in granulomas.

CASE 11

A 27-year-old man who is stabbed in the chest in a bar fight is taken to the emergency department by ambulance. He is conscious with rapid breathing (tachypnea), hypotension, and pleuritic chest pain. Other findings include tracheal deviation to the left, jugular venous distintion, right-sided hyperresonance to percussion, and decreased breath sounds over the right lung. A chest x-ray shows decreased vascular markings on the right side. A needle thoracostomy is performed immediately to decompress the lung, and then a chest tube is inserted to stabilize breathing.

1. What is the diagnosis?

Pneumothorax. More specifically, because the patient has tracheal deviation, he probably has a tension pneumothorax. This type of pneumothorax is typically caused by penetrating injuries to the chest wall that cause defects in either parietal or viscera pleura, allowing air into the pleural cavity during inspiration. In a tension pneumothorax, the defect serves as a one-way valve, allowing air to enter but not to exit. As a result, intrathoracic pressures increase to supraatmospheric levels. This increased intrathoracic pressure results in mediastinal shifting and compression of the superior vena cava and inferior vena cava (reducing venous return), explaining the signs of tracheal deviation, jugular venous distension, and hypotension, respectively.

2. Why should the chest tube be inserted immediately superior to the lower rib in the intercostal space in which it is inserted?

To avoid the neurovascular bundle that runs on the inferior aspect of each rib.

3. What is the pressure inside the pleural cavity (intrapleural space) normally?

The pleural pressure is normally negative, which helps maintain the lungs in expanded form. When either the visceral or parietal pleura is punctured, the influx of air under atmospheric pressure abolishes the vacuum and results in a positive intrapleural pressure, which collapses the lung.

4. How does hypoxia-induced vasoconstriction help compensate, to some extent, for the respiratory dysfunction caused by pneumothorax?

The blood that would ordinarily go to the collapsed (hypoxic) lung is shunted to the opposite lung, where it can be oxygenated and reduce the level of hypoxemia that develops.

5. Is this patient more likely to experience respiratory acidosis or respiratory alkalosis? Explain.

Decreased effective ventilation secondary to a collapsed lung causes hypercapnia and respiratory acidosis.

Note: A pneumothorax can cause a mixed respiratory and metabolic acidosis because of both impaired ventilation, which increases plasma CO_2 levels, and increased anaerobic metabolism in the tissues due to reduced oxygen delivery, which increases plasma levels of acids such as lactic acid.

6. What effect will a pneumothorax have on the serum ionized calcium level?

A pneumothorax increases the serum ionized calcium level because acidosis causes displacement of calcium from binding sites on albumin (via increased competition with hydrogen ions for these binding sites).

13. GENITOURINARY SYSTEM

Dave Brown and Thomas Brown

BASIC CONCEPTS

1. What forces govern the glomerular filtration rate (GFR) at the level of the glomerulus?
The forces governing GFR at the level of the glomerulus are the same as the forces that affect fluid movement across the systemic capillaries. Forces that drive fluid across the glomerular membrane include the hydrostatic pressure in the glomerular capillaries and the oncotic pressure in Bowman's space. Because there is usually very little protein in Bowman's space, the oncotic pressure contribution from protein is typically negligible. Forces that oppose fluid movement across the glomerular membrane are the hydrostatic pressure in Bowman's space and the plasma oncotic pressure.

Note: By constricting or dilating the efferent arteriole, the glomerular hydrostatic pressure can be increased or decreased. An increase in glomerular hydrostatic pressure leads to an increase in GFR, whereas a decrease in glomerular hydrostatic pressure leads to a decrease in GFR.

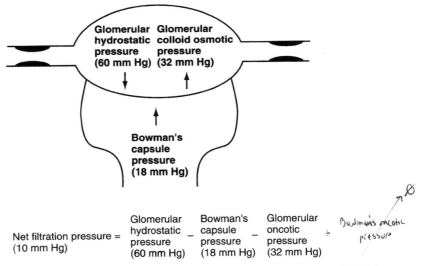

Forces governing glomerular filtration rate. (From Guyton AC, Hall JE: Textbook of Medical Physiology, 10th ed. Philadelphia, W.B. Saunders, 2000, p 487, with permission.)

2. How does the glomerular membrane affect GFR?
Although not forces, the surface area and integrity of the glomerular membrane are also important determinants of GFR. In certain disease states in which the glomerular membrane is damaged, the filtration forces are less effective; thus, the overall GFR is reduced.

3. Define filtration fraction. How does increasing the glomerular capillary oncotic pressure (without changing any other factor) affect the filtration fraction?
The filtration fraction (FF) is the percentage of plasma passing through the glomerular capillaries that is actually filtered by the glomerulus. It can be calculated as shown below and is normally approximately 20%:

$$FF = \frac{GFR}{RPF}$$

where RPF = renal plasma flow. Because the glomerular oncotic pressure opposes filtration, the net filtration pressure will decrease if glomerular oncotic pressure is increased; thus, the fraction of plasma that is filtered across the glomerulus also decreases.

4. What are the three layers of the glomerular filter? How do they contribute to the process of renal filtration at the glomerulus?

The three layers of the glomerular filter include the endothelial cells of the glomerular capillaries, the underlying basement membrane, and the glomerular epithelial cells. These layers contribute to renal filtration in unique ways. The **endothelium of the glomerular capillaries** is fenestrated. Along with the high hydrostatic pressure in the glomerular capillaries, the fenestrated capillaries allow the filtration of large volumes of plasma across the capillary bed. The **underlying basement membrane** is negatively charged, which helps prevent filtration (and subsequent loss in the urine) of large negatively charged plasma proteins. The **glomerular epithelial cells** or podocytes compose the final layer of the glomerular filter. These specialized cells "send out" cytoplasmic extensions (so-called foot-processes or slit-pores) that envelope the glomerular capillaries and form a final barrier for filterable molecules to traverse before entering the capsular space of the glomerulus.

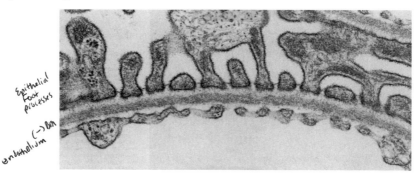

Layers of the glomerular filter. (From Cotran, Kumar, Collins (eds): Robbins Pathologic Basis of Disease, 6th ed. Philadelphia, W.B. Saunders, 1999, p 933, with permission.)

5. What is the significance of creatinine clearance? How is it measured?

The clearance of any substance is defined simply as the volume of plasma that has been "cleared" of that substance within 1 minute. For example, a creatinine clearance of 125 ml/min implies that creatinine has been completely removed and excreted (by the kidneys) from 125 ml of plasma within 1 minute. As shown by the equation below, the clearance of a substance can be calculated by dividing the urinary excretion of the substance by its plasma concentration. Because creatinine is neither reabsorbed nor secreted (for the most part), its clearance closely approximates that of the actual GFR and is therefore an important indicator of renal function.

$$C = \frac{V \times UCr}{P_{Cr}}$$

where C = clearance, V = urinary flow rate/minute, UCr = urinary creatinine concentration, and P_{Cr} = plasma creatinine concentration.

6. Why is net renal acid excretion necessary to maintain acid-base homeostasis?

Daily metabolism generates a large quantity of nonvolatile acids (e.g., lactate, sulfate, phosphate) that cannot be excreted by the lungs. These nonvolatile acids must be excreted by the kidneys; otherwise metabolic acidosis develops.

Note: Nonvolatile acids are derived primarily from the metabolism of dietary proteins. The metabolic breakdown of carbohydrates and fats, in contrast, yields largely carbon dioxide, which is easily excreted by the lungs.

7. What mechanisms does the kidney use to prevent the development of acidosis?

The ability of the kidney to prevent acidosis depends on its ability to efficiently reabsorb filtered bicarbonate (which depends on hydrogen ion secretion into the tubular fluid), synthesize de novo bicarbonate from the deamination of glutamine, secrete titratable buffers such as ammonia (which bind hydrogen ions and increase the acid excretory capacity of the urine without allowing a precipitous drop in urine pH), and to actively secrete acid (in the form of hydrogen ions) into the tubular fluid.

8. How do the kidneys reabsorb filtered bicarbonate?

Hydrogen ions are secreted in the proximal tubule. They react with bicarbonate to form carbonic acid, which dissociates into carbon dioxide and water, both of which can diffuse back into the cell. In the cell the reverse reaction takes place: carbon dioxide reacts with water to generate bicarbonate, which is then reabsorbed into the systemic circulation.

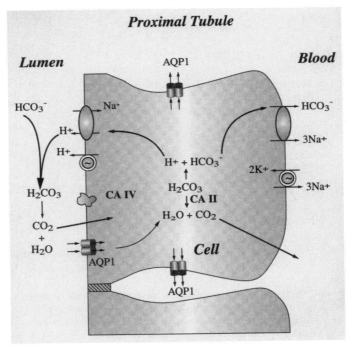

Mechanisms of proximal tubule bicarbonate reabsorption. (From Brenner (ed): Brenner and Rector's The Kidney, 6th ed. Philadelphia, W.B. Saunders, 2000, p 1675, with permission.)

9. How does acetazolamide function as a diuretic? What effect does it have on the acid-base balance of the body?

Acetazolamide, a carbonic anhydrase inhibitor, inhibits the conversion of bicarbonate to carbonic acid, a reaction normally catalyzed by the enzyme carbonic anhydrase in the proximal tubule of the nephron. This enzyme is anchored to the luminal surface of the plasma membrane of tubular epithelial cells. Because carbonic acid normally dissociates rapidly in the tubular fluid to carbon dioxide and water, with the carbon dioxide diffusing into the epithelial cells and reforming bicarbonate, the net effect of inhibiting carbonic anhydrase is the increased urinary excretion of bicarbonate. The increased bicarbonate excretion promotes an osmotic diuresis.

Note: This pharmacotherapeutic mechanism of action essentially mimics the pathophysiology seen with proximal tubular acidosis, in which bicarbonate reabsorption by the tubular epithelium is impaired. The result of decreased bicarbonate reabsorption is a mild metabolic acidosis. This "side effect" of acetazolamide can be used therapeutically—for example, in the treatment of the respiratory alkalosis that can develop at elevated altitudes (e.g., mountain sickness).

10. How is bicarbonate generated de novo by the kidney?

The deamination of glutamine in the kidney generates two ammonium (NH_4^+) molecules and two bicarbonate (HCO_3^-) molecules. The ammonium molecules are secreted into the tubular lumen and the bicarbonate molecules are reabsorbed into the systemic circulation

Note: Glutamine deamination is stimulated by hydrogen ions and increased carbon dioxide levels. These stimuli increase renal bicarbonate generation in acidotic conditions.

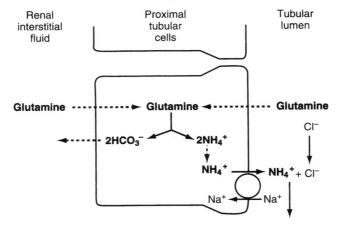

De novo bicarbonate generation. (From Guyton AC, Hall JE: Textbook of Medical Physiology, 10th ed. Philadelphia, W.B. Saunders, 2000, with permission.)

CASE 1

A 48-year-old man is admitted to the hospital for an elective cholecystectomy, and a presurgical work-up reveals a serum sodium level of 125 mEq/L (normal = 135–145 mEq/L). He complains of some fatigue, anorexia, and mild confusion. He denies any recent vomiting or diarrhea and has not used any diuretics; he has a normal albumin level and no signs of heart failure. Vital signs were within normal limits, as is the physical exam. Urinalysis reveals a urine osmolality of 620 mOsm/kg.

1. What is the diagnosis?

Syndrome of inappropriate secretion of antidiuretic hormone (SIADH).

2. What is the function of antidiuretic hormone (also known as vasopressin)?

This hormone of the posterior pituitary has two primary functions: to maintain plasma osmolarity and to maintain plasma volume/blood pressure. To maintain plasma osmolarity, antidiuretic hormone (ADH) is secreted in response to increased plasma osmolarity and reduces the osmolarity by increasing water reabsorption in the collecting ducts of the kidneys. It does so by stimulating the insertion of water channels (aquaporins) into the luminal membranes of the collecting ducts. To maintain plasma volume and blood pressure, ADH is secreted in response to low blood pressure. In addition to increasing water reabsorption in the kidney to expand extracellular fluid volume, it also causes arterial vasoconstriction.

Note: Desmopressin is a synthetic analog of ADH that has the same renal effects but causes significantly less vasoconstriction. It is used to treat central diabetes insipidus, in which the pituitary does not secrete ADH.

3. How is SIADH diagnosed?

Too much ADH causes excessive water retention, which dilutes plasma osmolarity (hyponatremia) and increases urine osmolarity because of the significant water reabsorption without solute. Thus, the diagnosis of SIADH is established by hyponatremia in a setting of increased urine sodium and osmolarity.

4. What are the principal causes of SIADH?

SIADH is usually secondary to another disease process. For the Step 1 exam, ectopic secretion of ADH by small-cell carcinomas of the lung is the classic cause of SIADH. However, lesions or tumors of the pituitary and/or hypothalamus also can cause SIADH as well as a variety of nonmalignant diseases of the lung (e.g., tuberculosis, pneumonia, pneumothorax).

5. How can hyponatremia contribute to central nervous system symptoms (fatigue, anorexia, confusion)?

Because serum sodium is an important determinant of plasma osmolarity, hyponatremia results in a fluid shift from the extracellular compartment to the intracellular compartment. In the brain, this shift can result in cerebral edema and a wide variety of neurologic effects. If the hyponatremia is sufficiently severe, coma and convulsions may occur.

6. Why must hyponatremia be corrected with great caution in this patient?

Overly rapid correction of hyponatremia (> 12 mEq/24 hr) is thought to place patients at high risk for the development of central pontine myelinolysis (CPM), a disorder characterized by flaccid quadriplegia, dysphagia, facial weakness, and perhaps coma. The pathophysiology of this disorder is believed to involve dehydration of the brain in response to a rapid increase in plasma osmolarity and demyelination of oligodendrocytes. Such demyelination is often readily apparent on magnetic resonance imaging (MRI) of the brain, but it is not typically detected until several weeks after the correction of hyponatremia.

Note: As shown by MRI, other areas of the brain are damaged with the overly rapid correction of hyponatremia, leading to symptoms such as cognitive and psychiatric dysfunction. Thus, the term *osmotic demyelination syndrome* is perhaps a better descriptor of the pathophysiology than the term *central pontine myelinolysis.*

7. Why is it important to ask about vomiting, diarrhea, or diuretic use?

All three are causes of sodium wasting and can all result in hyponatremia. Note that in these cases significant fluid losses result in *hypovolemic* hyponatremia. Although in these cases both water and salt can be lost, the hyponatremia occurs because of fluid replacement with pure water without salt.

8. Why is it important to examine the albumin level and look for evidence of heart failure to determine the cause of hyponatremia?

Both liver disease and heart failure cause fluid retention and hyponatremia, resulting in *hypervolemic* hyponatremia.

9. How are levels of plasma ADH, plasma osmolarity, and serum osmolarity expected to differ in SIADH, diabetes insipidus, and psychogenic polydipsia?

SYNDROME	PLASMA ADH	PLASMA OSMOLARITY	URINE OSMOLARITY	PATHOPHYSIOLOGIC EXPLANATION	CLASSIC STEP 1 ASSOCIATION
SIADH	High	Low	Inappropriately high	ADH causes excessive water reabsorption by the kidneys, creating an inappropriately concentrated urine for the level of plasma hypoosmolarity	Small-cell carcinoma
Central diabetes insipidus	Low	High	Low	Lack of hypothalamic ADH secretion causes water diuresis, resulting in plasma hyperosmolarity secondary to the preferential renal excretion of water over sodium	Head trauma
Nephrogenic diabetes insipidus	High	High	Low	Inability of the kidneys to respond to ADH, resulting in plasma hyperosmolarity secondary to the preferential renal excretion of water over sodium	Lithium toxocity
Psychogenic polydipsia	Low	Low	Maximally dilute	Kidneys work normally and, in an attempt to remove the excessive ingested water, create a maximally dilute urine of approximately 50 mOsm	Crazy person

CASE 2

A 78-year-old man comes to the emergency department because he has not been able to urinate for the past two days and is experiencing lower abdominal pain. For the previous few years, he admits to some difficulty in initiating the urinary stream, a weak stream, nocturia, and dribbling after voiding. He denies taking any tricyclic antidepressants, antipsychotics, or sympathomimetic agents. On physical exam his bladder seems palpably enlarged, and a digital rectal examination reveals an enlarged prostate. Urinalysis shows no hematuria or crystalluria. Routine lab tests show significantly elevated levels of blood urea nitrogen (BUN) and creatinine but a normal level of prostate-specific antigen (PSA). An abdominal ultrasound reveals a markedly distended bladder and enlargement of both kidneys.

1. What is the probable diagnosis?

Acute urinary retention, most likely secondary to occlusion of the bladder neck by benign prostatic hyperplasia (BPH).

2. What are the three etiologic classifications of acute renal failure? Which is associated with BPH?

Renal failure is classified as having a prerenal, renal, or postrenal (obstructive) etiology. This patient's renal failure clearly has an obstructive etiology. Acute bladder distention caused by longstanding BPH has resulted in bilateral hydronephrosis and acute renal failure.

3. Why is the absence of hematuria on urinalysis helpful in establishing the diagnosis?

Urinary calculi can cause lower urinary tract obstruction and often are associated with hematuria as well as with microscopic crystals in the urine. Tumors of the bladder can likewise cause lower tract obstruction and hematuria.

4. Why is looking at the urethral meatus also important in establishing the diagnosis?

Other causes of obstruction of the lower urinary tract (bladder or urethra), such as meatal stenosis or urethral stricture, can also cause acute urinary retention with resultant renal failure. Obstruction of the lower urinary tract can back up urine and expand the dimensions of both kidneys (bilateral hydronephrosis).

5. Why may an uncircumcised man be predisposed to a similar form of urinary retention?

He may have paraphimosis, in which a restricted, uncircumcised prepuce (foreskin) is forcibly retracted behind the glans penis, where it becomes stuck and compresses the penis, possibly causing urethral constriction (plus considerable pain).

Note: In general, paraphimosis is preceded by phimosis, in which the prepuce cannot be easily retracted behind the glans penis. Repeated bouts of infection and consequent scarring of the prepuce are usually responsible for phimosis.

6. Why is it important to ask this patient about tricyclic antidepressants, antipsychotics, and sympathomimetics?

These classes of drugs can cause urinary retention. The tricyclic antidepressants (e.g., *amitriptyline*) and antipsychotics (e.g., phenothiazines) have significant anticholinergic properties. Recall that the detrusor muscle of the bladder is stimulated to contract by parasympathetic (cholinergic) innervation. The sympathomimetics can cause retention by increasing the tone of the internal urethral sphincter.

Note: The anticholinergic atropine has a similar effect, as do *oxybutinin* and *tolterodine*, both of which are widely used for urge incontinence.

CASE 3

A 68-year-old man experiences a ruptured abdominal aortic aneurysm and is rushed to the hospital and into the operating room. During the procedure the surgeons had to clamp the abdominal aorta at a level superior to the renal arteries for a little over an hour. Although the patient survived the operation, the next morning he was found to have a severe acute decline in renal function with a BUN level of 75 and a creatinine level of 3.2. His GFR was depressed to about 10 ml/minute, his urine output diminished to about 200 ml in 24 hours (despite being normotensive), and microscopic urinalysis revealed renal epithelial cell casts.

1. What is the probable diagnosis?

Acute tubular necrosis (ATN) secondary to prolonged renal ischemia during surgery.

2. What is the site of the lesion in ATN?

The renal tubular epithelial cells are damaged and slough off the basement membrane. These cells can be damaged by either ischemia (as in this patient) or by various nephrotoxins such as lead, mercury, and cisplatin.

Note: The aminoglycosides and amphotericin B are well known for causing renal epithelial cell damage and ATN, as are radiographic contrast media.

3. Explain the origin of the decreased GFR in ATN.

The sloughed tubular epithelial cells block the lumen of the renal tubules into which they are released, impeding urine flow. Note that this patient had casts of renal epithelial cells in his urine. In addition, the denuded areas of basement membrane allow back leakage of filtered fluid.

Although this back leakage does not change the amount of fluid that flows across the glomerular membrane, it does change the amount of waste products that are excreted, which consequently changes the *calculated* GFR. Both obstruction to flow and back leakage explain why overall urine output is frequently reduced in ATN.

4. What are the three phases of ATN?

Initiation phase, in which the injurious agent or condition that will eventually cause renal failure is present but renal functional deterioration has not yet begun or is just beginning.

Maintenance phase, in which GFR is reduced and oliguria persists. Uremic complications are likely to manifest.

Recovery phase, in which renal tubular epithelial cells proliferate and repopulate the denuded areas.

5. How does prerenal azotemia due to ischemia differ from ATN due to ischemia?

The differences are based on the severity of insult. In prerenal azotemia, inadequate renal perfusion reduces the GFR, but the reduced perfusion is not so severe as to cause cellular damage. In contrast, in ischemia-induced ATN the ischemia is significant. Generally, if the ischemia is so severe as to cause acute tubular necrosis, a component of prerenal azotemia is also present.

6. What is rhabdomyolysis? How can it cause ATN?

Rhabdomyolysis is acute destruction of skeletal muscle cells, which can occur with trauma, drugs (e.g., statins), and a whole host of other scenarios. The released myoglobin can precipitate in the renal tubules and obstruct urine flow. Myoglobin is also directly toxic to renal tubular epithelial cells.

CASE 4

A 65-year-old African-American woman with a longstanding history of severe and uncontrolled hypertension is evaluated as a new patient. She has no history of other medical conditions. Routine lab tests are notable for a significant elevation of both BUN and creatinine, but fasting plasma glucose is normal. Previous records from several months ago show a similar elevation in BUN and creatinine. A microscopic urinalysis reveals no hematuria, red blood cell casts, or white blood cell casts. Additional laboratory findings include hypocalcemia, hyperphosphatemia, and metabolic acidosis.

1. What is the most likely cause of the elevations in BUN and creatinine?

Hypertensive nephrosclerosis (also known as benign nephrosclerosis and hyaline arteriolar nephrosclerosis). In African-Americans, hypertension is one of the most common causes of renal failure; therefore, hypertension should be aggressively managed in such patients.

2. What is the value of the normal fasting glucose in the differential diagnosis?

Diabetic nephropathy is the most common cause of chronic renal failure.

3. What is the difficulty in establishing that the patient's renal failure was definitely due to hypertension, even if no other specific disease processes can be identified on renal biopsy?

Often, if renal failure is chronic, renal biopsy findings are nonspecific and cannot distinguish among various precipitating insults. For example, the patient's renal failure may have been due to a bout of glomerulonephritis that permanently damaged the kidneys, and her hypertension could be a result of kidney damage. Nevertheless, hypertension, regardless of its origin, also contributes to progressive loss of renal function.

4. How could the patient's renal failure explain her hypocalcemia?

Several insults contribute to this process. First, the kidney is the site of 1,25-dihydroxyvita-min D3 synthesis from 25-hydroxyvitamin D3 via the activity of renal 1-alpha hydroxylase. Loss of renal parenchyma reduces synthesis of 1,25-dihydroxyvitamin D, which is the active form that stimulates intestinal calcium absorption. Thus, intestinal calcium absorption is reduced. Second, as the GFR declines, renal phosphate excretion declines, leading to hyperphosphatemia. Elevated serum phosphate can complex with serum calcium and reduce levels of ionized calcium; the increased phosphate also inhibits the synthesis of 1,25-dihydroxyvitamin D3.

5. Would parathyroid hormone levels in this patient be increased or decreased? Explain.

Because parathyroid hormone is released in response to hypocalcemia (or hyperphos-phatemia), the parathyroid hormone level would be increased. This process is called compensatory or secondary hyperparathyroidism. However, in severe renal failure compensatory hyperparathy-roidism cannot correct the low serum calcium. Note the difference between this condition and primary hyperparathyroidism, in which serum calcium levels are consistently elevated.

6. What are the potential pathologic manifestations of the hyperparathyroidism that develops in renal failure?

Parathyroid hormone also stimulates bone resorption, which can cause osteoporosis as well as cysts in areas of demineralized bone (osteitis fibrosa cystica).

7. Why is the patient also predisposed to osteomalacia?

Osteomalacia is a disease characterized by impaired mineralization of newly deposited osteoid matrix in bone. As a result, the bones are more malleable (malacia). Hypocalcemia and reduced 1,25-dihydroxyvitamin D3 synthesis by the kidneys in this disease reduce bone mineralization.

Note: If this impaired mineralization occurs in prepubertal persons before closure of the epiphyseal plates, it is referred to as rickets.

Note: Renal osteodystrophy includes the spectrum of bony changes that result from renal failure, such as osteitis fibrosa cystica due to secondary hyperparathyroidism, osteomalacia due to decreased mineralization, and bone loss due to buffering of excessive acid in the metabolic acidosis that accompanies renal failure.

8. How can renal failure explain metabolic acidosis?

The kidneys normally excrete a large quantity of nonvolatile acids, such as ammonium and hydrogen ions. Metabolic acidosis may develop as this critical function of the kidneys becomes compromised in renal failure and acids accumulate in the body.

This effect is due in part to impaired renal synthesis of ammonia, which buffers secreted acid, and in part to reduced renal acid secretion. Because the damaged renal parenchyma synthesizes and secretes less ammonia, less acid can be buffered; the decreased GFR also reduces the amount of acid that can be secreted into the tubules.

9. Explain the relationship between renal failure and hyperkalemia.

Under normal conditions, in the presence of aldosterone, the kidneys are responsible for efficient sodium reabsorption (which maintains plasma volume) and excretion of excessive potassium. In renal failure, the ability to excrete potassium is compromised; in conjunction with a decreased GFR, this results in hyperkalemia.

Note: Marked hyperkalemia, which can cause fatal cardiac arrhythmias, is an indication for emergent renal dialysis.

10. How can renal failure lead to anemia? Would you expect a microcytic, normocytic, or macrocytic anemia?

Renal erythropoietin synthesis is likewise compromised in severe renal failure and results in anemia. We would expect a normocytic anemia, because lack of erythropoietin simply reduces the rate of erythropoiesis. Insufficiencies of iron or folate/vitamin B12 would cause a microcytic or macrocytic anemia, respectively.

11. Is this woman suffering from azotemia or uremia?

Azotemia refers to increased levels of BUN and creatinine in an asymptomatic person. If this patient had symptoms developing from her renal failure, she would be described as suffering from uremia (i.e., she would be uremic).

Note: Clinical symptoms of uremia include nausea, pruritus, seizures, and encephalopathy.

12. If the patient is uremic and a friction rub is detected on exam, what might you suspect?

Uremic pericarditis, characterized by a fibrinous exudate within the pericardial space.

Note: For the Step 1 exam, you can spot pericarditis by the presence of a friction rub on physical examination and chest pain that is relieved by sitting forward.

CASE 5

A 35-year-old woman complains of flank pain and blood in her urine. She denies any urinary symptoms such as dysuria, urgency, or frequency. The past medical history is notable only for hypertension, which she developed at an unusually young age (in her 20s). Urinalysis reveals hematuria and mild proteinuria, but no white blood cell or red blood cell casts. Lab tests show elevated levels of BUN and creatinine. Renal ultrasound reveals no stones but shows enlarged kidneys with numerous cysts bilaterally. The patient then remembers that her mother also had a kidney disease with cysts

1. What is the diagnosis?

Autosomal dominant (adult) polycystic kidney disease (ADPKD)

2. How does this diagnosis explain the early onset hypertension?

The kidney damage that occurs in ADPKD elicits hypertension via similar mechanisms as renal artery stenosis (the angiotensin-aldosterone system). Note that she already has elevated levels of BUN and creatinine.

3. What is the main danger of this disease?

Renal failure. In approximately 10% of patients with chronic renal failure, the cause is ADPKD.

4. Why are urinary tract infections treated aggressively in patients with this disease?

If the infection ascends into the kidney, it is extremely difficult to eradicate from the cysts, which are essentially urine cesspools that do not drain.

5. If the patient develops a severe headache, what vascular abnormality may be detected on an MRI of the brain?

An intracranial aneurysm, which often develops in ADPDK. Presumably, the mutations in the polycystin gene that allow tissue to separate in the kidneys and form cysts also make it easier for vascular connective tissue to separate and form aneurysms.

6. How does ADPKD differ from autosomal recessive polycystic kidney disease (other than the pattern of inheritance)?

The autosomal recessive form occurs more commonly in children and is associated with hepatic fibrosis.

7. What is tuberous sclerosis? How can it be differentiated from ADPKD?

Tuberous sclerosis is a genetic disease that is inherited in an autosomal dominant manner. Multiple cysts form on the kidneys. The disease is also characterized by a variety of central nervous system abnormalities (e.g., mental retardation, seizure disorders) as well as dermato-logic lesions.

8. What is medullary cystic disease (MCD)? How can it be differentiated from ADPKD?

In MCD the cysts are confined to the medulla and do not develop throughout the kidney as in ADPKD.

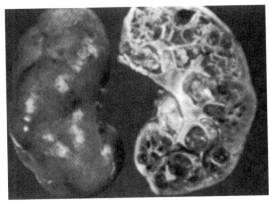

Outer and cut surface of kidney with severe medullary cystic disease. (From Brenner (ed): Brenner and Rector's The Kidney, 6th ed. Philadelphia, W.B. Saunders, p 1716, with permission.)

9. Cover the right side of the table and list the characteristic feature of each of the cystic kidney diseases.

	SITE OF CYSTS IN KIDNEY	INHERITANCE	AGE OF ONSET	KEY ASSOCIATED FEATURES
ADPKD	Throughout	AD	Adult	Intracranial aneurysm Asymptomatic hepatic cysts
ARPKD	Throughout	AR	Childhood	Hepatic Fibrosis
Tuberous sclerosis	Throughout	AD	Childhood	Mental retardation Seizure disorder Angiomyolipoma of kidney
Medullary cystic disease	Medulla		Childhood	

AD = autosomal dominant, AR = autosomal recessive.

10. Why is medullary sponge kidney omitted from the above chart?

Typical cysts do not form in medullary sponge kidney. Rather, segments of the collecting tubules become abnormally dilated in the medulla and renal papillae. The main problem is that the dilations predispose to nephrolithiasis.

CASE 6

A 5-year-old boy is brought to the clinic by his parents, who are concerned because he has been lethargic recently and appears "swollen" to them. Marked peripheral edema is noted on physical exam. Lab tests reveal hyperlipidemia and hypoalbuminemia. Urinalysis reveals the presence of proteins and lipids in the urine, but no red blood cells.

1. What is the likely diagnosis? Why?

Nephrotic syndrome, characterized by massive proteinuria (> 3gm/24 hr), hypoalbuminemia and edema, and hyperlipidemia and lipiduria. Although slight hematuria is sometimes seen in nephrotic syndrome, it is typically transient and much less severe than that associated with the nephritic syndrome.

2. What is the likely cause of nephrotic syndrome in this patient?

Minimal change disease (also known as lipoid nephrosis), which is the most common cause of nephrotic syndrome in children and commonly occurs following infections.

Note: Membranous glomerulonephritis (membranous nephropathy) is the most common cause of nephrotic syndrome in adults. It is characterized by electron-dense, immunoglobulin-containing deposits on the subepithelial side of the basement membrane on renal biopsy.

3. Assuming that minimal change disease is the underlying pathology, what should you expect gross histology to reveal if a renal biopsy is performed?

Next to nothing, explaining the term *minimal change* disease. However, electron microscopy and immunofluorescence studies may show flattening of the glomerular foot processes and IgM deposition within the renal mesangium.

4. Why might the boy be susceptible to infections?

Because of hypogammaglobulinemia due to loss of immunoglobulins in the urine.

5. How should the boy be managed? Is a renal biopsy necessary?

Nephrotic syndrome caused by minimal change disease typically responds well to steroids and is usually treated with prednisone. Because the majority of nephrotic cases in children are secondary to minimal change disease (roughly 80%), a renal biopsy is not needed. If, however, the boy's condition does not respond well to steroids, a renal biopsy may be necessary to determine the precise pathogenesis of the nephrotic syndrome.

6. What condition should you suspect in a 6-year-old girl who complains of extreme abdominal pain and joint pain if her work-up is significant for hematuria and a maculopapular rash on the lower extremities?

Henoch-Schonlein purpura (HSP), a vasculitis that typically affects the blood vessels in the gastrointestinal tract, kidneys, and skin. This pattern of organ involvement explains the abdominal pain, hematuria, and rash, respectively.

CASE 7

A 42-year-old man presents for a pre-employment physical. He has no current complaints but mentioned that he has recently recovered from a bad sore throat. Physical exam is significant for mild hypertension. Blood work reveals elevated BUN and creatinine levels, and urinalysis is significant for hematuria and microscopic proteinuria. Antistreptolysin O (ASO) titers are markedly elevated. Lab tests from a visit 3 months ago showed no elevation of BUN or creatinine.

1. What is the likely diagnosis?

Acute nephritic syndrome (also known as acute glomerulonephritis), which is characterized by a relatively sudden onset of mild proteinuria (< 3gm/24 hr), hematuria, renal insufficiency, and hypertension.

Note: Urinalysis also typically shows dysmorphic red blood cells and red blood cell casts in glomerulonephritis.

2. What sore throat did this patient probably have? What is its relationship to the renal dysfunction?

Streptococcal pharyngitis, caused by group A beta-hemolytic streptococci (particularly *Streptococcus pyogenes*). He is now suffering from poststreptococcal glomerulonephritis (PSGN).

This condition is caused by antibody-antigen complex deposition in the glomerulus, which results in inflammatory destruction of the glomerulus (primarily mediated via complement activation).

Note: Of interest, cutaneous streptococcal infections can also cause poststreptococcal glomerulonephritis.

3. What is the most common cause of nephritis worldwide?

IgA glomerulonephritis (Berger's disease). Although the pathogenesis of this disorder is poorly understood, it is commonly seen after an upper respiratory illness, and renal biopsy typically shows immune complex deposition (composed of IgA and complement C3) within the mesangium.

4. How might the treatment be affected if renal biopsy revealed glomerular crescents?

Glomerular crescents are the hallmark of a rapidly evolving glomerulonephritis and therefore indicate the need for aggressive treatment to prevent irreversible renal damage. Crescents are formed by clusters of rapidly proliferating epithelial cells and infiltrating leukocytes.

Note: Pauci-immune glomerulonephritis is the most common cause of rapidly progressive glomerulonephritis. Its name derives from the fact that on renal biopsy, very few immune complexes can be seen. Pauci-immune glomerulonephritis is commonly associated with vasculitic conditions (e.g., Wegener granulomatosis, microscopic polyarteritis nodosa) as well as autoimmune disorders (e.g., Goodpasture syndrome).

5. Cover the left-hand column and diagnose the cause of the glomerulonephritis based on the lab tests and history provided on the left.

IF TESTS AND HISTORY REVEAL	SUSPECT AS CAUSE OF GLOMERULONEPHRITIS
Antiglomerular basement membrane antibodies, hematuria, and hemoptysis	Goodpasture syndrome (anti-GMB nephritis)
c-ANCAs with a history of hemoptysis	Wegener granulomatosis
Defect in type IV collagen and congenital hearing difficulty	Alport syndrome
p-ANCAs and hepatitis B antigenemia	Polyarteritis nodosa
Hematuria, episodic abdominal pain, joint pain, and a lower extremity purpuric rash	Henoch-Schonlein purpura (HSP)

ANCA = antineutrophilic cytoplasmic antibody.

CASE 8

A 45-year-old man comes into the emergency department (ED) complaining of severe left flank pain that radiates into his groin. He does not complain of nausea, vomiting, diarrhea, or abdominal pain. On exam his abdomen is tender to deep palpation on the left side. Urinalysis reveals gross hematuria with no red cell or white cell casts, and microscopy shows calcium oxalate stones. An intravenous pyelogram (visualization of the kidneys, ureters, and bladder with contrast media) reveals a stone in the left ureter. Routine lab tests done in the ED also show hypercalcemia.

1. What is the diagnosis?

Nephrolithiasis, most likely secondary to hypercalcemia.

2. What are the most common types of kidney stones?

The vast majority are calcium stones; struvite stones (magnesium ammonium phosphate) are next, followed by uric acid stones and cystine stones.

3. How can nephrolithiasis cause renal failure?

Complete obstruction of a ureter or the ureteric pelvis increases the hydrostatic pressure in the ureters and/or renal tubules. The increased hydrostatic pressure substantially diminishes the net filtration pressure at the glomerulus, causing an acute decline in the GFR. However, if the other kidney is intact and healthy, it can compensate for the decreased GFR in the obstructed kidney.

Note: Obstruction of urine flow from a kidney causes hydronephrosis, in which the renal pelvis and calyces dilate significantly.

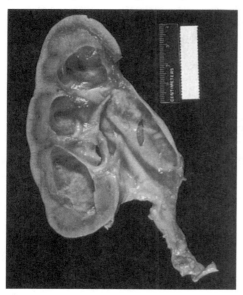

Hydronephrosis of the kidney, with marked dilation of the pelvis and calyces and thinning of the renal parenchyma. (From Cotran, Kumar, Collins (eds): Robbins Pathologic Basis of Disease, 6th ed. Philadelphia, W.B. Saunders,1999, p 989, with permission.)

4. What are the most commons cause of hypercalcemia in the community vs. in the hospital?

Primary hyperparathyroidism predominates in the community, whereas malignancy-induced hypercalcemia predominates in hospitalized patients. Malignancies produce hypercalcemia by metastasizing to bone and causing lysis or by secreting an ectopic hormone known as parathyroid hormone-related peptide (PTHrP). Other causes of hypercalcemia include hypervitaminosis D and the milk-alkali syndrome, in which excessive calcium and absorbable alkali (e.g., calcium carbonate) are ingested.

5. Why is hypercalcemia secondary to hyperparathyroidism less likely to cause renal calculi formation than other causes of hypercalcemia?

In general, the risk of calcium oxalate stone formation in the urine is proportional to the urine calcium concentration. Although both hyperparathyroidism and other causes of hypercalcemia increase urine calcium concentration, hyperparathyroidism increases urine calcium concentration to a lesser extent, because parathyroid hormone also stimulates renal tubular calcium reabsorption.

6. How does hyperparathyroidism cause hypercalcemia?

Parathyroid hormone stimulates bone resorption, renal tubular calcium reabsorption, and renal 1,25-dihydroxyvitamin D3 synthesis. The latter is the metabolically active form of vitamin D and stimulates intestinal calcium absorption.

Note: In *hypo*calcemia secondary to *hypo*parathyroidism, 1,25-dihydroxyvitamin D_3 is often given to facilitate intestinal calcium absorption. This approach bypasses the renal defect in the synthesis of this hormone that occurs during hypoparathyroidism.

7. How does urinary tract infection with *Proteus mirabilis* or *Klebsiella* species predispose to struvite stone formation?

Struvite stones, which consist of magnesium ammonium phosphate, precipitate at higher urinary pH. *P. mirabilis* and *Klebsiella* species elaborate the enzyme urease into the urinary tract, where it cleaves urea to form ammonia and carbon dioxide. The ammonia increases urinary pH and also precipitates as part of the stones.

8. How does urinary pH influence the precipitation of uric acid stones?

Uric acid is less soluble than its urate salt, and decreasing the urinary pH increases the concentration of the uric acid form, thereby facilitating crystallization.

Note: Because *acetazolamide* increases urinary pH, it can also be used to help dissolve uric acid stones.

9. What is cystinuria? How does it lead to cystine stones?

Cystinuria is a genetic disease in which renal tubular reabsorption of cystine (and a few other amino acids) is impaired. Cystine is not as soluble as the other amino acids that are not reabsorbed; thus, it precipitates selectively in this disease. Like uric acid stones, cystine stones are "organic" and typically radiolucent.

Note: Cystinuria is distinct from homocystinuria, in which a genetic defect in homocysteine catabolism causes extreme elevations in plasma and urine homocysteine concentrations.

CASE 9

A 38-year-old woman complains of dysuria, frequent urination, urgency, and the feeling that she does not completely empty the bladder. She also complains of nausea, vomiting, back pain, and high fever. On exam she has a fever of 102.5°F, costovertebral angle tenderness, and suprapubic tenderness. Urinalysis reveals numerous white blood cells, bacteruria, and white blood cell casts. She is admitted to the hospital and prescribed trimethoprim-sulfamethoxazole (TMP-SMX), ciprofloxacin, and pyridium. She is also told to drink plenty of fluids.

1. What is the most likely diagnosis?

Acute pyelonephritis.

Note: White blood cell casts are virtually pathognomic of acute pyelonephritis.

2. What is the most common source of infection in pyelonephritis?

The vast majority of these infections are due to ascending infection from the bladder/urinary tract, whereas a minority result from hematogenous dissemination. Most of the infectious agents are fecal floras that have colonized the vaginal introitus. *Escherichia coli* is the predominant pathogen. In sexually active young women, infection with *Staphylococcus saprophyticus* is the second most common pathogen.

3. Why are pregnant women with asymptomatic bacteruria treated more aggressively than nonpregnant women with the same condition?

Although asymptomatic bacteruria (bacteria in the urine) rarely causes problems in nonpregnant women, a large percentage of pregnant women with this condition go on to develop pyelonephritis. Aside from the obvious dangers of developing bacteremia and sepsis, pyelonephritis also increases the risk of premature delivery.

4. What is acute interstitial nephritis? How does it differ from acute pyelonephritis?

Interstitial nephritis, or inflammation of the renal interstitium, is predominantly due to an immunologic hypersensitivity reaction (e.g., drug hypersensitivity). Although infectious agents can precipitate interstitial nephritis, the infectious process itself is minimally involved in the pathogenesis; the immunologic hypersensitivity to the infectious agent is paramount. Interstitial nephritis may also cause renal failure.

5. Why are urinary tract infections (UTIs) in men younger than 50 often worked up aggressively?

Ordinarily younger men are quite resistant to UTIs (with the exception of sexually transmitted diseases). When UTIs occur in younger men, they are usually due to urologic abnormalities. Women are presumably more predisposed to UTI's because of the shorter length of the urethra.

6. Why are men older than 50 predisposed to UTIs?

The benign prostatic hyperplasia that commonly develops in older men causes greater urinary retention and stasis of bladder urine, both of which facilitate bacterial overgrowth.

14. IMMUNE SYSTEM

Robin Parmley, Ph.D.

BASIC CONCEPTS

1. What is hematopoiesis?

Hematopoiesis is defined as the generation of blood cells, including erythrocytes (RBCs), leukocytes (white blood cells [WBCs]), and platelets (which are actually fragments of cells). All of the blood cells develop in the adult bone marrow from a common stem-cell precursor.

2. What are the two lineages along which blood cells differentiate?

A small number of multipotent stem cells have the ability to differentiate along two lineages: myeloid and lymphoid. The **myeloid lineage** gives rise to nonlymphocytic cell types, including monocytes/macrophages, granulocytes (neutrophils, eosinophils, basophils), dendritic cells, RBCs, and platelets. The **lymphoid lineage** gives rise to T cells, B cells, and natural killer (NK) cells. Various cytokines (e.g., interleukin-3, granulocyte-macrophage colony-stimulating factor, erythropoietin) are required for the proliferation and differentiation of the different hematopoietic cells.

3. Define the innate immune system. What are its components?

Innate or natural immunity is a nonspecific type of immunity that is the body's first line of defense against insult and injury. Components of innate immunity include anatomic barriers, such as skin and mucus membranes, in addition to physiologic barriers, such as the low pH of gastric secretions. All of these components hinder entry of pathogens into the tissues. These defense mechanisms are always present, regardless of the presence or absence of pathogens. The innate responses of phagocytosis and inflammation occur rapidly (within hours) and are mediated by cells such as macrophages and neutrophils and by chemical mediators such as complement and acute-phase proteins. Once activated the same mechanism occurs with the same magnitude of response, regardless of the challenge or previous exposure.

Note: Complement may be activated by either the innate or adaptive immune system.

4. What is adaptive immunity?

Adaptive immunity develops in response to the stimulation and proliferation of antigen-specific B and T lymphocytes. Thus, only B cells and/or T cells with a given specificity respond to a particular antigen at the time of exposure. In addition to this high degree of specificity, an adaptive response is a source of immunologic memory. Subsequent exposure to the same pathogen engenders a more powerful immunologic response. That is, response to a second (or third, etc.) challenge is more rapid, stronger, and usually more efficient at clearing the pathogen.

5. Summarize the differences in the effector cells, chemical mediators, and response characteristics of the innate and adaptive immune systems.

Characteristics of Innate and Acquired Immunity

	INNATE (NATURAL)	ACQUIRED (ADAPTIVE)
Effector cells	Neutrophils (polymorphonuclear), macrophages, eosinophils, basophils, mast cells, natural killer cells	B cells, T helper cells (TH), cytotoxic T cells (CTLs)

(Cont'd.)

Characteristics of Innate and Acquired Immunity (Continued)

	INNATE (NATURAL)	ACQUIRED (ADAPTIVE)
Chemical mediators	Complement, lysosomal enzymes, interferons, acute-phase proteins (e.g., mannose-binding protein and C-reactive protein)	Antibodies (immunoglobulins), cytokines, complement
Response characteristics	Rapid, nonspecific; same intensity against all antigens, no memory	Slow, antigen-specific, long-term memory with enhanced response after first exposure (e.g., more rapid and intense)

6. Distinguish between the primary and secondary immune responses.

The primary and secondary immune responses refer to the activity of the adaptive immune system. The **primary response** is the activity of the adaptive immune system after first exposure to the pathogen, whereas the **secondary response** occurs after immunologic memory has been generated from a previous exposure. The secondary response is more rapid and powerful.

7. What are the major primary and secondary organs that make up the human lymphoid system?

Primary lymphoid organs (the sites at which lymphocytes mature) include bone marrow, thymus, and fetal liver. In adults, B cells mature in the bone marrow, and T cells mature in the thymus. Maturation in these organs occurs in the absence of stimulating antigen and involves a stringent selection process that eliminates autoreactive lymphocytes.

Secondary lymphoid organs include lymph nodes, spleen, and mucosa-associated lymphoid tissue (MALT). MALT ranges from poorly organized clusters of lymphoid cells to highly organized structures such as the appendix, tonsils and Peyer's patches (in the small intestines). These secondary lymphoid organs trap antigen and provide a site for mature lymphocytes to respond.

8. What are the basic characteristics of cell-mediated and humoral immunity?

Cell-mediated immunity involves direct interactions between target cells and immune cells, including T lymphocytes, macrophages, neutrophils, and NK cells. The cell-mediated response is effective against virally infected cells, tumor cells, fungi, mycobacteria, and tissue grafts. **Humoral immunity** is mediated by soluble factors that are secreted by cells. These mediators, which include antibodies, complement, and lysozyme, are highly effective at eliminating bacteria.

Note: Effective immunity involves innate and acquired responses as well as the cooperation of cell-mediated and humoral components.

INNATE IMMUNITY		ACQUIRED IMMUNITY	
Cell-mediated	**Humoral**	**Cell-mediated**	**Humoral**
Macrophages	Complement	T lymphocytes	Antibody
Neutrophils	Lysozyme		
Natural killer cells	Interferon		

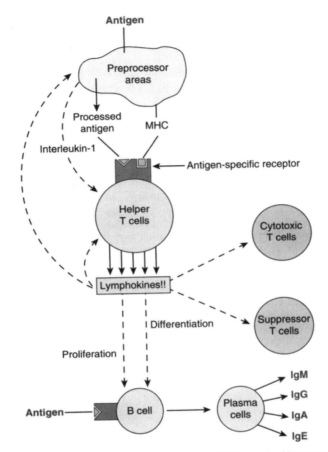

Cooperation of cell-mediated and humoral immune responses. MHC = major histocompatibility complex. (From Guyton AC, Hall JE: Textbook of Medical Physiology, 10th ed. Philadelphia, W.B. Saunders, 2000, p 409, with permission.)

9. How does antigen presentation by major histocompatibility complex (MHC) class I elicit an immunologic response? MHC class II?

T lymphocytes are MHC-restricted. They become activated only when the T-cell receptor (TcR) binds to antigen presented by MHC molecules. Specifically, $CD8^+$ cytotoxic T lymphocytes (CTLs) respond to immunogenic peptides that have been endogenously processed and presented by **MHC class I** molecules found on the surface of most nucleated cells in the body. For example, activated CTLs kill virally infected cells that display foreign viral antigen in association with surface MHC class I molecules. Specific recognition of antigen in the context of class I by the TcR on $CD8^+$ cells leads to differentiation of the mature CTLs into effector cells that directly kill target cells. Because the T cell receptor and CD8 on CTLs interact with antigen and MHC class I, these cells are MHC class I-restricted.

T_H cells, which are $CD4^+$, are **MHC class II**-restricted. They respond to immunogenic peptides that have been exogenously (via phagocytosis, endocytosis) processed and presented by MHC class II molecules found on the surface of professional antigen-presenting cells (APCs), which include macrophages, dendritic cells, and B cells. Specific recognition of antigen in the context of class II by the TcR on $CD4^+$ cells leads to differentiation of the mature T_H cells into effector cells that produce high levels of cytokines.

10. How does the immune system respond to extracellular pathogens?

Extracellular pathogens (e.g., bacteria, free virions) commonly induce production of humoral antibodies. Extracellular pathogens that are coated with opsonizing antibodies (IgG) are efficiently phagocytized by macrophages and neutrophils. Following phagocytosis and processing of extracellular antigens, expression of antigenic peptides in association with MHC class II on the surface of APCs stimulates CD4$^+$ T$_H$2 cells, which further enhance the humoral response. Keep in mind that certain antibodies activate complement (IgG, IgM) that may lyse, neutralize, or opsonize extracellular pathogens.

11. How does the immune system respond to intracellular pathogens?

In contrast to extracellular pathogens, intracellular pathogens (e.g., intracellular bacteria and protozoa and virally infected cells) stimulate a cell-mediated response characterized by activation of CD8$^+$ CTLs. This response is due to activation of CTLs after presentation of foreign antigen in association with MHC class I on infected cells. CTLs subsequently destroy the infected cells using perforins, granzymes, and *fas* binding.

12. What are the five classes of immunoglobulins? Describe their respective distributions in the body.

IgA, IgD, IgE, IgG, and IgM. Dimeric IgA and (infrequently) IgM are found in external secretions; IgE is commonly bound to FcεR1 receptors on the surface of tissue mast cells and blood basophils; IgD, IgG, monomeric IgA , and IgM are found in the blood.

IMMUNOGLOBULIN ISOTYPE	LOCATION	BIOLOGIC ACTIVITIES
IgA (two subclasses; can exist as a monomer, dimer, trimer, or tetramer)	External secretions (e.g., tears, saliva, breast milk, and mucus of bronchial, genitourinary, and digestive tracts)	Dimeric form important in protection of mucosal epithelia (prevents attachment of pathogens to mucosal cells—neutralization)
IgD (monomer)	Blood	Present on membrane of mature B cells Secreted function unknown
IgE (monomer)	Surface of mast cells and basophils	Mediates immediate (type I) hypersensitivity reactions Plays a beneficial role in parasitic infections
IgG (monomer, 4 subclasses with slightly different biologic functions)	Blood	Crosses placenta Acts as an opsonin by binding to Fc receptors of phagocytes Activates classical complement pathway Primarily secreted during a memory (secondary) response
IgM (pentameric with valence of 10)	Blood	Important in primary immune response Activates classical complement pathway Present on membrane of mature B cells (monomeric form)

13. What are complement proteins? How do they function in an immune response?

Complement proteins are a network of soluble plasma proteins that become activated as a cascade by IgM and IgG (classical pathway) or by surface molecules of microorganisms (alternative and lectin pathways). The complement proteins have many important biologic activities. The membrane attack complex (MAC) mediates cell lysis, whereas other components participate in the inflammatory response, opsonization and neutralization of pathogens, and clearance of immune complexes.

BIOLOGIC ACTIVITY	COMPLEMENT COMPONENT(S)
Cell lysis	C5b–C9 (membrane attack complex)
Degranulation of mast cells and basophils	C3a, C4a, C5a (anaphylatoxins)
Opsonization of particulate antigens	C3b, C4b, iC3b (opsonins)
Chemotaxis of leukocytes (mainly polymorpho-nuclear neutrophils)	C5a, C3a, C5b67 (chemotactic factors)
Viral neutralization	C3b, C5b–C9
Solubilization and clearance of immune complexes	C3b

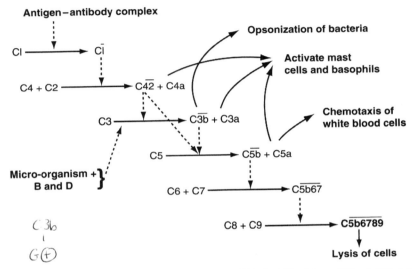

Complement cascade. (From Guyton AC, Hall JE: Textbook of Medical Physiology, 10th ed. Philadelphia, W.B. Saunders, 2000, p 408, with permission.)

14. Discuss the symptopms of complement protein deficiencies.

Deficiencies in complement proteins involve a range of symptoms, depending on which complement proteins are lacking. Patients with C1, C2, and C4 deficiencies have an increased incidence of immune complex diseases (e.g., systemic lupus erythematosus, glomerulonephritis). Because gram-positive organisms are typically resistant to complement lysis, most are cleared by opsonization with antibody and C3b. Thus, C3-deficient patients are prone to infections with encapsulated pyogenic organisms (e.g., *Streptococcus pyogenes*, *Staphylococcus aureus*, *Streptococcus pneumoniae*, *Hemophilus influenzae*). Most gram-negative organisms are susceptible to complement lysis, especially when they lack a capsule. Accordingly, when the terminal components of the lytic cascade are lacking (e.g., C5–C8), susceptibility to neisserial infections greatly increases.

15. Describe the leukocytes and their effector functions.

CELL	GENERAL DESCRIPTION	EFFECTOR MECHANISM
Monocyte	Phagocytic cell that constitutes 4–10% of WBCs in peripheral blood. Several hours after release from the bone marrow, monocytes will die or migrate into the tissue and differentiate in macrophages.	Phagocytosis

(Cont'd.)

CELL	GENERAL DESCRIPTION	EFFECTOR MECHANISM
Macrophage	Highly phagocytic tissue dwelling cells. Major functions include phagocytosis of particulate material, antigen presentation to T cells, and secretion of certain factors. *TNF α*	Antimicrobicidal activity includes generation of both oxygen-dependent mediators (e.g., superoxide anion, hydrogen peroxide, hypoclorous acid) and oxygen-independent mediators (e.g., tumor necrosis factor alpha, lysozyme, defensins, hydrolytic enzymes).
Dendritic cell	Potent antigen-presenting cells that form an extensive web in lymphoid tissue for trapping antigen (e.g., Langerhan cells in the epidermis).	Phagocytosis
Neutrophil	Type of granulocyte that makes up ~70% of WBCs in peripheral blood. Neutrophils are active phagocytes that are the first cell to arrive at sites of inflammation.	Like macrophages, they employ both oxygen-dependent and oxygen-independent pathways to generate antimicrobial substances.
Eosinophil	Type of granulocyte that makes up 2–5% of WBCs in peripheral blood. It is a phagocytic cell that migrates into tissue spaces, where it plays a role in defense against parasitic organisms.	Exocytosis of granules containing extremely basic proteins *major basic protein*
Basophil	Nonphagocytic granulocyte that makes up 0.5–1% of peripheral WBCs. Basophils play a major role in allergic responses.	Release of pharmacologically active substances from cytoplasmic granules (histamine and other vasoactive amines) upon crosslinking of surface-bound IgE by allergen.
Mast cell *CD14*	Tissue-dwelling cell that plays a similar role in allergic responses to basophils. Mast cells have surface receptors for IgE and histamine-containing granules.	Release of pharmacologically active substances from cytoplasmic granules (histamine and other vasoactive amines) upon crosslinking of surface-bound IgE by allergen.
Helper T cell *CD4*	$CD4^+$ lymphocyte that matures in the thymus and functions in cytokine production. TH cells play a central role in the immune response by regulating the function of cells such as CTLs, B cells, NK cells, and macrophages. TH cells are activated by foreign antigen in the context of MHC class II molecules.	Secretion of various cytokines that may stimulate cell-mediated immunity (from T_H1 cells) or humoral immunity (from T_H2 cells).
Cytotoxic T cell *CD8*	A $CD8^+$ lymphocyte that matures in the thymus and functions in direct cell killing upon activation by foreign antigen presented by MHC class I molecules.	Perforins, granzymes, interferon gamma, tumor necrosis beta, *fas* ligand
B cell *CD 19 20*	A $CD20^+$ lymphocyte that has membrane-bound immunoglobulin. Upon activation by soluble antigen, B cells differentiate into plasma cells. By presenting endocytosed antigen in the cleft of class II, B cells also function as antigen presenting cells in the activation of T_H cells.	Antibody

CD3x

(Cont.d)

CELL	GENERAL DESCRIPTION	EFFECTOR MECHANISM
Natural killer cell $CD\ 16,56$	A large granular lymphocyte that has no markers in common with B or T cells and is not MHC-restricted. NK cells act to lyse virally infected cells and tumor cells with decreased levels of MHC class I.	Perforins, granzymes, interferon gamma, tumor necrosis factor alpha

CASE 1

Shortly after taking the first dose of a course of amoxicillin, a two-year-old boy becomes acutely short of breath, has audible wheezing, and develops pruritic hives. He also has a bout of nausea and diarrhea. His mother takes him to the emergency department, where he is found to be dangerously hypotensive with severe tachycardia and tachypnea. The child is immediately given a subcutaneous injection of epinephrine as well as intravenous diphenhydramine (Benadryl) and methylprednisolone. It is explained to the mother that this acute episode was most likely due to the amoxicillin, but she seems confused because he had taken amoxicillin previously to treat an ear infection and had no problems with it.

1. What is the diagnosis?
Acute systemic anaphylaxis (anaphylactic shock).

Note: The most serious result of drug hypersensitivity is anaphylaxis (i.e., systemic involvement causing acute shortness of breath, wheezing, and hypotension). However, the most common drug reaction involves cutaneous symptoms, such as generalized flushing, urticaria, or angioedema.

2. What type of hypersensitivity disorder is anaphylaxis? Describe its immunopathogenesis.
Anaphylaxis is the systemic form of the immediate hypersensitivity response (type I). Circulating allergen binds to IgE that is present on mast cells and basophils, triggering the release of preformed histamine and the de novo synthesis and release of lipid mediators (e.g., leukotrienes, prostaglandins, platelet-activating factor). The short-lived effects of histamine include a widespread increase in vascular permeability and smooth muscle contraction. Leukotrienes elicit prolonged bronchoconstriction, mucus secretion, and an increase in vascular permeability. There can also be a late-phase inflammatory response after exposure to an allergen that involves leukocyte migration and activation.

Note: Penicillin is the most common cause of medication-induced anaphylaxis, but such reactions are still quite rare with this class of antibiotics.

3. What is the pathophysiologic explanation for the wheezing and diarrhea that developed?
Release of mast-cell mediators, such as histamine and leukotrienes, causes an increase in vascular permeability and contraction of certain smooth muscle types in multiple organ systems. In the airways this process leads to laryngeal edema, bronchoconstriction, and mucus hypersecretion, resulting in wheezing. In the gastrointestinal tract, smooth muscle contraction and edema result in nausea, vomiting, and diarrhea.

Note: Allergic asthma is also a type I hypersensitivity reaction, causing bronchospasm for the same reasons as anaphylaxis.

4. How does anaphylaxis cause urticaria?
The widespread vasodilation and increased vascular permeability that develop in anaphylaxis allow fluid to accumulate in the superficial dermis, producing little wheals with a pale

center encircled by a red flare. This same mechanism is responsible for edema in the deep dermis (angioedema) and laryngeal edema, which can develop in anaphylaxis.

5. Why was the child immediately given epinephrine?

Epinephrine reverses anaphylaxis through its positive adrenergic effects. By stimulating beta-2 receptors, it relaxes bronchial smooth muscles to make breathing easier; by stimulating peripheral alpha-1 receptors, it constricts small blood vessels, thereby reducing vascular leakage and raising blood pressure.

6. Why was the child given diphenhydramine and methylprednisolone?

Diphenhydramine is an H_1 receptor antagonist that ameliorates the histamine-mediated components of anaphylaxis. Methylprednisolone is an anti-inflammatory corticosteroid that blocks the late-phase allergic response involving recruitment of neutrophils and eosinophils.

7. Why did the child have no reaction to amoxicillin when it was first administered for his previous ear infection?

He was not sensitized to the allergen at that time. Several days after initial exposure, an allergen generates allergen-specific IgE antibodies, which become bound to receptors on the mast-cell surface (sensitization). Repeat exposure to the same allergen crosslinks the IgE-bound mast cells and causes degranulation (release of histamine and other vasoactive amines).

8. What clinical testing can be performed to confirm that the immediate hypersensitivity reaction was caused by amoxicillin?

A few days after the attack, a skin test for amoxicillin and other common drug allergens can be performed. If the child is allergic, intradermal injections of amoxicillin will cause degranulation of local mast cells at the site of injection. The resultant release of histamine and other mediators causes a large wheal and flare to develop within 30 minutes. The wheal is a central raised area reflecting leakage of plasma from venules (edema), and the flare is a surrounding red area caused by vasodilation (erythema).

9. What was the motivation for developing the second-generation H_1 receptor antagonists such as fexofenadine (Allegra)?

These agents do not cross the blood-brain barrier like the first generation H_1 receptor antagonists and do not cause as much drowsiness. They are generally used for allergic rhinitis, another (milder) type I hypersensitivity response.

Note: Cromolyn sodium and nedocromil are used to prevent type I hypersensitivity reactions by inhibiting mast-cell degranulation and are referred to as mast-cell stabilizers.

10. List the common classes of drugs that are used to treat type I hypersensitivity disorders along with their general mode of action and clinical indications.

TYPE OF DRUG	MODE OF ACTION	CLINICAL INDICATION	COMMENTS
Antihistamines	Block H_1 and H_2 receptors on target cells	Allergic rhinitis, atopic dermatitis, allergic conjunctivitis	Second-generation histamine receptor antagonists have fewer adverse side effects (e.g., they are nonsedating)
Mast-cell stabilizers	Prophylactic inhibitors of mast-cell mediator release	Allergic rhinitis and asthma	Include cromolyn sodium and nedocromil
Corticosteroids	Anti-inflammatory; block production of inflammatory cytokines	Allergic asthma, atopic dermatitis	Include prednisone, beclamethasone, triamcinolone, flunisolide

(Cont'd.)

TYPE OF DRUG	MODE OF ACTION	CLINICAL INDICATION	COMMENTS
Sympatho-mimetics	Adrenergic effects	Acute and chronic asthma	Epinephrine has both alpha- and beta-adrenergic effects; albuterol, metaproterenol, and isoetharine are selective beta-adrenergic bronchodilators
Leukotriene pathway inhibitors	Prophylactic inhibitors of leukotriene synthesis or receptor antagonists	Asthma	Include cysteinyl leukotriene receptor antagonists (e.g., zafirlukast, montelukast) and 5-lipoxygenase inhibitors (e.g., zileuton)

CASE 2

A 43-year-old man with uncomplicated pneumococcal pneumonia is prescribed a 10-day course of penicillin G. On the ninth day, he appears a little jaundiced, and his hematocrit has dropped significantly from when he was first seen. He denies any hemoptysis, hematemesis, melena, or hematochezia. Additional tests reveal an elevated reticulocyte count, elevated indirect bilirubin, and a positive direct Coombs' test.

1. What is the probable diagnosis?
Autoimmune hemolytic anemia.

2. What is the significance of a positive Coombs' test? How does it support the diagnosis in this patient?
A Coombs' test is an antiglobulin assay that detects both immunoglobulin attached to the surface of RBCs (direct test) and the presence of circulating immunoglobulin against RBCs (indirect test). A positive Coombs' test supports but does not prove the presence of an immune-mediated hemolytic process.

3. How do medications such as penicillin cause immune hemolytic anemia?
Certain antibiotics (e.g., penicillin, cephalosporins, streptomycin, tetracycline) and other small molecules may nonspecifically adsorb to proteins on red blood cell surfaces, forming a complex similar to a hapten-carrier complex. These drugs are generally too small to elicit an immune response by themselves; however, they can become immunogenic when combined with larger molecules such as cell membranes. This complex can induce the formation of antibodies, which then bind to the adsorbed drug on RBCs. The presence of these autoantibodies is detected in the direct Coombs' test.

Note: This is an example of a type II hypersensitivity reaction, in which IgM or IgG antibodies bind to cell surface antigens. Other examples of type II hypersensitivity include blood transfusion reactions, Graves' disease, myasthenia gravis, hyperacute rejection of organ transplants, and hemolytic disease of the newborn.

4. What is the mechanism by which hemolysis occurs in drug-induced immune hemolytic anemias?
Both IgG and IgM can induce complement-mediated lysis of red blood cells. In addition, IgG can damage red blood cells by binding and activating effector cells carrying Fc_ receptors (e.g., neutrophils, macrophages and NK cells).

Note: In some people the extended use of certain drugs, including methyldopa, levodopa, and procainamide, can stimulate production of anti-RBC antibodies. The mechanism by which the autoantibodies are induced is unknown, and the antibodies do not cross-react with the drug that appears to elicit their production.

CASE 3

A 12-year-old boy who stepped on a nail in Zimbabwe was given horse antitetanus immune serum. The next week he had puffy eyes, swelling around the mouth, a tight feeling in his throat, and widespread urticaria. Later he developed a fever, swollen lymph nodes and spleen, and swollen and painful ankles. Laboratory tests of a blood sample revealed an elevated white blood cell count with the majority of the cells being lymphocytes. Plasma cells were detected in a peripheral blood smear. His total serum complement level and his C1q and C3 levels were decreased. Urinalysis revealed proteinuria and hematuria. The patient was started on prednisone, and all of his symptoms progressively improved.

1. What is the diagnosis?
Serum sickness.

2. Describe the pathogenesis of serum sickness.
Serum sickness is a type III hypersensitivity reaction caused by the formation of immune complexes and their deposition in the tissues, eventuating in activation of the complement cascade. Immune complexes form when antigen and antibody bind together. In this case, the antibody is most likely the patient's IgG with specificity for the highly immunogenic horse serum proteins (e.g., horse immunoglobulins). These complexes may deposit in tissues if large amounts of antigen and antibody are present, creating more immune complexes than the mononuclear phagocyte system can clear from the circulation. In addition, some of the smaller immune complexes that are not cleared effectively by phagocytosis are taken up by endothelial cells in various parts of the body and deposited in tissues. Local activation of the complement system by these complexes provokes an inflammatory response.

Note: Systemic lupus nephritis is a type III hypersensitivity disorder with the same pathogenesis, but the antigens are from the patient's own cells.

3. What is the significance of decreased serum levels of complement?
This finding indicates consumption of complement, most likely due to activation of the classical pathway by immune complexes.

Note: IgG- and IgM-containing complexes activate the classical pathway. IgG-, IgA-, and IgE-containing complexes, although less efficient, can activate the alternative pathway.

4. What caused the hives and facial swelling?
The production of complement components C3a, C4a, and C5a (anaphylatoxins) elicits mediator release from mast cells. Histamine and leukotrienes cause vasodilation and increased vascular permeability that lead to localized and systemic edema.

5. What is the significance of RBCs and protein in the urine?
One potential site of immune complex deposition in type III hypersensitivity is the renal glomeruli. Inflammation at this site (nephritis) is likely to result in proteinuria and hematuria.

Note: Most causes of glomerulonephritis (e.g., poststreptococcal status, IgA nephropathy) are also caused by a type III hypersensitivity reaction. When the complexes deposit in synovial tissue, the resulting inflammation of the joints produces the arthritis seen in rheumatoid arthritis, an autoimmune disease that is also classified as type III hypersensitivity.

6. Does manifestation of a type III hypersensitivity reaction require previous exposure (sensitization) to antigen?
No. If an exogenous antigen is given in large excess on first exposure it can cause formation of large numbers of immune complexes. Their subsequent deposition in tissue leads to activation of the complement cascade.

7. Why has the increasing use of antibody therapy lead to a greater incidence of immune complex-mediated illness?

Therapeutic antibodies are typically synthesized in other species and are thus highly immunogenic in humans. Recipients may mount a humoral immune response to the drug, forming immune complexes that can activate complement. Serum sickness after the administration of snake antivenom (horse antibody to venom) is a good example of this phenomenon. Recent advances in recombinant technology allow the production of chimeric antibodies (part human) that are much less immunogenic.

CASE 4

A 23-year-old woman uses Solarcaine Aerosol (benzocaine 20%, triclosam 0.13%) to relieve the pain of sunburn. She applies the anesthetic to her arms and upper chest. After 2 days a rash covers both arms, her torso, and her face. She takes diphenhydramine (Benadryl) to control the itching. When the rash does not improve within 1 week, she visits her dermatologist. Physical examination reveals large patches of raised, red blisters filled with clear fluid on her body and extremities. She also has swollen eyelids. There is no history of fever, fatigue, or any other symptom. She is given a corticosteroid-containing cream to apply to the skin lesions and oral diphenhydramine. Within 1 week the rash has almost disappeared.

1. What is the diagnosis?

Contact dermatitis.

2. What is the causative agent? Describe the mechanism by which it induced an immune response.

Benzocaine and other ingredients in topical drugs constitute a major cause of contact dermatitis, a type IV or delayed-type hypersensitivity (DTH) response. Antigen-presenting cells in the skin (dendritic Langerhans cells) internalize self-proteins to which exogenous molecules are bound (haptenated self-proteins). This process renders the self-proteins immunogenic and results in activation of sensitized T_H1 (T_{DTH}) cells, release of cytokines, and subsequent activation of tissue macrophages. The release of lytic enzymes by the macrophages results in the redness and pustules that characterize the patient's reaction to benzocaine.

3. Why is the correct diagnosis contact dermatitis rather than atopic dermatitis?

The appearance of a rash 48–72 hours after topical application of the anesthetic is typical of a delayed hypersensitivity reaction (assuming the person has already been exposed and sensitized). In a sensitized person, IgE-mediated dermatitis (atopic dermatitis) manifests symptoms within minutes of exposure to allergen, and they may persist for up to 24 hours. Another good example of contact dermatitis is the poison ivy-induced eczematous reaction that occurs several hours after contact with the plant.

4. Why did the patient have lesions in areas other than her arms and upper chest (where she applied the lotion)?

The topical drug can be transferred from the initial point of contact to other areas of the skin by the fingernails after scratching the itchy lesions at the primary site. Therefore, unexpected sites can be affected (e.g., eyelids and genitals).

5. Why is it important for the patient to avoid the use of benzocaine in the future?

Once a person is sensitized, each subsequent exposure not only produces the hypersensitivity reaction but also generates more effector and memory T cells. Thus the reaction becomes worse with each exposure. Memory T cells can persist for the person's lifetime.

Note: The first contact with an allergen does not typically result in a type IV allergic response (as is also the case in type I reactions). Accordingly, a contact hypersensitivity has a sensitization stage, in which a clonal population of memory CD4⁺ T cells is produced, and an elicitation stage, in which the memory T cells become activated on subsequent exposure to antigen. In addition, a person may be able to touch the material (allergen) for many years without adverse reaction.

6. Summarize hypersensitivity reactions.

CLASSIFI-CATION	DEFINITION	MEDIATOR	MECHANISM OF DESTRUCTION	CLINICAL PRESENTATION	DETECTION
Type I	IgE-mediated immediate hypersensitivity	IgE	Mast-cell degranulation induced by allergen cross-linked IgE	Systemic anaphylaxis, allergic rhinitis, bronchial asthma, atopic dermatitis, food allergies	Skin testing RIST, RAST
Type II	Antibody-mediated cytotoxic hypersensitivity	IgM, IgG	Antibodies directed against cell-bound antigens induce destruction of cells or tissues	Transfusion reactions, hemolytic disease of the newborn, autoimmune hemolytic anemia	Direct and indirect Coombs' test and specific antibody tests
Type III	Immune complex-mediated hypersensitivity	IgG	Antibodies directed against soluble serum antigen form circulating complexes that deposit nonspecifically in tissue and activate complement	Serum sickness, glomerulonephritis, rheumatoid arthritis, systemic lupus erythematosus	Serum complement levels, specific tests (anti-DS DNA, rheumatoid factor), biopsy (glomerulonephritis)
Type IV	Cell-mediated delayed hypersensitivity	T$_{DTH}$ cells	Antigen-specific T$_H$1 cells activate tissue macrophages and stimulate a local inflammatory response over 24–78 hours	Contact dermatitis, tuberculin-type hypersensitivity, granulomatous hypersensitivity, acute tissue graft rejection	Patch test

RIST = radioimmunosorbent test, RAST = radioallergosorbent test.

CASE 5

A 4-month-old boy is evaluated for a runny nose and cough that have persisted for over 1 month. Examination reveals oral thrush and failure to thrive, as indicated by a fall from the 50th percentile in weight to the 10th percentile. Chest x-ray demonstrates a diffuse, symmetric interstitial infiltrate. Lab tests reveal marked lymphopenia with normal numbers of CD20⁺ cells (B lymphocytes) and an absence of CD3⁺ cells (T lymphocytes). Further specialized testing reveals that blood lymphocytes are unresponsive to the B- and T-cell mitogen, pokeweed (PWM). A diagnosis of *Pneumocystis carinii* pneumonia (PCP) is made, with a silver stain of sputum. The boy responds well to intravenous trimethoprim-sulfamethoxazole. Testing to rule out HIV infection was negative.

1. What is the most likely diagnosis, given the fact that specialized testing revealed defects in both cellular and humoral function?

Severe combined immunodeficiency (SCID). This condition is invariably fatal in infants unless recognized and treated by bone marrow transplant. Typically, babies with SCID become ill within the first 3 months of life, suffering from recurrent respiratory infections, pneumonia, thrush, diarrhea, and failure to thrive. Opportunistic infections with intracellular pathogens such as *Candida albicans*, *Pneumocystis carinii*, *Cryptococcus neoformans*, and *Mycobacteria* spp. are commonly observed in such infants.

Note: These are the same opportunistic organisms that commonly affect patients with AIDS.

2. Why is a bone marrow transplant from an appropriate donor likely to cure this boy?

The pathogenesis of SCID involves abnormal production and function of mature T cells. After transplantation of normal T-cell precursors (with no genetic defect), the infant's immune system will reconstitute with mature, functional CD3$^+$ T cells.

3. What is the significance of the marked lymphopenia and complete lack of CD3$^+$ cells?

SCID is a family of primary immune disorders characterized by low numbers of circulating lymphocytes; myeloid and erythroid cells appear normal in number and function. Within the lymphocyte population, T-cell numbers are typically low to absent, B-cell numbers are fairly normal, and NK-cell numbers may be low to normal. The affected infant fails to mount an immune response mediated by T cells, and this lack of cell-mediated immunity makes patients with SCID highly susceptible to opportunistic infection with intracellular organisms.

4. Since B cell numbers are normal, why is SCID classified as a combined immune deficiency?

Activation of B cells requires the involvement of T_H cells. An absence of T cells means that B cells cannot function even if they are not directly affected by the defect. Thus humoral and cell-mediated functions are deficient.

5. Why are B-cell defects not evident in many infants when they are first diagnosed with SCID?

The infants have antibodies in their circulation that have been passively obtained from transplacental circulation (IgG) or mother's milk (IgA). As these antibodies are cleared over time and the infant becomes responsible for its own immunoglobulin synthesis, all levels will be low to absent.

6. What are the most common causes of SCID?

Several forms of SCID arise from different genetic defects. The most common form is due to an X-linked mutation leading to several defective interleukin receptors that are responsible for activation and proliferation of lymphocytes. Another common cause is deficiency of the enzyme adenosine deaminase. Absence of this enzyme leads to accumulation of metabolic byproducts that are toxic to lymphocytes.

7. What primary immunodeficiency should be suspected in a baby boy with normal cell-mediated immunity but almost completely absent plasma immunoglobulins?

Bruton's agammaglobulinemia is an X linked immunodeficiency syndrome. Affected boys have few or no B cells in their blood or lymphoid tissue, and their serum usually contains no immunoglobulins except for small amounts of IgG. The defect involves a tyrosine kinase that is crucial to the maturation of pre-B cells.

8. Hypogammaglobulinemia is also seen in common variable immunodeficiency (CVID). How does CVID differ from Bruton's agammaglobulinemia?

Common variable immunodeficiency typically manifests later in life and affects males and females equally. CVID is also characterized by decreased numbers of antibody-producing plasma cells and extremely low levels of most immunoglobulin isotypes.

CASE 6

A 14-year-old boy is admitted to the hospital with severe shortness of breath, persistent cough, and chest pain. A chest x-ray reveals the presence of large fuzzy densities in both lungs. Aspirate from one of the lesions grows *Aspergillus fumigatus*. The white cell count is normal with normal proportions of neutrophils, lymphocytes, and monocytes. Serum antibody levels are in the high normal range. In a white cell function test, monocytes and neutrophils fail to reduce nitroblue tetrazolium (NBT), a test of the adequacy of the oxidative respiratory burst. The child is started on intravenous amphotericin B and given a tracheotomy to assist with ventilation. He slowly improves over a 2-month period. However, during this time in the hospital he contracts two bacterial respiratory infections that are treated with antibiotics. The patient is started on treatment with injections of interferon-gamma (IFN-γ) and subsequently released from the hospital.

1. What is the diagnosis?

Chronic granulomatous disease (CGD), a disease of monocyte/macrophage and neutrophil dysfunction.

2. What are the two mechanisms by which a macrophage may kill bacteria following phagocytosis?

Destruction of internalized pathogens by macrophages (and neutrophils) involves both oxygen-dependent and oxygen-independent mechanisms. During phagocytosis a metabolic process known as the respiratory burst occurs. This process depends on the activity of reduced nicotinamide adenine dinucleotide phosphate (NADPH) oxidase and results in the generation of reactive oxygen intermediates. The macrophage may also kill ingested pathogens using lysozyme, various hydrolytic enzymes, and cytotoxic peptides. The degradative activities of these factors do not require oxygen.

3. What is the genetic basis of CGD?

The most common form of CGD involves mutations in the X-linked gene encoding NADPH oxidase. A deficiency in this enzyme results in an inability of phagocytes to kill ingested pathogens; hence, the formation of granulomas following bacterial and fungal infections.

4. What may account for the large fuzzy densities in both lungs?

These densities are characteristic of a fungal infection that cannot be cleared by phagocytic cells in the lung (alveolar macrophages). The cells attempt to "wall off" the infection by forming multinucleated giant cells (fused macrophages) surrounded by CD4+ T cells. The sustained activation of chronically infected macrophages results in a persistent localized inflammation called a granuloma; hence, the designation chronic *granulomatous* disease.

Note: Select other diseases that result from failure of macrophages to clear infection, resulting in granuloma formation, include tuberculosis and coccidiomycosis.

5. What agents are most commonly responsible for infections in CGD?

Intracellular fungi and bacteria most often cause the infections and granuloma formation observed in CGD since most of these organisms reside in macrophages.

6. How does Chediak-Higashi syndrome (CHS) differ from CGD?

CHS is also a primary immunodeficiency of the myeloid lineage. It is an autosomal recessive disorder that renders lysosomes incapable of lysing intracellular bacteria. Recurrent infections with organisms similar to those seen in CGD are common. In contrast to CGD, an NBT test is normal for CHS because oxygen consumption and hydrogen peroxide formation in phagocytes do occur.

7. **Compare and contrast monocytes and macrophages with respect to origin, location, lifespan, and function.**

Both monocytes and macrophages are phagocytes derived from myeloid stem cells in the bone marrow. Monocytes circulate in the blood stream for several hours, during which time many enlarge, migrate into various tissues, and differentiate into macrophages. Monocytes that remain in the blood survive for 1–2 days, whereas those that become tissue-dwelling macrophages have longer life spans of 4–15 days. Macrophages serve different functions in different tissues and are named according to their location (see table, next page).

MACROPHAGE TYPE	TISSUE LOCATION	FUNCTION
Kupffer cells	Liver	Removal of senescent RBCs and debris
Splenic macrophages	Spleen	Removal of senescent RBCs and debris
Mesangial cells	Kidney	Phagocytosis
Microglial cells	Central nervous system	Ingest degenerated myelin
Histiocytes	Connective tissue	Phagocytosis
Alveolar macrophages	Lung	Phagocytosis of inhaled particles

CASE 7

A 12-week-old girl is evaluated by a pediatric cardiologist for a congenital heart defect. The mother notes that a neurologist is also evaluating the girl for repeated muscle "seizures." Physical exam reveals several facial abnormalities, including low-set ears, wide-set eyes (hypertelorism), a small jaw (micrognathia), and a fish-shaped mouth. Laboratory evaluation is remarkable for hypocalcemia, and a chest x-ray reveals absence of a thymic shadow.

1. **What is the likely diagnosis? Describe the pathophysiology of this disorder.**

DiGeorge syndrome (also known as DiGeorge anomaly, congenital thymic aplasia). This genetic disorder is caused by microdeletions of DNA on chromosome 22, resulting in dysmorphogenesis of the third and fourth pharyngeal pouches during embryologic development. Because the thymus and lower two parathyroids normally arise from this tissue, these structures may be absent in DiGeorge syndrome. For the same reason, the heart and aorta may also be affected.

Note: DiGeorge syndrome is typically detected early in life after evaluation of infants suffering from hypocalcemia-induced seizures (due to hypoparathyroidism).

2. **To what type of infections may the child be vulnerable, given that thymic development is abnormal?**

The thymus is a primary lymphoid organ that is responsible for the maturation of progenitor T cells. When the thymus is underdeveloped or lacking, there is a dramatic decrease in all populations of T cells and a corresponding lack of cell-mediated immunity. Patients with DiGeorge syndrome who survive the immediate neonatal period are susceptible to recurrent or chronic fungal and viral infections that normally would be eradicated by cytotoxic T cells. In addition, because T helper (T_H) cells and their cytokines (e.g., IL-2, IL-4, IL-5) are critical to the proliferation and differentiation of B cells, humoral immunity deteriorates over time as the maternal antibodies are degraded. Thus, the patient also becomes susceptible to infection with extracellular pathogens such as bacteria, which are normally defended against by the humoral system.

3. **Would you expect the humoral response to be normal in this infant?**

Because DiGeorge anomaly is typically diagnosed shortly after birth, immunoglobulin levels may appear normal at this time due to passive transfer of maternal antibodies.

4. What may a lymph node biopsy in this infant reveal?

Thymic absence or hypoplasia in DiGeorge syndrome results in inadequate production of functionally mature T cells. Histologic analysis of lymph nodes, therefore, reveals nearly complete absence of T cells in the normal T cell-dependent zones of lymph nodes.

5. What does the process of "thymic education" involve?

The education of thymocytes involves both positive and negative selection and ensures that mature T cells will be MHC-restricted and self-tolerant, respectively. During positive selection, T cells able to recognize (bind) MHC molecules are selected to survive. Negative selection involves apoptosis of T cells that avidly bind self-peptide in association with MHC molecules (self-reactive T cells). Less than 5% of the thymocytes survive these selection processes.

6. Summarize the primary immunodeficiencies.

CLASSIFICATION	EXAMPLES OF IMMUNO-DEFICIENCY SYNDROMES	IMMUNE DEFECT	SUSCEPTIBILITY
B-cell deficiencies	Bruton's agammaglobulinemia (also known as X-linked agammaglobulinemia [XLA])	Few to no B cells; only Ig found in serum is IgG at very low levels	Recurrent pyogenic infections
	IgA deficiency	B cells fail to produce IgA and often IgG2 and IgG4	Recurrent pyogenic infections; immune complex disease
	X-linked hyper-IgM syndrome	No B-cell class switching from IgM to other isotypes	Recurrent pyogenic infections; auto-immune disease
	CVID _(Adult)_	Late onset agammaglobulinemia that has acquired and inherited characteristics; commonly follows viral infection	Recurrent pyogenic infections
T-cell deficiencies*	SCID	Few to no lymphocytes in blood or lymphatics	Opportunistic infections
	DiGeorge syndrome	Variable T-cell numbers resulting from thymic maldevelopment	Opportunistic infections; viral infections
	Wiskott-Aldrich syndrome (WAS)	X-linked defect in T cells and platelets; normal IgG, decreased IgM, and increased IgA and IgE	Opportunistic infections; pyogenic infections
Complement deficiencies	Deficiencies in early components of classical pathway	C1q, C1r, C1s, C2, and C4 deficiency	Immune complex disease (lupus, glomerulonephritis, vasculitis)
	C3 deficiency	Complement component is absent	Recurrent pyogenic (gram-negative) bacterial infection; immune complex disease

(Cont'd.)

CLASSIFICATION	EXAMPLES OF IMMUNO-DEFICIENCY SYNDROMES	IMMUNE DEFECT	SUSCEPTIBILITY
Complement deficiencies (cont'd.)	Deficiencies in terminal components of classical pathway	C5, C6, C7, and C8 deficiency	Recurrent meningo-coccal and gono-coccal infections caused by *Neisseria* species
	Deficiencies in comple-ment regulatory proteins	C1 inhibitor deficiency	Hereditary angio-edema
		Deficiencies in decay-accelerating factor (DAF) and homologous restric-tion factor (HRF)	Paroxysmal nocturnal hemoglobinuria (PNH)
Phagocyte deficiencies	Chronic granulomatous disease (CGD)	Defective oxidative killing pathway of phagocytes	Increased susceptibil-ity to intracellular bacteria and fungi; malignant granu-loma formation
	Chediak-Higashi syndrome	Defective lytic pathway of phagocytes	Recurrent bacterial infections
	Leukocyte adhesion deficiency (LAD)	Defective phagocyte membrane protein, resulting in defective phagocytosis and tissue migration	Severe gram-positive and gram-negative bacterial infections

* Since B-cell function is largely T cell-dependent, primary T-cell deficiencies result in combined deficiency of cell-mediated and humoral immunity.

CASE 8

A 42-year-old woman complains to her physician of a "run-down" feeling, recurrent low-grade fevers, and swollen lymph nodes in her neck. One year earlier she had a hysterectomy, from which she recovered quickly, but due to blood loss during the surgery she was given 2 units of blood. Results of her current blood work reveal that she has antibodies to human immunodeficiency virus (HIV). Subsequently, her husband also tests positive for antibodies to HIV. The woman is started on a combination of retroviral drugs (highly active antiretro-viral therapy [HAART]). Her CD4+ T-cell count is below 200 μl^{-1}, and she develops *Pneumocystis carinii* pneumonia. Despite treatment with trimethoprim and sulfamethoxa-zole, the infection recurs, and she dies 5 months later. Her husband remains asymptomatic despite the persistence of HIV antibodies in his serum.

1. Describe the disease caused by infection with HIV.

Acquired immunodeficiency syndrome (AIDS) is a secondary immunodeficiency that in-volves a decrease in cell-mediated immunity, resulting in recurrent opportunistic infections and a high incidence of certain cancers.

2. What is the major cause of death in AIDS?

Opportunistic infections and malignancies are the end result of the severe immunosuppres-sion of patients with HIV infection. Respiratory infection with *Pneumocystis carinii* is the most prominent cause of death. Other opportunistic pathogens and malignancies that are a major cause of mortality in AIDS are listed in the table below.

PARASITES	BACTERIA	FUNGI	VIRUSES	MALIGNANCIES
Toxoplasma spp.	*Mycobacterium*	*Pneumocystis carinii*	Herpes	Kaposi's
Cryptosporidium	*tuberculosis*	*Cryptococcus*	simplex	sarcoma
spp.	*Salmonella* spp.	*neoformans*	Cytomegalovirus	Burkitt's
Leishmania spp.		*Candida* spp.	Varicella zoster	lymphoma
Microsporidium		*Histoplasma*		Non-Hodgkin's
spp.		*capsulatum*		lymphoma
		Coccidioides immitis		

3. Briefly describe HIV and its life cycle.

HIV is an encapsulated retrovirus. Two viral envelope glycoproteins, gp120 and gp 41, allow the virus to infect CD4+ host cells that express an appropriate coreceptor, CXCR4 or CCR5. Host targets of HIV-1, and less frequently HIV-2, include T lymphocytes, monocytes-macrophages, follicular dendritic cells, Langerhans cells, and microglial cells. Upon entry into the cell, the virus efficiently copies its RNA genome into double-stranded DNA using the viral enzyme, reverse transcriptase (RT). The viral DNA copy is integrated into the host cell genome, aided by the viral enzyme integrase. The proviral form of the virus may remain latent in the cell until its expression is signaled. Expression of functional proteins by the virus involves a virally encoded protease that cleaves polyproteins into smaller functional proteins. When the provirus is expressed to form new virions, the host cell typically lyses.

4. What is the mechanism of CD4+ T cell depletion in HIV infection?

Infected cells can be killed by the cytotoxic effects of the virus (excessive budding of viruses causes host membrane lysis) or by activation of cytotoxic T lymphocytes.

5. What classes of drugs are used in HAART?

The first class of antiretroviral drugs includes two types of reverse transcriptase inhibitors. Nucleoside analog reverse transcriptase inhibitors (NRTIs) are incorporated by RT into the transcribed DNA strand, where they block further extension of the strand and thereby inhibit viral replication. Nonnucleoside reverse transcriptase inhibitors (NNRTIs) inhibit the action of the RT enzyme. A second class of drugs called protease inhibitors has proven effective when used in combination with NRTIs and NNRTIs. This type of combination therapy is designated HAART. The following table contains some anti-HIV drugs (common names) that are in clinical use.

REVERSE TRANSCRIPTASE INHIBITORS		
NUCLEOSIDE ANALOGS	NONNUCLEOSIDE ANALOGS	PROTEASE INHIBITORS
Zidovudine (AZT)	Delavirdine	Indinavir
Lamivudine (3TC)	Nevirapine	Ritonavir
Stavudine (d4T)	Efavirenz	Saquinavir
Didanosine (ddl)		Nelfinavir
Zalcitabine (ddC)		Amprenavir
Abacavir		
Combivir (3TC and AZT)		

6. Define the four stages of HIV infection.

The person with **acute HIV infection** may remain asymptomatic or develop an acute illness that resembles the flu or infectious mononucleosis. Symptoms usually develop within 2–6 weeks after infection. During this stage, antibodies to HIV are generally undetectable. **Clinical latency** is an asymptomatic period that varies greatly in duration. Persistent infection and replication of HIV gradually cause a decrease in CD4+ cells. Seroconversion (the appearance of anti-HIV antibodies) occurs during this stage. During **AIDS-related complex (ARC)** more chronic symptoms of infection (lymphadenopathy, weight loss, fever, malaise) develop as T cell counts further decline.

AIDS is defined in a person who is HIV positive and has a T cell count below 200 μl^{-1} or who presents with one of the AIDS-defining opportunistic infections/malignancies.

7. What is the most important determinant of the progression of HIV infection?

When monitoring patients, the CD4 count should be measured in conjunction with viral load. CD4 numbers indicate the damage that has occurred to the immune system and thus the risk of progression to AIDS. Viral load is an indication of the pace at which the damage is occurring.

8. Explain why certain individuals remain infected with HIV for up to 12 years with no symptoms.

Following seroconversion is a variable stage of asymptomatic infection (latency). The length of this latency period seems to be extended in patients whose virus burden is low. In addition, patients infected with HIV strains containing mutations in genes that are vital to its replication have a longer latency period. In both situations, patients seem to better handle (with cytotoxic T lymphocytes) the limited viral replication for longer periods. In addition, rare individuals are resistant to infection with HIV due to mutations in the coreceptor for the virus.

CASE 9

A 55-year-old man develops end-stage renal disease due to poorly controlled type I diabetes mellitus. He has undergone hemodialysis twice weekly for 6 months while waiting for a kidney transplant. Since he has no living blood relatives, he is in need of a cadaveric donor. His blood is type B, Rh-positive. A cadaveric kidney is found from a 28-year-old woman who was fatally injured in a car accident. The donor is blood type B positive, with one matched HLA-A allele to the recipient. Before the transplantation, a final crossmatch reveals that the recipient is nonreactive. Immunosuppressive therapy after the transplant procedure involves administration of azathioprine, cyclosporin A, methylprednisone, and antithymocyte globulin (ATG). Two weeks after the procedure, the patient is discharged from the hospital on azathioprine, cyclosporin A, and prednisone. His blood pressure and serum creatinine are normal. At 1-week follow-up, the patient complains of decreased urine output and has high levels of serum creatinine. The area around the graft is enlarged and tender to the touch. Renal biopsy shows the presence of many lymphocytes in the transplant. The patient is given high-dose steroids (500 mg of methylprednisone) and OKT3. This immunosuppressive regimen proves successful, and within 1year of transplantation the patient is doing well. He continues to take low doses of azathioprine, prednisone, and cyclosporin A.

1. What is the diagnosis?

Transplant rejection.

2. Discuss the genetics of the major histocompatibility complex (MHC) and the role of class I and II glycoproteins in histocompatibility.

In every human a set of MHC glycoproteins is expressed on the surface of most cells. These molecules are referred to as human leukocyte antigens (HLAs). Class I glycoproteins are known as HLA-A, HLA-B, and HLA-C antigens. Class II glycoproteins are known as HLA-DR, HLA-DP, and HLA-DQ antigens. A large number of genes (multiple alleles) code for each of the class I and II glycoproteins. At the genetic locus for each of these HLA proteins (for example, at the genetic locus for HLA-A), there are numerous different alleles in the population. Consequently, people can inherit different alleles for the HLA proteins coded for on the maternal and paternal chromosomes. Because of these molecular differences, transplanted tissues between genetically different members of the same species (allogeneic) are likely to be antigenically different and therefore stimulate an immune response.

Note: Even when a tissue is transplanted between genetically different people with a perfect ABO and MHC match, rejection can occur because of differences at various minor histocompatibility loci. Although the rejection is usually less vigorous, successful transplantation between MHC-matched people still requires some immunosuppression.

3. What types of rejection may occur in transplant patients?

Hyperacute rejection is mediated by preexisting serum antibodies (against ABO or major MHC antigens of the graft) in the recipient and occurs rapidly within hours to a few days of the transplantation procedure. Hyperacute rejection is untreatable.

Acute rejection is a T cell- and macrophage-mediated attack of the graft based on HLA and other tissue antigen mismatches. It typically occurs 10–14 days after transplantation and is treatable with immunosuppression.

Chronic rejection occurs several months to years after transplantation. The mechanisms of chronic rejection include both humoral and cell-mediated responses by the recipient. This form of rejection is resistant to therapy.

4. What type of rejection did this patient experience? Why was the graft swollen and tender?

Acute rejection. The graft became infiltrated with lymphocytes and macrophages. The resulting immune response involved specific attack of the graft by cytotoxic T lymphocytes and nonspecific release of lytic enzymes by activated macrophages. Inflammatory mediators produced by T cells and macrophages, as well as swelling of renal capsule induced by edema and cellular infiltrate, can induce pain.

5. What is the significance of the fact that the patient had no living blood relatives?

It is much easier to identify good HLA matches in blood relatives. Identical twins have the same histocompatibility type (HLA-identical). The probability is approximately 0.25 that two siblings with the same parents are HLA-identical and approximately 0.50 that they are one-half HLA-matched (haploidentical). Furthermore, parents and children are almost always haploidentical. Because the patient had no living relatives, a cadaveric donor was his option. A cadaveric donor that is blood-group-compatible is often considered even with a poor MHC match.

6. What does a nonreactive final crossmatch indicate?

It indicates that the recipient has no antibodies against the white blood cells of the potential donor. Sensitizing events, including blood transfusions, pregnancies, and previously failed transplant, may elicit the production of anti-HLA antibodies in the recipient. The presence of such preformed antibodies (as indicated by a positive crossmatch) is highly likely to cause hyperacute rejection of the transplanted tissue.

Note: Hyperacute rejection of transplanted tissue is a type II hypersensitivity response.

7. How does azathioprine work as an immunosuppressive agent? Cyclosporin A? Methylprednisone? Antithymocyte globulins? OKT3?

Azathioprine is a purine analog that is incorporated into DNA and inhibits replication. It targets rapidly dividing cells, such as activated lymphocytes. Mycophenolate mofetil is an antimetabolite drug that inhibits the synthesis of purines. Due to its increased specificity for lymphocytes, it has replaced azathioprine in many protocols.

Cyclosporin A inhibits gene transcription of IL-2 and other cytokines that are essential to the clonal expansion and activation of T cells.

Methylprednisone is a corticosteroid anti-inflammatory agent that functions by reducing the number circulating lymphocytes as well the killing ability of macrophages. It also causes decreased chemotaxis of cells so that fewer inflammatory cells are attracted to the site of activation (graft).

Antithymocyte globulins (ATGs) are antibodies against human lymphocytes that are produced in laboratory animals (heterologous antibodies). The antithymocyte (T cell) fraction is isolated and used in transplant recipients to decrease T cell numbers.

OKT3 is a murine monoclonal antibody that is specific for CD3 on the surface of T cells. It not only has the ability to inhibit T cell recognition of alloantigen but in vivo also leads to the elimination of T cells.

Note: ATGs and OKT3 are effective in reversing steroid-resistant rejection.

CASE 10

A 55-year-old woman receives a bone marrow transplant in an attempt to cure multiple myeloma. Fortunately, the patient has an HLA-identical brother who agrees to be the bone marrow donor. The patient is admitted to the hospital and given a course of busulfan to eradicate her own lymphocytes. She is then intravenously administered bone marrow removed from the donor's iliac crest. Her hospital recovery goes smoothly, and she is sent home, only to return 4 weeks after transplant. She presents with a skin rash on her upper trunk, palms, and soles and severe diarrhea. The patient is treated with topical corticosteroids and tacrolimus (FK506). Her skin rash fades, but the intestinal symptoms persist. The diarrhea finally disappears after treatment with weekly injections of a monoclonal antibody to CD2. One month later, the patient is released from the hospital on low doses of corticosteroid.

1. **What caused the adverse reaction in the patient 3 weeks after transplant?**
    Graft-versus-host disease (GVHD).

2. **Describe the pathogenesis of GVHD.**
    In GVHD mature T cells in the transplanted tissue (e.g., donor's bone marrow) react against antigens in the immunosuppressed recipient. Immunocompetent T_H cells from the graft are activated by allogeneic host molecules and produce high levels of cytokines that recruit and activate other T cells, macrophages, and NK cells to create the inflammation seen in GVHD. This inflammation typically results in a pruritic rash covering the face, neck, trunk, and limbs. Gastrointestinal symptoms resulting from the inflammatory response may include nausea, vomiting, and diarrhea caused by destruction of the normal architecture of the colon.

3. **Why did the donor's cells react against the recipient when they were haploidentical?**
    People who are haploidentical share the same MHC haplotypes. In other words, they have MHC class I and class II molecules that are genetically and antigenically identical. However, even in HLA-matched people, disparities in minor histocompatibility antigens exist. These allogeneic molecules, which are probably present in all donor-recipient pairs other than identical twins, have the potential to activate mature T cells of the donor. Unlike MHC antigens that are recognized directly by T cells, minor histocompatibility antigens are recognized only when presented by self-MHC molecules. Thus, tissue rejection due to minor histocompatibility differences takes longer to develop (several weeks) and is usually less vigorous.

4. **Why are the skin and intestinal tract the major sites of GVHD?**
    The skin and intestinal tract express a high level of histocompatibility antigens. Recall that the skin and intestinal tract are major portals of entry for infectious organisms. In addition, the intestinal tract may have also been damaged by the bulsulfan, which targets rapidly dividing cells.

5. **What is the mechanism of action of tacrolimus? Anti-CD2?**
    Tacrolimus blocks activation of resting T cells in the same way as cyclosporin A: by inhibiting transcription of interleukin-2. CD2 is an antigen found on thymocytes and mature T cells. Anti-CD2 (antibody against CD2) is effective at decreasing T-cell numbers by eliciting clearance by the reticuloendothelial system.

6. What laboratory test may have predicted that this patient would develop GVHD?

One-way mixed lymphocyte reaction (MLR). This test measures proliferation (activation) of donor white blood cells in response to irradiated recipient white blood cells. Proliferation of the cells in vitro is a good prediction of GVHD in vivo.

7. How may the donor's marrow have been treated to prevent GVHD?

Partial T-cell depletion of donor marrow before infusion can reduce the incidence of GVHD. Monoclonal antibodies against T-cell antigens (e.g., OKT3) are useful in the removal of T cells.

8. List the major transplant-related immunosuppressive drugs and summarize their mode of action.

See the following table.

AGENT	MODE OF ACTION	COMMENTS
Cyclosporin A (CsA) and FK-506 (tacrolimus)	Blocks IL-2 synthesis and thus prevents T-cell activation	CsA is nephrotoxic; FK-506 can be administered at lower doses and has fewer side effects than CsA.
Rapamycin	Blocks IL-2-dependent activation of T cells	Rapamycin can be administered at lower doses and has fewer side effects than CsA.
Mycophenolate mofetil	Mitotic inhibitor (blocks lympho-cyte nucleotide synthesis and cell division)	Greater selectivity and therefore fewer side effects than its predecessors azathioprine and cyclophosphamide. Commonly used in combination with CsA.
Corticosteroids	Block cytokine production by macrophages (TNF, IL-1); decrease number of circulating lymphocytes	Side effects include hypertension, osteoporosis, and muscle wasting
Antilymphocyte globulin (ALG)/antithymocyte globulin (ATG)	Decreases lymphocyte numbers and T cell numbers, respectively	Heterologous sera (from another species); therefore, adverse reactions include serum sickness, immune complex-induced glomerulonephritis, and anaphylactic reactions.
Anti-CD3 (OKT3)	Elimination of T cells	Mouse monoclonal antibody; fairly immunogenic in humans. Side effects include serum sickness and immune complex-induced glomerulonephritis.
Anti -CD25	Blocks binding of IL-2 to its receptor; elimination of T cells	Human-mouse chimeric form is less immunogenic in humans.

15. GENETIC AND METABOLIC DISEASES

Y. Gloria Yueh, Ph.D.

BASIC CONCEPTS

1. What is an enzymopathy? How does it result in clinical symptoms?

An enzymopathy is a genetic disease in which a deficiency in enzyme activity or concentration leads to a metabolic block in a pathway. The altered (usually reduced) enzymatic activity can be due to reduced cellular expression of the enzyme or to expression of a dysfunctional enzyme. All of the pathologic manifestations of an enzyme deficiency are a result of the accumulation of substrate and/or its alternate derivatives, lack of the product(s), or a combination of both.

Note: When a physiologic pathway is blocked due to an enzyme deficiency, the accumulated substrate can sometimes enter alternate pathways, leading to accumulation of potentially toxic substrate derivatives.

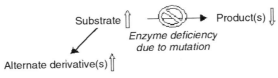

Mechanisms by which an enzymopathy produces clinical symptoms. ↑ = increased, ↓ = decreased.

2. What is the typical pattern of inheritance in enzymopathies?

Almost all enzymes are produced in excess of minimal requirements. Thus, even though heterozygotes usually only produce 50% of normal enzyme levels, they are phenotypically normal. Almost all enzymopathies, therefore, have an <u>autosomal recessive</u> pattern of inheritance, in which a phenotypic abnormality manifests only when there is close to no enzyme production or no functional enzyme (an extremely useful generalization for the boards).

3. Explain why the pathologic consequences of X-linked enzymopathies are manifested almost exclusively in males and rarely in females.

As mentioned in the above question, these diseases require substantial loss of functional enzyme. Males have only a single X chromosome. If the male inherits a defective copy of an X-linked gene for an enzyme from his mother, it will be the only source of this enzyme. He will then exhibit the pathologic consequences of this enzyme deficiency/abnormality. Females, however, have two X chromosomes and generally exhibit the disease only if they are homozygous for the mutated alleles (rare event).

Note: Selected examples of X-linked recessive enzymopathies are hemophilia A (factor VIII deficiency), hemophilia B (factor IX deficiency), glucose-6-phosphate dehydrogenase deficiency, and Lesch-Nyhan syndrome (deficiency of hypoxanthine-guanine phosphoribosyltransferase [HPRT]).

4. What is the process of lyonization? Why may it cause the manifestation of X-linked diseases in females?

Because females have two X chromosomes, they would have twice the level of expression of genes located on the X chromosome if it were not for random inactivation (lyonization) of one X chromosome in each cell. However, because of the normally random nature of the X-chromosome inactivation process, some females may happen to have the mutated allele on the active X chromosome of a large number of cells and thus may exhibit some pathologic symptoms. This rare event is termed *manifesting heterozygotes.*

5. Why do some diseases show an autosomal dominant pattern of inheritance? Why do the genetic diseases of connective tissue usually fall within this category?

In autosomal dominant diseases, the pathology manifests even though a normal copy of the gene produces 50% of the gene product. The dominance of the defective gene can be attributed to one of the following reasons: more than 50% of normal gene product is needed for a nondiseased physiologic state; the defective protein adversely affects the normal gene product (dominant negative effect); or the defective protein has acquired a novel detrimental property.

For most nonenzymatic structural proteins (e.g., collagen, fibrillin) or membrane receptors (e.g., low-density lipoprotein [LDL] receptor), mutations in these genes are usually inherited in an autosomal dominant manner. This also is a useful generalization to remember for the boards.

6. What is the general relationship between the function of a protein and its pattern of inheritance?

FUNCTION	PATTERN OF INHERITANCE	EXAMPLE DISEASES
Enzymes	Autosomal recessive	Phenylketonuria (phenylalanine hydroxylase) Galactosemia (galactose-1-phosphate uridyltransferase) Medium-chain acyl CoA dehydrogenase (MCAD) deficiency Tay-Sachs disease (hexosaminidase A)
Transport protein	Autosomal recessive	Thalassemias (alpha or beta hemoglobin) Cystic fibrosis (chloride channel)
Structural proteins	Autosomal dominant	Osteogenesis imperfecta (type I and II collagen) Marfan's syndrome (fibrillin) Hereditary spherocytosis (spectrin)
Developmental gene expression	Autosomal dominant	Achondroplasia (FGFR3 receptor)
Metabolic receptors	Autosomal dominant	Familial hypercholesterolemia (LDL receptor)

Note: Keep in mind that the above information contains the general pattern. A few exceptions can be found in each category.

7. What are the following molecular biologic diagnostic methods used for? Explain briefly how they work.

Southern blotting. This technique involves detecting a sample of a specific DNA sequence from patients by hybridizing it with a complementary DNA strand that can be detected. In the laboratory, it is typically used to detect the presence of large unique DNA sequences within the genome.

Northern blotting. This technique is similar to Southern blotting except that a specific strand of the patient's RNA is detected with complementary DNA. Northern blotting is commonly used to measure *expression* of a gene, as determined by its production of messenger RNA (mRNA).

Polymerase chain reaction (PCR). PCR allows detection of a specific DNA sequence (e.g., mutant allele) by making billions of copies of that allele from a single DNA molecule. This test is performed by using two complementary primer sequences that span the ends of the sequence of interest that is to be amplified. The target DNA is then amplified via multiple rounds of DNA denaturation, primer hybridization, and extension catalyzed by a temperature-insensitive DNA polymerase.

Western blotting. This test measures the expression of the final gene product, the protein. This is important because many diseases are caused by translational problems, in which transcription of the gene into mRNA occurs normally but the translation of this mRNA is defective.

CASE 1

A 2-day-old boy tests positive for a relatively rare but easily treatable medical condition. The diagnosis is based on the presence of markedly elevated serum levels of an essential amino acid. A second positive test is obtained during his 2-week check-up at the hospital. His family history is remarkable for a 45-year-old aunt who is mentally retarded, but who appeared to be healthy when she was born.

1. What is the most likely diagnosis? How is this condition typically inherited?

Phenylketonuria (PKU), which is typically inherited in an autosomal recessive manner. It is caused by the defective conversion of phenylalanine to tyrosine, which is caused by mutations in the phenylalanine hydroxylase (PAH) gene.

2. Describe the major defect and underlying pathology.

tyrosine is converted to DA

The PAH deficiency leads to an accumulation of phenylalanine (substrate) and phenylpyruvic acid (derivative via an alternate reaction) and a reduced tyrosine (product) and its derivatives. The pathology results primarily from substrate (phenylalanine) accumulation, which causes severe neuronal damage and mental retardation.

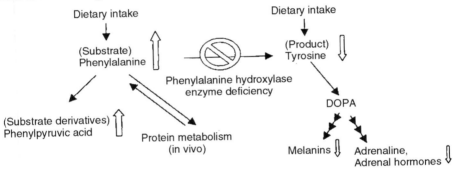

Pathologic mechanisms of phenylketonuria.

3. How is PKU treated?

Patients with PKU need to follow a strict diet that restricts phenylalanine intake and is supplemented with tyrosine. If started within the first month of life, this diet can be highly effective in preventing mental retardation.

4. Given the fact that PKU is a relatively rare condition (prevalence rates range from 1 in 2600 to 1 in 200,000 live births), why does it make sense to screen all neonates for this condition?

The screening test (Guthrie test) is inexpensive and simple (measurement of plasma phenylalanine levels), and the disease (PKU) is easily treated by dietary modifications. Furthermore, early screening detects the disease before irreparable damage (particularly to the central nervous system) has occurred (i.e., early intervention affects outcome).

5. If the parents have a female child with this disease, why is it crucial to advise her about the risks to her baby if she becomes pregnant when she is older?

Most women with PKU at childbearing age have abandoned the diet therapy by their early teens. This termination of diet therapy seems to have limited ill effects on the women themselves at this age but can cause irreparable harm to the developing fetus. High levels of phenylalanine can diffuse across the placenta, causing brain damage of the developing offspring. Therefore, even though the infants are heterozygous for the mutated PAH and are born without PKU, they can exhibit severe mental retardation, a condition termed *maternal PKU*.

6. Why is screening for hypothyroidism and galactosemia also routinely performed in newborns?

These diseases are preventable causes of mental retardation. In general, screening is performed for diseases in which treatment is available, a rapid and low cost laboratory test is available, or the condition is frequent and serious enough to justify the screening cost.

CASE 2

A woman and her husband just gave birth to a child with cystic fibrosis. Both the woman and her husband are in their thirties and are completely asymptomatic.

1. If the parents decide to have another child, what is the probability of that child having cystic fibrosis?

Because cystic fibrosis is an autosomal recessive disease, the chance of the second child having cystic fibrosis is still 25%. Because each parent is a carrier of the mutant allele, each parent has a 50% chance of passing it to offspring. Thus, the chance of a baby getting both mutant alleles is $0.5 \times 0.5 = 0.25$ or 25%.

2. If the parents want to have another child, what kind of genetic screening methods might they consider?

Several genetic screening methods are available. The first involves preimplantation diagnosis using the in-vitro fertilization method. A single cell is removed from an 8-cell or 16-cell blastomere, and the DNA from that cell is isolated. PCR is then applied to screen for the CFTR locus (CFTR = cystic fibrosis transmembrane conductance regulator). Only the unaffected embryos (wild type or carrier status) are implanted.

Other genetic screening methods involve prenatal diagnosis using amniocentesis (the withdrawal of 20–30 ml of amniotic fluid between 15–17 weeks' gestation) and chorionic villus sampling (aspiration of several milligrams of villus tissues between 10–11 weeks' gestation).

3. Despite mutations in the same gene, why do patients with cystic fibrosis often show significant clinical heterogeneity in terms of disease severity?

1. Different patients may have different mutations of the same gene, causing less severe phenotypes. For example, if a certain mutation causes only mild abnormalities of the chloride channel, clinical manifestations will be milder. This phenomenon, in which there are different mutations of the same allele, is known as *allelic heterogeneity*. Of interest, in most patients with cystic fibrosis the exact same locus is not mutated on each copy of the CFTR genes, making them *compound heterozygotes*.

2. Even in patients with identical mutations, some degree of clinical heterogeneity may be due to other genetic differences or to environmental variables.

Note: Many genetic diseases have allelic heterogeneity, leading to significant heterogeneity in clinical manifestations.

4. Assuming a prevalence rate of 1 in 2500, what is the carrier frequency for cystic fibrosis?

The Hardy-Weinberg equation can be used to describe the phenotypic distribution of a disorder $(p^2 + 2pq + q^2 = 1)$ and the genotypic distribution of the abnormal allele $(p + q = 1)$.

p^2 = unaffected individuals
$2pq$ = carriers (usually asymptomatic in autosomal recessive diseases)
q^2 = affected individuals
p = frequency of normal allele
q = frequency of abnormal allele $(1 - p)$

Assuming a prevalence of 1 in 2500 for cystic fibrosis, $q^2 = 1/2500$; thus, $q = 0.02$. Since $p + q = 1$, $p = 0.98$. Therefore, the carrier frequency for cystic fibrosis can be calculated as follows:

$$2pq = 2 \, (0.98) \, (0.2) = 0.039$$

or approximately 4% of the population. Thus, 1 in every 25 is a carrier.

CASE 3

A 9-month-old baby is brought to the hospital by her parents. The parents mentioned that she is having trouble with feeding and appears to be lethargic and easily startled. The baby's rigid movements continue to worsen, and she becomes blind by 12 months. A cherry-red spot is observed at the center of the macula. Both parents are Ashkenazi Jews.

1. What is the most likely diagnosis?

Tay-Sachs disease, a lysosomal storage disease. It is an autosomal recessive disorder of ganglioside (sphingolipid) catabolism that is caused by a deficiency of hexosaminidase A.

Note: Tay-Sachs disease is predominantly found among Ashkenazi Jews and their descendants.

2. Describe the pathogenesis of the disease.

Hexosaminidase A is a lysosomal enzyme that cleaves a cerebral ganglioside (GM_2, a sphingolipid). Mutations make this enzyme less effective, causing massive accumulation of GM_2 and its byproducts within the lysosomes of neurons. As these lysosomes become enormously enlarged, they begin to interfere with normal cell function and ultimately cause neuronal death. Neuronal death that overlies the fovea centralis of the retina is responsible for the cherry-red spot seen on fundoscopic exam.

Note: The pathogenesis of other lysosomal storage disorders (e.g., Gaucher's disease, Niemann-Pick syndrome) is similarly due to accumulation of substrates of lysosomal enzymes.

3. What are the mucopolysaccharidoses?

Mucopolysaccharidoses (MPS) are also lysosomal storage diseases, but the substrates that accumulate in the lysosomes are extracellular matrix molecules such as glycosaminoglycans (a mucopolysaccharide). These diseases are caused by hereditary deficiency of lysosomal enzymes required for the breakdown of mucopolysaccharides (glycosaminoglycans). The two main examples are Hurler syndrome and Hunter syndrome (see below).

MUCOPOLYSACCHARIDOSES	INHERITANCE GENE MUTATION	HIGH YIELD PATTERN	ASSOCIATIONS
Hurler syndrome (MPS I H)	Alpha-l-iduronidase	Autosomal recessive	Coarse facial features, mental retardation
Hunter syndrome (MPS II)	Iduronate sulfatase	X-linked recessive	Coarse facial features, mental retardation

I-cell disease,   no mucopolysaccharides in urine

4. Cover the right-hand column and describe the gene mutation, pathophysiology, and any high-yield associations for the following lysosomal storage disorders.

LYSOSOMAL STORAGE DISEASES	SPECIFIC GENE MUTATIONS/ENZYME DEFICIENCY	PATHOPHYSIOLOGY	HIGH-YIELD ASSOCIATIONS
Tay-Sachs disease	Hexosaminidase A	Cerebral ganglioside accumulation	Cherry-red spot on retina
Gaucher's disease	Glucocerebrosidase	Lipid-laden macrophages (Gaucher cells) in bone, liver, and spleen.	Massive hepatosplenomegaly
Niemann-Pick disease	Sphingomyelinase	Sphingomyelin accumulation in cells throughout body, especially neurons	Extensive neurologic dysfunction

CASE 4

A 2-year-old boy is brought to the clinic with choreoathetosis (constant and involuntary writhing movements of the legs and arms), spasticity (muscular hypertonicity with increased tendon reflexes), impaired cognitive development, and self-mutilation (compulsive biting of the fingers, lips, tongue, and inside of the mouth). The parents also report observation of orange "sand" in the diapers when the boy was a few months old.

1. What is the most likely diagnosis?

Lesch-Nyhan syndrome (LNS), a rare X-linked recessive disease that is caused by a defective hypoxanthine-guanine phosphoribosyl transferase (HPRT)) enzyme. The HPRT enzyme is present in most cell types and is involved in the salvage pathway of purine metabolism. The most striking neurologic symptom of this disease is self-mutilation, which is characteristic.

Note: The purine bases are adenine and guanine, and their respective nucleosides are adenosine and guanosine. A nitrogenous base linked to a sugar ribose or deoxyribose is referred to as a **nucleoside,** whereas a phosphorylated nucleoside is referred to as a **nucleotide.**

2. Summarize the normal function of the purine "salvage" pathway.

The purine salvage pathway functions to "salvage" purine metabolites such as hypoxanthine and guanine from being degraded and then excreted via the kidneys as uric acid. Instead, it normally recycles these metabolites to replenish the purine nucleotides guanine and adenine by the action of the HPRT enzyme. Physiologically, the de novo pathway (*smaller dark arrows*) synthesizes roughly 10% of the daily purine requirement, and the salvage pathway (*large curved arrows*) makes up the remaining 90% by salvaging the degradation intermediates. The amount of net degradation to uric acid (*open arrows*) is always balanced with the amount of purines synthesized via the de novo pathway.

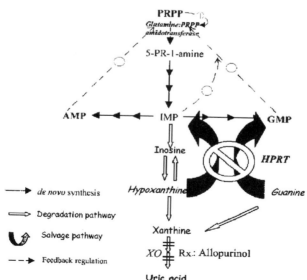

3. How do defects in the purine salvage pathway cause hyperuricemia?

In Lesch-Nyhan syndrome (LNS), HPRT activity is less than 1% of normal. Due to the absence of HPRT, the ability to reutilize hypoxanthine and guanine to make the purine nucleosides—inosine-5'-monophosphate (IMP) and guanosine monophosphate (GMP)—is lost. Therefore, these intermediates are degraded to uric acid. In addition, because of the reduced levels of

IMP and GMP, the normal feedback inhibition by IMP and GMP on the de novo pathway is lost (broken arrows in figure in question 2), greatly promoting the de novo synthesis pathway. Purines made from the de novo pathway are also degraded to uric acid, further exacerbating the hyperuricemia. Therefore, both excessive activation of the de novo pathway and insufficient HPRT salvage of purine metabolites contribute to the hyperuricemia in LNS.

4. Why was the orange "sand" in the boy's diapers?

Uric acid crystals. Because of its highly insoluble nature, uric acid precipitates from urine, forming the orange "sand." It can also precipitate from the plasma and accumulate in the joints, potentially causing gouty arthritis. Of interest, most patients with LNS do not develop gout, presumably because of their short life span (about 20 years).

Note: Patients with only a partial deficiency of HPRT (having 1–20% of activity) have a normal life span but are susceptible to developing severe gout.

5. Why do boys with LNS typically present with renal dysfunction?

Most kidney pathologies in LNS are associated with hyperuricemia, which leads to uric acid kidney stones and urinary tract obstruction. Remember, LNS is an X-linked recessive disease, seen primarily in males.

Note: The cause of the neurologic symptoms in LNS is not established.

6. How might this patient be managed pharmacologically?

With allopurinol, which prevents uric acid production by inhibiting xanthine oxidase (XO) (see figure in question 2).

CASE 5

A 4-year-old boy presents with profound hypoglycemia and seizures. The exam is remarkable for nontender hepatomegaly. He has a history of multiple hospitalizations for seizures and hypoglycemia since he was 6 months old. His parents have noticed that he does not tolerate well even short periods of fasting, and his blood sugar levels are typically low within a few hours after each feeding. In his previous hospital stays, lactic acidosis, hyperlipidemia, and hyperuricemia were also consistently observed. A liver biopsy indicates excessive accumulation of glycogen and fat. Specialized enzymatic analysis of the biopsy tissue indicates extremely low activity of the enzyme glucose-6-phosphatase.

1. What is the diagnosis?

Type 1 glycogen storage disease (glucose-6-phosphatase deficiency or von Gierke disease), an autosomal recessive disorder caused by deficiency of the enzyme glucose-6-phosphatase (G6Pase).

2. What type of enzymatic deficiency is present in all types of glycogen storage diseases?

A defect either in an enzyme required for glycogen synthesis (i.e., glycogenesis) or an enzyme required for glycogen catabolism (i.e., glycogenolysis). Glycogen storage diseases can affect mainly either the liver or skeletal muscle. When they affect the liver, they may cause hepatomegaly and can predispose to hypoglycemia and its attendant complications (e.g., seizures). When they affect the skeletal muscles, they may cause muscle pain and exercise intolerance, but they do not result in hypoglycemic episodes, because skeletal muscle plays a minor role in plasma glucose homeostasis.

3. How is glycogen normally synthesized and degraded in the liver?

Within the liver, glucose is first prevented from diffusing out of the cell by phosphorylation to glucose-6-phosphate, a reaction catalyzed by the enzyme glucokinase (hexokinase in nonhepatic tissues). Glucose-6-phosphate is then converted into glucose-1-phosphate by phosphoglucomutase and then into uridine diphosphate (UDP) glucose prior to attachment to glycogen by the enzyme glycogen synthetase. Glycogen degradation depends primarily on the activity of the enzyme glycogen phosphorylase (see diagram of tricarboxylic acid [TCA] cycle in question 6).

4. What is the function of glucose-6-phosphatase?

This enzyme cleaves phosphate from glucose, thus enabling glucose to diffuse out of the cell. This reaction is important in blood glucose homeostasis because a final common product of both glycogenolysis and gluconeogenesis is glucose-6-phosphate.

5. Why is hepatomegaly seen on exam?

The deficiency of glucose-6-phosphatase causes accumulation of glucose-6-phosphate, which stimulates glycogen synthesis and thus enlarges the liver.

6. Explain the severe fasting hypoglycemia and lactic acidosis.

During short-term fasting, liver glycogenolysis is the major pathway that maintains blood glucose homeostasis. When G6Pase activity is deficient, glycogenolysis is not effective at releasing glucose into the bloodstream; thus, hypoglycemia results. In addition, the release of glucose made from gluconeogenesis during fasting is also impaired, further contributing to hypoglycemia. In regard to the lactic acidosis, because of an excessive accumulation of G6P, glycolytic flux is greatly promoted, leading to high levels of pyruvate production. The pyruvate is then converted into lactate when the mitochondrial uptake of pyruvate is saturated.

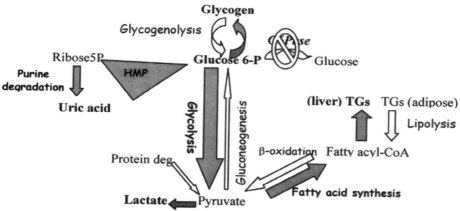

Tricarboxylic acid (TCA) cycle. During the postabsorptive phase, *open arrows* indicate the physiologic direction, whereas *filled arrows* indicate the pathologic direction.

7. Why is the patient susceptible to hypertriglyceridemia?

Due to an excessive accumulation of glucose-6-phosphate, the hepatic glycolysis becomes exaggerated, supplying substrates to the pathways downstream from glycolysis. These pathways include fatty acid (de novo) synthesis and triacylglycerol synthesis. Because the hypoglycemia causes a low insulin-to-glucagon ratio, lipolysis is promoted, providing abundant fatty acids for oxidation in many tissues for energy production. A portion of these fatty acids enters the mitochondria to be oxidized, but the excess is repackaged in the liver to form very-low-density lipoproteins (VLDLs).

8. What causes the hyperuricemia?

1. As mentioned previously, a lack of G6Pase activity leads to an accumulation of glucose-6-phosphate in the cell. Glucose-6-phosphate is shunted into the hexose-monophosphate-shunt, leading to accumulations of ribose 5-phosphate and PRPP (5'-phosphoribosyl 1-pyrophosphate).

PRPP is the major allosteric activator of the rate-limiting enzyme (glutamine:PRPP amido-trasferase; see the figure in case 3) for the purine de novo synthetic pathway. An increase in de novo synthesis leads to an increase in purine degradation and thus to uric acid/urate production.

2. Because of hypoglycemia, the increase in cytosolic adenosine monophosphate (from degradation of adenosine triphosphate and adenosine diphosphate) also results in an increase in uric acid production.

3. In addition, the excessive plasma lactate competes with uric acid for urinary excretion.

9. Explain how type 1 glycogen storage disease affects the activity of the rate-limiting enzymes in the following pathways.

PATHWAY	RATE-LIMITING ENZYME	EFFECT	BASIS OF EFFECT
Glycolysis	Phosphofructokinase (PFK)-1	Increase	Increased substrate concentration (G6P).
Glycogenesis	Glycogen synthetase	Increase	Increased substrate concentration
Fatty acid synthesis	Acetyl-CoA carboxylase	Increase	Increased substrate (citrate) concentration due to exaggerated glycolysis and tricarboxylic acid (TCA) cycle
Hexose monophosphate shunt	G6P dehydrogenase	Increase	Increased substrate (G6P) concentration
Triacylglycerol synthesis		Increase	Increase substrates (glycerol and fatty acids from de novo synthesis or from lipolysis)

10. Explain why a deficiency of muscle glycogen phosphorylase, as in McArdle disease, does not result in hypoglycemia.

Although muscle glycogen phosphorylase is required for glycogenolysis in muscle, muscle glycogenolysis does not play an important role in blood glucose homeostasis.

11. Summarize high-yield information about glycogen storage diseases.

GLYCOGEN STORAGE DISEASE	ENZYME DEFICIENCY	CLINICAL HALLMARK
Type I (von Gierke disease)	Hepatic and renal G6Pase	Hepatomegaly, fasting hypoglycemia
Type II (Pompe disease), also a lysosomal storage disease	Lysosomal glucosidase	Cardiomegaly, cardiorespiratory failure
Type V (McArdle disease)	Muscle glycogen phosphorylase	Exercise-induced muscle cramps

CASE 6

An 8-month-old girl is brought to the emergency department by her parents. She has been vomiting and irritable for the past 2 days, and in the past 8 hours she has become very lethargic. Laboratory findings indicate moderate hypoglycemia, hyperammonemia, and abnormally low serum ketones (given the degree of hypoglycemia). Additional laboratory findings indicate a defect of fatty acid oxidation.

1. What is the most likely diagnosis?

Medium-chain fatty acyl-CoA dehydrogenase (MCAD) deficiency, the most common genetic disorder of fatty acid oxidation.

2. What are the three classifications of fatty acids based on length?

A mixture of three types of fatty acids based on their length can be found in most edible fats: short-chain, medium-chain, and long chain fatty acids. These fatty acids (in fatty acyl-CoA form) are oxidized in the mitochondria of peripheral cells that metabolize fatty acids by long-chain acyl-CoA dehydrogenase (LCAD), medium-chain acyl-CoA dehydrogenase (MCAD), and short-chain acyl-CoA dehydrogenase (SCAD), depending on the length of the hydrocarbon chain.

3. Why is the patient susceptible to hypoglycemia and hyperammonemia during fasting?

Physiologically, most tissues rely on fatty acid oxidation as the primary fuel source for production of adenosine triphosphate (ATP) during fasting.

When MCAD is deficient, medium-chain fatty acyl-CoA accumulates in cytosol as well as mitochondrial matrix, leading to hepatic resynthesis of triacylglycerides in the cytosol (fatty liver). ATP production and ketogenesis are then greatly decreased. Without adequate supply of energy, the rate of both the urea cycle and gluconeogenesis is decreased, leading to hyperammonemia and hypoglycemia. The tissues also exhaust the endogenous glucose supply (liver glycogen) to meet the energy demand.

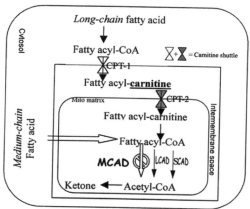

Summary of metabolism of fatty acids.

4. How should this child be treated?

Avoidance of fasting and medium-chain fatty acids is the key. By not allowing the child to rely on peripheral lipolysis and beta-oxidation for energy needs, hypoglycemia and accumulation of intermediates due to the metabolic block will be minimized. Frequent small meals high in carbohydrate and low in fat (< 20% of calories) are recommended. Patients with MCAD deficiency should take carnitine supplements to promote efficient long-chain fatty acyl-CoA transport into the mitochondria.

Note: Because the carnitine shuttle is the rate-limiting step for long-chain fatty acid oxidation, promoting this route by supplementing carnitine can reduce the energy deficiency caused by MCAD deficiency.

5. How are the following pathways/cycles affected by MCAD deficiency?

PATHWAY OR CYCLE	ACTIVITY OF THE PATHWAY	CAUSES
Hepatic gluconeogenesis	Decreased, causing hypoglycemia	Low ATP levels
Hepatic urea cycle	Decreased, causing hyperammonemia	Low ATP levels
Beta-oxidation of medium-chain fatty acids	Decreased	Enzyme deficiency
Hepatic ketogenesis	Decreased	Low acetyl-CoA production

CASE 7

A woman with acute intermittent porphyria seeks advice on how to avoid exacerbations of her disease.

1. What are the porphyrias?

These diseases are characterized by an enzymatic defect in the heme biosynthesis pathway. The enzymatic block leads to an accumulation of intermediates in the heme biosynthetic pathway, and many of these intermediates have toxic effects at high levels. In contrast to the majority of enzymopathies, most of the porphyrias have an autosomal dominant mode of inheritance.

Note: Defects in the later steps of heme biosynthesis cause accumulation of photoreactive intermediates, which makes these people photosensitive.

2. Why may anticonvulsants such as phenytoin and phenobarbital trigger porphyrias?

These medications induce hepatic cytochrome p450 enzymes, which require heme and thus promote heme biosynthesis. The increased heme biosynthesis results in an increased accumulation of various intermediate porphyrins, depending on the site of the metabolic block due to the respective enzyme deficiency.

3. Why is hemin given to patients with porphyrias?

Hemin is an oxidized form of heme that, via a negative feedback mechanism, decreases the synthesis of aminolevulinate (ALA) synthase (the rate-limiting enzyme of heme biosynthesis). This negative feedback mechanism can be exploited therapeutically in the porphyrias.

4. How does lead poisoning affect heme synthesis?

Lead poisoning inhibits the heme synthesis enzymes ALA dehydrase and ferrochelatase, resulting in anemia. For step 1, know that red blood cells on a peripheral blood smear demonstrate *basophilic stippling*.

5. What are the sideroblastic anemias?

Sideroblastic anemias are also caused by defects in the heme biosynthesis pathway. Unlike the porphyrias, the clinically apparent pathology results from insufficient heme production rather than the accumulation of toxic heme precursors. Because substantial amounts of bodily iron are stored in heme, defects in heme synthesis lead to iron deposition in "siderotic" granules in cells. Because these anemias involve a defect in the heme moiety of hemoglobin synthesis, they are often hypochromic and microcytic.

CASE 8

A 7-week-old girl is brought to the office with vomiting, diarrhea, dry skin, pallor, hepatomegaly, jaundice, and hypoglycemia. The mother notes that the baby starts to vomit or has diarrhea after milk ingestion. Laboratory findings include the following: elevation in serum galactose, serum galactose-1-phosphate, hypergalactosuria, albuminuria and unconjugated hyperbilirubinemia.

1. What is the diagnosis?

Galactosemia. Left untreated, this disease can lead to severe mental retardation. It is due to defective galactose metabolism characterized by elevated levels of serum galactose. Typically, galactosemia is a result of deficiency in galactose kinase or galactose-1-phosphate uridyltransferase. Since both galactose and galactose-1-P were elevated in the blood, this child is likely to suffer from a deficiency of Gal-1-P uridyltransferase , a disease termed classic galactosemia.

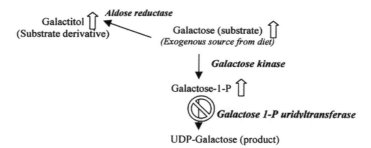

Pathophysiology of galactosemia.

2. Why does gal-1-P uridyltransferase deficiency manifest jaundice? What type of jaundice?

As in other tissues such as nerves, lens, and kidney, the pathologic manifestations in the liver and red blood cells are also due to the accumulation of galactose-1-phosphate and galactitol. The premature destruction of red blood cells (hemolysis) increases the concentration of serum unconjugated bilirubin, leading to prehepatic (hemolytic) jaundice.

3. Why do people with galactosemia tend to develop cataracts if left untreated?

When galactose (substrate) accumulates due to a metabolic block, it enters an alternate reaction, catalyzed by aldose reductase and leading to production of galactitol (a substrate derivative). Accumulation of galactitol leads to an increased cellular osmolarity, causing other cellular proteins (such as lens crystallins) to denature and thus resulting in cataracts.

4. Describe the treatment for classic galactosemia.

The patient needs to follow a strict diet that eliminates all galactose-containing compounds, which include lactose (milk and dairy products) and galactose-containing supplements. Avoidance of dietary galactose intake quickly eliminates the potential for or reverses the development of poor growth, jaundice, anemia, liver disease, and cataracts.

CASE 9

A newborn presents with somewhat ambiguous external genitalia. The genitalia seem more like an enlarged clitoris than a penis, but there is a scrotum-like structure that appears to result from labial fusion. An ultrasound reveals seemingly normal ovarian development. The karyotype is 46,XX.

1. What is the most likely diagnosis?

Congenital adrenal hyperplasia, most commonly due to a deficiency of 21-alpha-hydroxylase.

2. How does a 21-hydroxylase-deficiency cause virilism of females?

The adrenal steroid biosynthetic pathways produce three major hormones: mineralocorticoids (such as aldosterone), glucocorticoids (such as cortisol), and sex hormones (androgens or estrogens). When 21-alpha-hydroxylase is deficient (usually partial deficiency), the production of aldosterone and cortisol decreases due to the metabolic block at two reactions depicted below. The precursors are then shunted into the pathway of sex hormone biosynthesis, leading to excessive accumulation of androgen, which causes masculinization of the external genitalia, as seen in this baby girl.

Note: **Male pseudohermaphrodites** are genetically (46XY) and gonadally (with testes) male but have female genitalia (as in testicular feminization syndrome). **Female pseudohermaphrodites** are genetically and gonadally female but have male secondary sex characteristics. Female pseudohermaphroditism usually results from congenital adrenal hyperplasia, which can be caused by deficiency of 21-alpha-hydroxylase or 11-beta-hydroxylase. Unlike true hermaphrodites, pseudohermaphrodites have gonadal tissue of only one sex.

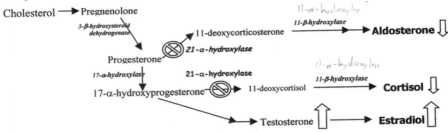

Pathophysiology of congenital adrenal hyperplasia.

3. Why may this patient exhibit hyperkalemia and hypotension?

Hyperkalemia is due to a decreased synthesis of aldosterone, which is known to stimulate renal reabsorption of sodium ions and excretion of potassium ions. Hypotension is primarily the result of sodium loss with loss of extracellular volume.

4. Why is bilateral adrenal hyerplasia present?

The low cortisol level reduces negative feedback on pituitary production of adrenocorticotropic hormone (ACTH); thus, ACTH production increases significantly and stimulates hyperplasia of the adrenal glands. Recall that ACTH also stimulates adrenal androgen synthesis, which further contributes to the virilization seen in this patient.

5. Why does 11-alpha-hydroxylase deficiency share similar virilizing manifestations as 21-beta-hydroxylase deficiency?

When 11-alpha-hydroxylase is deficient, aldosterone and cortisol synthesis are also decreased. Overproduction of precursors occurs, and the precursors are then shunted into androgen production. In addition, low cortisol causes increased pituitary ACTH production, which further stimulates androgen production.

Note: In this disease the accumulation of 11-deoxycorticosterone, which has mineralocorticoid activity, causes fluid retention and hypertension.

6. Why are patients with 17-alpha-hydroxylase deficiency phenotypically female?

All fetuses are female by default; it is production of androgen that makes fetuses male. However, with low levels of 17-alpha-hydroxylase, insufficient levels of these androgens are produced in fetuses that are genetically male, making them phenotypically female.

Note: Such patients also have low estrogen production, which inhibits their maturation.

7. Why are patients with 17-alpha-hydroxylase deficiency often hypertensive?

The block in the pathway to make androgens or cortisol increases flux through the metabolic pathway that makes aldosterone. The ensuing high levels of aldosterone cause significant salt and water retention, expanding the extracellular volume and increasing the blood pressure.

8. Summarize the metabolic pathways, symptoms, and primary causes of symptoms in congenital metabolic disorders.

METABOLIC PATHWAY	GENETIC DISEASES	PRIMARY REASON(S) FOR CLINICAL SYMPTOMS	MAJOR SYMPTOMS
Glycogenolysis	Glucose-6-phosphatase deficiency (Von Gierke disease)	Hypoglycemia	Hypoglycemic episodes

(Cont'd.)

METABOLIC PATHWAY	GENETIC DISEASES	PRIMARY REASON(S) FOR CLINICAL SYMPTOMS	MAJOR SYMPTOMS
Glycogenolysis *(cont'd.)*	Muscle glycogen phosphorylase deficiency (McArdle's disease)		Muscle pain exercise intolerance
Hexose monophosphate shunt/pentose phosphate pathway	Glucose-6-phosphate dehydrogenase (G6PD) deficiency	Susceptibility to oxidative stresses	Hemolytic anemia
Fatty acid oxidation	MCAD	Hypoglycemia	Hypoglycemic episodes
Urea cycle		Hyperammonemia	Encephalopathy
Amino acid metabolism	PKU, maple syrup urine disease		Encephalopathy
Heme synthesis	Porphyrias	Accumulation of porphyrin intermediates	Anemia, episodic abdominal pain, neurologic symptoms
Peroxisomal diseases	Neonatal adrenoleukodystrophy		
Adrenal corticosteroid synthesis	CAH (21-beta-hydroxylase deficiency	Deficient aldosterone and cortisol	Virilization, weakness, fatigue, hypotension
	17-Alpha-hydroxylase deficiency)	High aldosterone Low cortisol Low androgens	Hypertension, lack of virilization

MCAD = medium-chain acyl-CoA dehydrogenase, PKU = phenylketonuria, CAH = congenital adrenal hyperplasia.

CASE 10

A tall, slim 14-year-old boy is referred to the genetic clinic by his ophthalmologist. He has ectopia lentis (detached lens), flat corneas, and hypoplastic irides. His mother, a tall, thin woman, had died of heart failure caused by aortic rupture while she was jogging. Physical examination reveals an arm span-to-height ratio of 1.5 (normal < 1.05), joint hypermobility, arachnodactyly (spider fingers), a diastolic murmur, and stretch marks on the shoulders and thighs. Echocardiogram shows dilation of the ascending aorta with aortic regurgitation.

1. What is the diagnosis?
Marfan syndrome, an autosomal dominant disorder. It is caused by mutations of the fibrillin gene.

2. Why does the patient exhibit multiple pathologic presentations in the ocular, skeletal, and cardiovascular systems?
Fibrillin is a component of microfibrils, which are part of the extracellular matrix that is prevalent in eye tissue, aorta, skin and periosteum. Detached lenses, aortic dilation, and stretchy skin are the pathologic consequences of defective fibrillin. The skeletal defects, such as arachnodactyly (long and skinny fingers and toes), tall stature, and joint hypermobility, are caused by the inability of periosteum to provide oppositional force in normal bone growth. Overgrowth of bone occurs when the periosteum has become too "flexible" due to defective fibrillin.

3. What are the major causes of death in this disorder?
The major causes of death in patients with Marfan syndrome are heart failure due to aortic dilation, which causes regurgitation, and aortic rupture and dissection. Pregnancy or heavy

exercise increases cardiac output greatly; both are particularly risky for patients with Marfan syndrome.

4. What structural protein is defective in the hereditary skeletal disease that predisposes to bone fractures from minor stresses?

In osteogenesis imperfecta, defects are present in type I collagen (the predominant collagen type in the extracellular matrix of bone). Patients often have blue sclera because the reduced collagen in the sclera allows the blue choroid coat to show through the sclera.

5. What is the genetic defect in Ehler-Danlos syndrome?

Ehler-Danlos syndrome can develop from multiple different genetic abnormalities in one of the collagen types. The syndrome is frequently characterized by hyperextensible skin and hypermobile joints.

CASE 11

A 6-year-old boy is brought to the hospital by his mother because of severe shortness of breath. He has a fever and leukocytosis, and a chest x-ray shows a right lower lobe infiltrate. His mother is really worried because he has had pneumonia already three times as a child. A sputum culture grows *Pseudomonas aeruginosa*. A sweat test shows significantly elevated sodium and chloride.

1. What is the most likely diagnosis?

Cystic fibrosis.

2. What causes this disease? How is it inherited?

Cystic fribrosis involves a mutation in the chloride transmembrane channel (CFTR gene or cystic fibrosis transmembrane conductance regulator gene). It is inherited in an autosomal recessive manner.

3. Why does the boy develop respiratory infections so easily?

In cystic fibrosis, the mucous secretions from the pulmonary epithelium are particularly thick. They impair mucociliary action and predispose to tracheobronchial infection. In fact, the most common cause of death in patients with cystic fibrosis is respiratory infection.

4. Why may the boy be susceptible to developing pancreatitis as he grows older?

Increased viscosity of the secretions from the exocrine pancreas predisposes to obstruction of the pancreatic duct, which can cause pancreatitis.

5. What is bronchiectasis? Why does it commonly develop in cystic fibrosis?

Bronchiectasis is an irreversible dilation of the bronchi that typically occurs secondary to subtotal obstruction of the airways (e.g., tumor, mucous impaction, necrotizing infection). The primary cause for the dilation (in all forms of bronchiectasis) is inflammation

6. How does Kartagener's syndrome produce similar clinical manifestations?

Kartagener's syndrome is associated with a primary disturbance in ciliary function due to dysfunction of the dynein arm of microtubules. This dysfunction also compromises sputum expectoration. Of interest, ciliary dysfunction in cystic fibrosis is due to abnormally thick secretions, whereas in Kartagener's syndrome it is due to an intrinsic defect in the microtubules. Both diseases, however, are associated with recurrent pulmonary infections as well as infertility in males.

Note: Situs inversus is commonly observed in Kartagener's syndrome. The internal organs are reversed in position or location; for example, the heart is on the right side of the thorax.

CASE 12

While playing basketball over the weekend, a 35-year-old college professor experiences severe chest pain that radiates to his left jaw and left arm. He is taken by ambulance to the emergency department, where an electrocardiogram confirms that he has suffered a myocardial infarction (MI). Physical examination is significant for the presence of xanthelasma (periorbital cholesterol deposit) and tendinous xanthomas, indicating the pathologic deposition of lipids. His family history is remarkable for two first-degree relatives who suffered from coronary heart disease when they were in their mid-forties. Blood work reveals total plasma cholesterol of 400 mg/dl, and a cardiac angiogram reveals complete occlusion (hence the infarction) of the left anterior descending artery and 90% occlusion of the right coronary artery. The patient responds well to coronary angioplasty and is discharged home after only 3 days. The fasting lipid profile is summarized below.

Lipid	Patient	Reference Range
Triacylglycerol	150 mg/dl	(60–160 mg/dl)
Total cholesterol	400 mg/dl	(< 200 mg/dl)
High-density lipoprotein (HDL)	31 mg/dl	(≥ 35 mg/dl)
Very-low-density lipoprotein (VLDL)	30 mg/dl	(20–40 mg/dl)
Low-density lipoprotein (LDL)	359 mg/dl	(< 100 mg/dl)

1. What is your diagnosis based on family history and fasting lipid profile?

Based on the relatively early onset of MI, family history of premature cardiovascular disease, significant hypercholesterolemia and elevated LDL levels with normal triacylglycerols, and the presence of xanthelasma and tendinous xanthomas, he most likely has familial hypercholesterolemia (FH). FH is caused by a defective LDL receptor in peripheral tissues, particularly the liver, which plays an important role in the clearance of cholesterol from the blood. FH is inherited in an autosomal codominant fashion; that is, homozygotes manifest more serious pathologic sequences than heterozygotes.

2. Based on clinical presentations, is the patient likely to be heterozygous or homozygous for this deficiency?

This patient is likely to a heterozygote. As mentioned previously, FH homozygotes exhibit more severe symptoms than heterozygotes, probably due to the concept of gene dosage. People who are homozygotes typically suffer their first heart attack before age 20, and the total cholesterol levels usually range between 500 and 1000 mg/dl. Cholesterol levels are usually between 300 and 500 mg/dl in heterozyotes, who usually do not suffer heart attacks until later in life. Occasionally a few xanthomas can be found on the Achilles tendon in heterozygous FH.

3. What are the primary mechanisms by which mutations in the LDL receptor can impair LDL uptake from the plasma?

Physiologically, serum LDL is constantly made from intermediate-density lipoprotein (IDL), which is derived from VLDL degradation. About 75% of LDL is cleared via LDL receptor-mediated endocytosis in the liver (primary site), adrenal cortex, and other tissues. The remainder of LDL is cleared via poorly understood LDL receptor-independent mechanisms, including the one that macrophages use to endocytose oxidized LDL.

Note: In FH, five classes of mutations on the LDL receptor result in the impairment of receptor-mediated uptake of LDL from the circulation. These mutations include prevention of protein synthesis (*null*), incorrect insertion into the plasma membrane (*transport defective*), abnormal clathrin-mediated endocytosis (*ligand receptor-binding defective* and *internalization defective*), or an inability to recycle LDL back to the membrane (*recycling defective*).

4. What is the pathological consequence of elevated plasma LDL in FH?

Atherosclerosis of arteries can lead to premature cardiovascular disease, even in the absence of other risk factors such as obesity and smoking.

5. Describe the mechanism by which FH results in atherosclerosis.

Because the LDL receptor is defective, plasma LDL clearing has to rely on scavenger receptors on macrophages that "scavenge" (endocytose) oxidized LDL (oxidized LDL levels are proportional to the levels of LDL). These macrophages then form foam cells and release cytokines, causing proliferation of arterial smooth muscle cells. At the beginning, the smooth muscle cells produce enough extracellular matrix proteins to form a fibrous cap over the foam cells. However, because the scavenger receptors are not downregulated by intracellular cholesterol concentration, the foam cells continue to endocytose oxidized LDL and eventually rupture from the fibrous plaque, initiating thrombus formation. The dislodging of these thrombi usually leads to myocardial infarction and strokes.

6. How should this patient be managed medically and pharmacologically to decrease his risk of future cardiovascular complications?

Like any patient with cardiovascular disease and associated risk factors. He should be encouraged to undertake dietary and lifestyle modifications (e.g., increased exercise, smoking cessation). Pharmacologic options include HMG CoA reductase inhibitors ("statins") and bile-sequestering agents (e.g., cholestyramine).

Note: HMG CoA reductase is the rate-limiting enzyme in cholesterol synthesis.

CASE 13

A 5-year-old boy is sent to a developmental pediatric clinic for evaluation of delay of intellectual development and hyperactivity. His 7-year-old sister was diagnosed with mild mental retardation and a learning disability last year. He has an unusually long face with a prominent jaw and large ears, and genital exam reveals large testes (macro-orchidism). His maternal aunt had learning disabilities when she was young. Both his mother and his father had normal intellect.

1. What is the diagnosis?

Fragile X syndrome, an X-linked dominant disorder that is the most commonly inherited form of mental retardation.

2. Explain briefly the pathogenesis of this disorder.

It is caused by a trinucleotide repeat expansion in the FMR1 gene (for familial mental retardation), resulting in deficient expression of the FMR protein (FMRp). This protein is thought to play an important role in transporting nuclear mRNA from the nucleus into the cytoplasm prior to translation.

3. Southern blotting indicates that the mother has 90 CGG (trinucleotide) repeats whereas he has 350 CGG repeats. Why are the child's repeats much higher than his mother's?

When a parent (e.g., the mother of this boy) transmits the mutation to offspring, there is often an **expansion of the trinucleotide repeat**. Patients manifesting symptoms have more repeats on average than those who do not manifest symptoms; this explains why the mother was normal but her son affected. The process in which a genetic disease is more pronounced or develops at an earlier age in subsequent generations is called **anticipation**. Generally, anticipation is due to expansion of trinucleotide repeats (i.e., **amplification**).

Anticipation due to expansion of trinucleotide repeats (amplification).

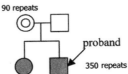

Note: The boy's sister was affected because she also had a higher number of trinucleotide repeats. However, since the disease is X-linked, the normal functioning FMR1 gene from her other X-chromosome attenuates the disease to some extent.

4. How are the genetics of fragile X syndrome similar to the genetics of Huntington's disease?

Huntington's disease is also due to a trinucleotide repeat expansion and exhibits anticipation because of the trinucleotide repeat in subsequent generations. However, it has an autosomal dominant rather than an X-linked dominant pattern of inheritance.

CASE 14

The newborn boy of a 42-year-old woman presents with upslanting palpebral fissures, excessive skin of the inner eyelid and at the back of the neck, a flattened maxillary and malar region, and palmar creases. Cytology reveals an abnormal karyotype.

1. What is the most likely diagnosis?

Down syndrome, or trisomy 21, an *aneuploid* condition (abnormal chromosome number due to either monosomy or trisomy), which leads to the most common genetic cause of moderate mental retardation. Generally speaking, maternal age older than 35 greatly increases the incidence rate.

Note: Although Down syndrome is the most common cause of congenital mental retardation, it is not the most common *hereditary* cause of mental retardation, because most cases of Down syndrome are due to meiotic nondysjunction during oogenesis.

2. How can a Robertsonian translocation in one of the parents cause Down syndrome in an offspring?

A Robertsonian translocation is caused by a translocation event in the germ line of either of the parents, such that the germ line cells (oocytes or sperm) contain three copies of material located on chromosome 21. This mechanism is different from the meiotic nondysjunction event in one of the parents that gives rise to most cases of Down syndrome. In this case, extra genetic material from the long arm of chromosome 21 attaches to another chromosome (typically, chromosome 14), resulting in an identical triple gene dosage of chromosome 21 material.

3. What mechanism gives rise to mosaic Down syndrome, in which only select tissues express the 21 trisomy?

Mosaic Down syndrome is caused by a *mitotic* nondysjunction phenomenon that occurs in the developing embryo or fetus. This mechanism is in contrast to the typical *meiotic* nondysjunction event responsible for most cases of Down's syndrome. In general, the earlier the event occurs, the more tissues are affected and the more severe the phenotype (although there are certainly exceptions to this rule).

4. What causes most of the deaths in infancy or childhood in Down syndrome?

Patients with Down syndrome have a high frequency of various congenital heart defects, which serve as the major cause of early mortality.

5. What characteristic neuropathologic findings are seen in the brain of older (> 40 years) people with Down syndrome?

Almost all patients of this age develop the characteristic manifestations of Alzheimer's disease, including neurofibrillary tangles and amyloid deposits.

Note: People with Down syndrome also have a substantially increased risk for developing acute leukemia (acute lymphoblastic or acute myelogenous).

6. What other two autosomal trisomies can sometimes produce liveborn infants?

Trisomy 18 (Edward syndrome; 47XX+18 or 47XY+18) and trisomy 13 (Patau syndrome; 47XX+13 or 47XY+13). Trisomy 18 is the most common chromosomal abnormality among stillborns. Both trisomies produce more severe symptoms than trisomy 21, causing death within the first few years of life, and most cases result from maternal nondysjunction during meiosis I of the respective chromosome pair.

Note: Both Edwards syndrome and Patau syndrome are associated with rocker-bottom feet, cardiac defects, and renal defects. An important distinction is that Edwards syndrome is associated with micrognathia (small mouth), whereas Patau syndrome is associated with micropthalmia (small eyes).

7. What two diseases are due to microdeletion of the same section of chromosome 15?

Angelman syndrome and Prader-Willi syndrome.

8. Why is the parental source of the chromosome significant in these microdeletion syndromes?

It has been a central dogma of genetics that phenotype is the same whether a given allele is from a paternal or maternal source. Like most dogmas, however, this one has not stood the test of time. It appears that the expression of a select number of genes depends on whether they are maternally or paternally derived. This phenomenon of gene expression based on parental origin is known as **genomic imprinting**.

Angelman syndrome usually is due to a deletion in the maternally derived chromosome 15, leading to a loss of function of many genes located in that region. Patients with this disease often exhibit insatiable laughter.

Prader-Willi syndrome is usually due to a microdeletion of the paternally derived chromosome 15. Patients are frequently obese.

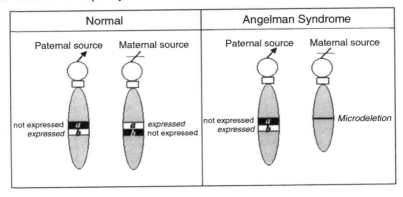

Maternal microdeletion in Angelman syndrome.

CASE 15

A 15-year-old girl is examined by an endocrinologist in the hospital. She has short stature, a webbed neck, and broad chest with widely spaced nipples. Secondary sexual characteristics, such as menses and breast development, are absent. She has normal intellect and seems to be a happy, healthy person. A pelvic ultrasound reveals streak ovaries. The laboratory test findings include a normal level of growth hormone and an elevated level of follicle-stimulating hormone (FSH). Her karyotype is 45XO.

1. What is the diagnosis?

Turner syndrome, a disorder of sex chromosome aneuploidy. Females with Turner syndrome are missing one X chromosome.

2. What causes the abnormal karyotype?

About 80% of the cases are caused by meiotic error in the father; that is, patients do not receive an X chromosome from their father.

3. Why are secondary sex characteristics absent?

Girls with Turner syndrome have ovarian dysgenesis. Instead of normal ovaries they have streaks of connective tissue that do not produce sufficient quantities of estrogen or progesterone, hormones that are required for secondary sexual characteristics.

4. How should the patient be managed medically and pharmacologically to correct the lack of secondary sexual characteristics?

Estrogen therapy for teenaged girls with Turner syndrome can promote development of secondary sexual characteristics.

5. Describe the reproductive fitness of females with Turner syndrome.

Ninety percent of females with Turner syndrome present with ovarian dysgenesis and are infertile. However, a small percentage (5–10%) of patients have sufficient ovarian development, and some of them are fertile.

6. Compare and contrast Turner syndrome with other examples of sex chromosome aneuploidies.

	TURNER SYNDROME	KLINEFELTER SYNDROME	TRISOMY X	TRISOMY XYY
Karyotype	45X female 45X/46XX mosaics	47XXY male 48XXXY	47XXX female	47XYY male
Characteristics	Short stature Sexual immaturity Ovarian dysgenesis	Tall with long extremities Hypogonadism	Usually tall	Tall Behavioral problems
Intelligence	Normal	Learning disability	Learning disability	Normal

CASE 16

A 16-year-old girl is concerned because she has not yet started her period, whereas all of her friends have had periods for at least 2 years. She also has no breast development. Physical exam reveals scant axillary and pubic hair, and the uterus is not palpable. On speculum examination no cervix is visible (i.e., the vagina ends in a blind pouch). A laparoscopy reveals no uterus or ovaries. Her karyotype is 46XY.

1. What is the syndrome?

Androgen insensitivity syndrome, also known as the testicular feminization syndrome. Patients are genetically and gonadally male, but phenotypically female.

2. What causes this syndrome?

Genetic alterations in testosterone receptors make the tissues unresponsive to testosterone's androgenic effects. Testicles are present and functional, producing testosterone, but the tissues do not respond.

3. Why is a vaginal pouch present?

The vaginal pouch and the penis are formed embryologically from the urogenital fold, which in the absence of testosterone (or testosterone action) forms a vagina instead of a penis.

4. Why is no uterus present?

The uterus is formed from the mullerian ducts. In males these structures are dissolved by mullerian-inhibiting substance, which is produced by the testicles. Since the testicles themselves are not abnormal in androgen insensitivity syndrome, mullerian-inhibiting substance is secreted and the ducts dissolve, forming no uterus.

5. Would testosterone levels be low or high in this patient?

They would be high since the nonfunctional receptors reduce negative feedback on pituitary production of luteinizing horone (LH), which in turn increases testosterone production.

6. Why should the patient's testicles be removed?

Generally, patients have undescended testes (cryptorchidism), which places them at increased risk for testicular cancer.

CASE 17

A 54-year-old male smoker is sent to the emergency department with complaints of severe chest pains. His cardiac enzyme work-up is negative after 24 hours, but an angiogram reveals severe atherosclerotic coronary artery disease. Triple bypass surgery is performed. After surgery he is in the hospital for two and a half weeks without substantial nutrient intake. The wound-healing process is slow, he has obvious skin peeling on the back and buttocks as well as pitting edema, and his hair can be plucked painlessly. Laboratory findings are remarkable for the following: serum albumin 1.9 gm/dl (normal = 3.4–5.0 gm/dl), transferrin of 130 mg/dl (normal = 250–390 mg/dl), and reduced numbers of WBCs (leukopenia). His daily urinary urea nitrogen excretion is about 15 gm/day (normal = < 5 gm/day).

1. What is the noncardiac diagnosis?

Kwashiorkor, a maladaptive state with protein calorie malnourishment and severely increased catabolic rate. In modern nations, it is typically caused by acute, life-threatening illnesses such as trauma and sepsis. It is also seen after major surgical operations.

Note: In third-world nations, kwashiorkor usually results when children are weaned off breast milk, a good protein source, and start a diet high in carbohydrate and very low in protein (the only diet available).

2. What is the reason for elevated urinary urea nitrogen excretion?

His body is going through a hypercatabolic state characterized by the breaking down of endogenous protein in an attempt to supply precursors for gluconeogenesis. Because urea is formed only from amino acid metabolism, elevated protein catabolism leads to a proportional increase in urea synthesis, and more urea is excreted in the urine.

3. What is the reason for the low serum albumin level?

The patient's dramatic serum albumin decrease is a result of catabolism of albumin (amid a generalized increase in protein catabolism) due to the severe stress (bypass surgery) and, to a lesser extent, poor feeding. In addition, inflammatory mediators may also reduce hepatic albumin production. Neither hepatic albumin production nor extravascular reservoirs of albumin can compensate for the degree of catabolism. The low albumin level also explains the pitting edema.

4. Would you expect this patient to have an obviously emaciated appearance and muscle wasting?

No. In fact, people with Kwashiorkor usually have unaltered or only slightly decreased fat reserves and muscle mass. The reasons are still a mystery. The lack of emaciation can be quite deceiving in terms of the severity of the patient's inadequate nutrition. These findings are in stark contrast to **marasmus**, in which malnutrition leads to severe muscle wasting.

5. Compare and contrast kwashiorkor and marasmus.

	KWASHIORKOR	MARASMUS
Cause	Stress-induced low protein intake (takes only weeks to develop)	Chronic low calorie intake (takes months to years to develop)
Basic characteristic	Loss of visceral protein	Loss of somatic protein
Presentations	Hair pluckability, pitting edema, well-nourished look	Emaciated appearance, weight lower than 80% of ideal weight
Laboratory tests	Very low serum albumin (< 2.8 mg/dl), decreased TIBC and lymphocytes	Low creatinine (from low muscle mass)
Mortality	High	Low (if there is no other underlying disease)

TIBC = total iron-binding capacity.

16. BACTERIAL DISEASES

Bahair Ghazi

BASIC CONCEPTS

Bacteriology

1. What makes an organism gram-positive or gram-negative?

Both gram-positive and gram-negative organisms have an internal cell membrane and cell walls made of peptidoglycan. However, gram-negative bacteria have much thinner cell walls and, in addition, an outer membrane outside the cell wall.

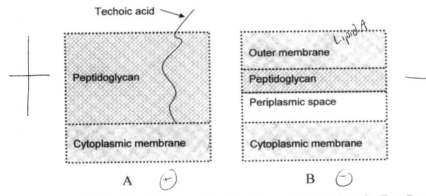

Structural differences in the cell wall of gram-positive (*A*) and gram-negative (*B*) bacteria (From Brochert A: Platinum Vignettes: Microbiology. Philadelphia, Hanley & Belfus, 2003, p 17, with permission.)

2. Why are gram-negative infections more likely to produce bacterial sepsis?

The outer membrane of gram-negative organisms (see above) contains lipid A, an endotoxin that is released on bacterial death and has potent proinflammatory effects.

3. Describe the mechanism by which lipid A causes toxicity.

Lipid A activates macrophages to secrete interleukin-1 (IL-1) and tumor necrosis factor (TNF) as well as stimulates the release of nitric oxide (NO) from endothelial cells. Large doses of lipid A lead to shock and intravascular coagulation via this stimulatory effect.

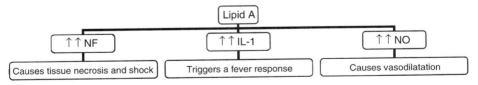

Mechanism by which lipid A causes toxicity.

4. Define exotoxin, enterotoxin, and neurotoxin.

Exotoxins are proteins released by both gram-positive and gram-negative bacteria during their normal life cycle. **Enterotoxins** are exotoxins that act on the GI system, and **neurotoxins** are exotoxins that act on the nerves or motor endplates. For example, infectious diarrhea is

259

caused by enterotoxins released by *Vibrio cholera*, *Escherichia coli*, *Campylobacter jejuni*, and *Shigella dysenteriae*. Exotoxins released into food can cause poisoning, as in *Bacillus cereus* and *Staphylococcus aureus* food poisoning. Pyrogenic exotoxins released by *S. aureus* and *Streptococcus pyogenes* can cause rash, fever, and toxic shock syndrome.

5. What is a capsule? What purpose does it serve?

Certain species of bacteria produce a slippery outermost covering called a capsule. This covering consists of high-molecular-weight polysaccharides, which help the bacteria to evade phagocytosis by neutrophils and macrophages. The capsule is not essential for growth and serves only in a protective capacity. The most common medically relevant encapsulated organisms are *Streptococcus pneumoniae*, *Neisseria meningitidis*, and *Haemophilus influenzae* type B.

Note: These encapsulated organisms are also the most common cause of sepsis in splenectomized patients and meningitis in adults, largely because of their ability to evade host defenses.

6. What is the quellung reaction?

The quellung reaction is a test for encapsulated bacteria. It causes encapsulated bacteria to swell when exposed to certain antibodies.

7. Test your knowledge of the properties of the bacteria listed in the left-hand column by covering the right-hand columns.

ORGANISM	DISEASES CAUSED BY	NOTES
Gram-positive cocci		Toxin-mediated diseases: staphylococcal toxic shock syndrome, scalded skin syndrome, staphylococcal gastroenteritis
Staphylococcus aureus	Cellulitis, osteomyelitis, necrotizing pneumonia, carbuncles, stye, furuncles	
Staphylococcus epidermidis	Prosthetic valve endocarditis	Normal skin flora
Staphylococcus saprophyticus	Cystitis in young women	
Streptococcus agalactiae	Neonatal meningitis, chorioamnionitis	Normal vaginal flora
Streptococcus pneumoniae	Sinusitis, otitis media, pneumonia	
Streptococcus pyogenes	Pharyngitis, cellulitis	Later sequelae of rheumatic fever, glomerulonephritis
Enterococcus species	Endocarditis, septicemia, urinary tract infection, abdominal abscess	Normal fecal flora (cause disease when host is compromised or integrity of GI tract is breached)
Gram-positive bacilli		
Bacillus anthracis	Pulmonary anthrax, cutaneous anthrax	
Corynebacterium diphtheriae	Diphtheria	Pseudomembrane in throat Secretes toxin that shuts down protein synthesis
Listeria monocytogenes	Neonatal and elderly meningitis	
Gram-negative cocci		
Neisseria meningitidis	Meningitis, septicemia	Common cause of meningitis in college dorms, military barracks Waterhouse-Friderichsen syndrome: adrenal crisis in meningococcal sepsis

(Cont'd.)

ORGANISM	DISEASES CAUSED BY	NOTES
Gram-negative cocci *(cont'd.)*		
Neisseria gonorrhoeae	Urethritis, epididymitis, pelvic inflammatory disease, pharyngitis, gonococcal arthritis, conjunctivitis	
Enteric gram-negative rods		
Campylobacter jejuni	Enteritis	
Escherichia coli	Enteritis	
Salmonella species	Enterocolitis	Typhoid fever from *Salmonella typhi*
Shigella sonei	Bacillary dysentery	
Helicobacter pylori	Peptic ulcer, acute gastritis, chronic gastritis, MALToma	
Other gram-negative rods		
Bordetella pertussis	Pertussis	
Brucella species	Brucellosis	From unpasteurized milk
Francisella tularensis	Tularemia	From tick bites, animal vectors
Haemophilus influenzae	Otitis media, sinusitis, pneumonia, cellulitis	Encapsulated type B was most common cause of pediatric meningitis and epiglottitis before vaccine
Pseudomonas aeruginosa	Bone and joint infections, endocarditis	Osteomyelitis in sickle-cell patients
Legionella pneumophila	Legionnaire's disease (acute pneumonia with multisystem involvement) Pontiac fever (similar to flu)	
Yersinia pestis	Bubonic plague	
Yersinia enterocolitica	Enterocolitis	
Anaerobes		
Clostridium perfringens	Anaerobic cellulitis, gas gangrene (myonecrosis), food poisoning	
Clostridium tetani	Tetanus	Immunization with tetanus toxoid
Clostridium botulinum	Botulism (food poisoning causing flaccid paralysis)	
Clostridium difficile	Pseudomembranous colitis	Usually due to antibiotic use
Spirochetes		
Borrelia burgdorferi	Lyme disease	
Borrelia recurrentis	Relapsing fever	Organism switches surface protein to evade immune response, causing intermittent fevers
Treponema pallidum	Syphilis	Nontreponemal tests VDRL and RPR for screening Treponemal tests: FTA-ABS for confirmation
Leptospira interrogans	Weil's disease (ictero-hemorrhagic fever)	Transmitted by animal urine

(Cont'd.)

ORGANISM	DISEASES CAUSED BY	NOTES
Intracellular organisms		
Mycoplasma pneumoniae	Atypical pneumonia (walking pneumonia)	No cell wall
Chlamydia trachomatis	Urethritis, pelvic inflammatory disease	Sexually transmitted disease
Chlamydia psittaci	Psittacosis (flulike syndrome)	Transmitted by bird droppings (*Chlamydia* shit attack)
Chlamydia pneumoniae	Atypical pneumonia	
Mycobacterium tuberculosis	Tuberculosis	
Mycobacterium leprae	Leprosy	Tuberculoid: milder form, few organisms in lesions Lepromatous: severe form, many organisms in lesions
Rickettsia rickettsii	Rocky Mountain spotted fever	Ascending maculopapular rash that begins on extremities

VDRL = Venereal Disease Research Laboratory test, RPR = rapid plasmin reagin, FTA-ABS = fluorescent treponemal antibody, absorbed test.

Antibacterial Pharmacology

8. What are the beta-lactam antibiotics? Describe their mechanism of action.

The beta-lactam antibiotics include the penicillins, cephalosporins, and carbapenems (imipenem, meropenem). By virtue of their beta-lactam chemical moiety, they inhibit bacterial cell wall synthesis. Resistance to these antibiotics is mediated by bacterially synthesized beta-lactamase enzymes that destroy the beta-lactam ring.

9. Why is clavulanic acid, sulbactam, or aztreonam added to some penicillins?

These agents inhibit beta-lactamase, thereby reducing resistance of bacterial species to the penicillins.

10. Summarize the antibacterial spectrum of the various subclasses of penicillins and cephalosporins.

ANTIBIOTIC CLASS	SPECTRUM
Natural penicillins (penicillin V, penicillin G, benzathine penicillin)	Mostly gram-positive coverage
First-generation cephalosporins (cephalexin, cefazolin, cefadroxil, cephalothin)	Mostly gram-positive coverage
Second-generation cephalosporins (cefotetan, cefoxitin, cefaclor)	Between first and third generation
Extended-spectrum penicillins (ampicillin, amoxicillin)	Gram-positive and increased gram-negative coverage
Third-generation cephalosporins (ceftriaxone, cefotaxime)	Gram-positive and increased gram-negative coverage
Antipseudomonal penicillins (ticarcillin, piperacillin)	Increased gram-negative overage, including *Pseudomonas* species

Note that the first-generation cephalosporins and natural penicillins have a similar spectrum and that the third-generation cephalosporins and extended-spectrum penicillins have a similar spectrum. Knowing this general pattern helps understand selection of antimicrobial therapy.

11. What is the antibacterial spectrum of the fluoroquinolones? Describe their mechanism of action.

This class of antibiotics has a broad spectrum of activity, including both gram-positive and gram-negative organisms. Fluoroquinolones also cover *Pseudomonas* species, making them fairly similar in spectrum to the antipseudomonal penicillins. They inhibit bacterial DNA synthesis by inhibiting the bacterial topoisomerase (DNA gyrase).

12. Describe the spectrum and mechanism of action of the macrolides.

Macrolides have good gram-positive coverage, and several members of this class are effective against intracellular organisms. They work by inhibiting bacterial protein synthesis.

13. What is special about the tetracyclines?

Tetracyclines are the most important agents for the treatment of intracellular organisms. They also work by inhibiting bacterial protein synthesis.

14. Describe the mechanism of action and spectrum of the aminoglycosides.

Aminoglycosides are irreversible inhibitors of protein synthesis that are generally effective only against gram-negative rods. However, they may be used in combination with penicillins for enterococcal endocarditis (a gram-positive organism).

15. How does chloramphenicol work? Why is it seldom used?

Chloramphenicol also inhibits protein synthesis, but because of the risk of aplastic anemia it is not commonly used in modern nations.

16. Cover the right-hand columns and describe the mechanism of action and adverse effects for the antimicrobials listed in the left-hand column.

ANTIMICROBIAL	MECHANISM OF ACTION	ADVERSE EFFECTS
Beta lactams	Inhibit transpeptidase and stimulate autolysins	Hypersensitivity, diarrhea (Cephalo-(sporins have ~ 20% cross-reactivity with penicillin-allergic patients)
Tetracyclines	Bind to the 30S subunit of bacterial ribosome, thus inhibiting protein synthesis	GI upset, discolored teeth in children, toxicity in renal impaired patients, photosensitivity
Aminoglycosides	Impair proper assembly of the ribo-some, causing the 30S subunit to misread genetic code	Nephrotoxicity and ototoxicity
Macrolides	Bind to 50S subunit of ribosome and inhibit translocation	GI distress
Fluoroquinolones	Inhibit DNA gyrase, preventing DNA replication	Damages cartilage in young children
Chloramphenicol	Reversibly inhibits protein synthesis	Aplastic anemia
Trimethoprim	Inhibit folic acid synthesis by inhibiting dihydrofolate reductase	Mimics folic acid deficiency (megaloblastic (anemia, leucopenia, granulocytopenia)
Sulfonamides	Inhibit folic acid synthesis by acting as structural analog (competitive inhibitor) of PABA, a precursor of folic acid in bacteria	Allergic reactions

PABA = para-aminobenzoic acid.

17. Why is trimethoprim (TMP) commonly given in combination with sulfamethoxazole (SMX)?

Because both these agents inhibit folic acid synthesis at different steps, the combination (TMP-SMX) is synergistic.

18. Summarize the selection of antimicrobial agents for the following organisms.

ORGANISM	TREATMENT	NOTE
Gram-positive cocci		
Streptococcus pyogenes	Penicillins	
Streptococcus agalactiae	Penicillins	
Streptococcus pneumoniae	Penicillins	In areas of resistance, use third-generation cephalosporin (e.g., ceftriaxone, cefotaxime)
Staphylococcus aureus	Penicillins	Use antistaphylococcal penicillins (oxacillin, cloxacillin)
		Use vancomycin for serious/resistant infections
Enterococcus species	Penicillins	Penicillin + aminoglycoside (synergistic)
Gram-positive bacilli		
Bacillus anthracis	Penicillins	Ciprofloxacin also first-line choice
Listeria monocytogenes	Penicillins	
Corynebacterium diphtheriae	Penicillins	
Anaerobes		
Clostridium perfringens	Penicillins	
Clostridium tetani	Penicillins	
Clostridium difficile	Metronidazole	Vancomycin second-line choice
Spirochetes		
Borrelia burgdorferi	Penicillins	
Treponema pallidum	Penicillins	
Leptospira interrogans	Penicillins	
Gram-negative cocci		
Neisseria meningitidis	Ceftriaxone/cefotaxime	Sensitivity testing mandatory
Neisseria gonorrhoeae	Ceftriaxone	
Enteric gram-negative rods		
Campylobacter jejuni	Ciprofloxacin	
Escherichia coli	Ciprofloxacin	Alternatives: ampicillin/cefotaxime/TMP-SMX
Salmonella typhi	Ciprofloxacin	Alternative: Ceftriaxone
Shigella sonnei	Ciprofloxacin	Alternative: ampicillin
Helicobacter pylori	Triple antibiotic treatment	
Other gram-negative rods		
Haemophilus influenzae	Ceftriaxone/cefotaxime	Alternative: ciprofloxacin
Pseudomonas species	Antipseudomonal penicillin (piperacillin, ticarcillin)	
Nasty gram-negative rods		
Yersinia pestis	Aminoglycoside	
Brucella species	Aminoglycoside	
Francisella tularensis	Aminoglycoside	
Intracellular organisms		
Mycoplasma species	Tetracyclines	Alternative: macrolide
Chlamydia pneumoniae	Tetracyclines-	Alternative: macrolide
Chlamydia trachomatis	Tetracyclines	Alternative:macrolide
Chlamydi psittaci	Tetracyclines	Alternative: macrolide
Rickettsia species	Tetracyclines	
Erhlichia species	Tetracyclines	
Coxiella species	Tetracyclines	
Legionella species	Macrolide	

TMP-SMX = trimethoprim-sulfamethoxazole.

CASE 1

A 64-year-old man presents with complaints of dyspnea and productive cough. The patient states that approximately two days ago he began experiencing high fevers and chills. He informs you that he began to worry when he started coughing up "rust-colored" phlegm. On exam you appreciate a febrile elderly man with dullness to percussion and decreased breath sounds in the left lower posterior fields. You promptly order a chest x-ray and, while awaiting the results, obtain a sample of sputum for Gram stain. Complete blood count shows significant leukocytosis, and a pulse oximeter shows low oxygen saturation of 89%.

1. What is the most likely diagnosis?

Fevers, chills, shortness of breath, pain with inspiration, and productive cough are classic signs of pneumonia.

2. Why is it important to distinguish between community-acquired and nosocomial pneumonia?

In general, a different spectrum of organisms causes these two types of pneumonia; therefore, empirical selection of antibiotics is different. In community-acquired pneumonia, the most common bacterial organism is *Streptococcus pneumoniae*, followed by *Haemophilus influenzae*, *Legionella pneumophila* and *Mycoplasma pneumoniae*, not necessarily in that order.

Note: The patient has a cough productive of rust-colored phlegm, a typical product of pneumococcal pneumonia. Gram stain of an adequate sputum sample often shows gram-positive, lancet-shaped diplococci. <u>*Streptococcus pneumoniae*</u> is also uniquely susceptible to optochinin.

α hemolytic / optochinin susceptible

3. What is the chest x-ray likely to reveal in this patient?

On a chest film classic pneumococcal pneumonia causes lung lobe consolidation. The consolidation classically appears as right middle lobe or lower left lobe opacification, meaning that a clearly demarcated part of the lung is clearly visible.

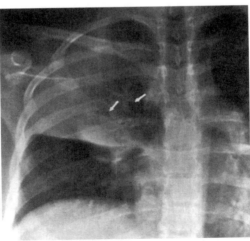

Lobar consolidation in a typical pneumonia. (From Brochert A: Platinum Vignettes: Internal Medicine. Philadelphia, Hanley & Belfus, 2003, p 1, with permission.)

4. How should the patient be treated pharmacologically?

Although penicillin G has been the first choice for community-acquired pneumonia, a rising incidence of penicillin resistance among strains of *S. pneumoniae* often necessitates the use of an alternative agent, such as ceftriaxone. Note that as a third-generation cephalosporin, ceftriaxone can cover the more common gram-positive organisms that cause community-acquired pneumonia (pneumococci) as well as the more common gram-negative organisms (*Haemophilus influenzae*).

5. The patient is hospitalized and takes a turn for the worse. He spikes a fever and becomes hypotensive and tachycardic, his skin becomes cool and clammy, plasma levels of blood urea nitrogen (BUN) and creatinine increase, urine output drops, and liver enzymes become elevated. What probably happened?

The patient has developed a feared complication of any serious bacterial infection: septic shock. To review, bacteremia is simply the presence of bacteria in the blood stream, whereas sepsis is an infection of the blood stream causing symptoms and illness. Shock is defined as inadequate end-organ perfusion, causing tissue damage. Therefore, septic shock is an infection that has caused a systemic state of end-organ starvation.

6. What defense mechanisms prevent pneumonia in healthy people?

The respiratory tract has many defenses in place to prevent access to the lung. The nasal hairs, mucosa, and dynamics of airflow all act early to prevent inhalation of microorganisms. The epiglottis and cough reflex help to prevent particulate matter from traveling into the deeper airways. The respiratory tract is lined with mucus until the terminal bronchioles are reached. This mucus is propelled upward by the ciliated epithelium, eliminating foreign material as expectorant. The last line of defense is in and around the alveolar complex and consists of macrophages, neutrophils, immunoglobulin, and complement. These components become hyperactive during an infectious process since many of their triggers are foreign antigen.

Note: Any state that alters consciousness (anesthesia, seizure, intoxication, sedation, and neurologic disorders such as coma) predisposes to aspiration pneumonia and its feared complication of lung abscess. This risk is due to the suppressed cough reflex and inability of the patient to respire normally. The organisms causing this type of infection are usually anaerobes from the mouth or refluxed gastric contents; other organisms that can cause lung abscesses include Staphylococcus aureus, mycobacteria, and *Klebsiella pneumoniae*, which produces the famous currant-jelly sputum.

7. Why may a mechanically ventilated (intubated) patient in the intensive care unit be at increased risk for developing nosocomial pneumonia?

Mechanical ventilation bypasses the normal host defenses for preventing contamination of the sterile lower respiratory segments (e.g., mucociliary clearance).

8. What is atypical or "walking" pneumonia? Explain the classic presentation and etiology.

Atypical pneumonia has a more insidious onset than typical pneumonia. "Walking" pneumonia is characterized by headache, nonproductive cough, and a nonspecific diffuse interstitial infiltrate on x-ray that looks worse than the patient. Atypical pneumonia is generally caused by viruses or intracellular bacteria, such as *Legionella pneumophila*, *Mycoplasma pneumoniae*, and species of *Chlamydia* (e.g., C. psitacci). *Mycoplasma pneumoniae* is the classic causative organism and can be differentiated from other causes based on a high titer of cold agglutinins (IgM). Most of the bacterial causes can be treated with a macrolide or tetracycline, our favorite drugs for intracellular bugs.

Note: The term *cold agglutinins* refers to the fact that specific IgM antibodies bind to red blood cells at low temperatures and cause them to agglutinate or stick together. This can be demonstrated at the bedside when a blood sample becomes clumpy when placed in ice and returns to a fluid state when rewarmed.

CASE 2

A 26-year-old woman complains of severe diarrhea for the past day. Her bowel movements are watery with small stool particles, but she denies the presence of any blood. She just returned from a weeklong trip to Mexico, where she drank only bottled water supplemented with ice from her hotel room. She worries that her symptoms may represent a more serious disease than traveler's diarrhea. She has no other complaints or problems. Exam is remarkable for tachycardia and dry mucous membranes.

1. **What is the most likely diagnosis?**
   Traveler's diarrhea. Despite her best efforts to drink only bottled water, she has made the common mistake of using ice made with local water.

2. **What is the difference between osmotic and secretory diarrhea? Name a cause for each.**
   Secretory diarrhea is caused by active secretion of fluids by the intestines. Examples include diarrhea due to the toxins of *Vibrio cholerae* and enterotoxigenic *E. coli* (ETEC), the cause of traveler's diarrhea.
   Osmotic diarrhea is caused by osmotically active agents within the gut lumen, which cause passive movement of water into the intestinal lumen along osmotic gradients. An example is nutrient malabsorption (e.g., in celiac sprue or pancreatic insufficiency), in which the osmotically active nutrients pull water into the intestines.

3. **What other types of diarrhea can be caused by *E. coli*?**
   Enterohemorrhagic *E. coli* (EHEC) and enteroinvasive *E. coli* cause a dysentery-like syndrome with fever and bloody stools. Enteropathogenic *E. coli* is a common cause of diarrhea in infants, and enteroadherent *E. coli* is another cause of traveler's diarrhea.

E. COLI TYPE	DISEASE
Enterotoxigenic	Traveler's diarrhea
Enteroadherent	Traveler's diarrhea
Enterohemorrhagic	Bloody diarrhea, hemolytic uremic syndrome
Enteroinvasive	Bloody diarrhea
Enteropathogenic	Diarrhea in infants

4. **How is diarrhea treated?**
   A good rule of thumb is that diarrhea is treated with supportive therapy, meaning that in the absence of systemic infection, dehydration and electrolyte replacement are the focus of therapy. For the more serious organisms, such as those causing bloody diarrhea, broad-spectrum antibiotics may be helpful.
   Note: The use of broad-spectrum antibiotics must be carefully monitored to avoid inducing *Clostridium difficile* colitis, also known as pseudomembranous colitis. Pseudomembranous colitis occurs when one of the normal intestinal flora (*C. difficile*) proliferates and causes a superinfection when its competitors have been reduced. *C. difficile* elaborates two exotoxins, referred to as A and B, that cause secretory diarrhea in addition to damage of the mucosa. Toxin B is used by laboratories to detect the infection. Pseudomembranous colitis is treated with metronidazole or oral vancomycin.

CASE 3

A 65-year-old woman complains of malaise, myalgias, and night sweats. She claims that for the past 2 weeks she has experienced the sudden onset of high feverish spells ranging from 102 to 104°F. Her past medical history is significant for hypertension, hyperlipidemia,

and several bouts of rheumatic fever. On exam you notice a slight weight loss since her last visit. A new murmur can be auscultated. Furthermore, you appreciate painful nodules on her fingers and toes coupled with subungual splinter hemorrhages. Fundoscopic examination reveals Roth spots, as shown below. A transesophageal electrocardiogram reveals vegetations on the mitral valve. Two sets of blood cultures are ordered; the results are pending.

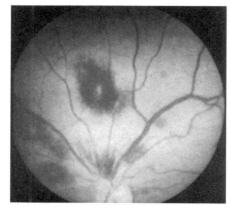

Roth spots revealed on fundoscopic examination. (From Brochert A: Platinum Vignettes: Internal Medicine. Philadelphia, Hanley & Belfus, 2003, p 31, with permission.)

1. What is the most likely diagnosis?
Acute bacterial endocarditis, an infection of the endothelial lining of the heart.

2. What are the major risk factors for endocarditis?
The major risk factor for the development of endocarditis is a structurally abnormal heart causing aberrant flow streams. Common structural abnormalities include prosthetic valves, native valve lesions, calcifications, rheumatic heart disease, congenital abnormalities, and heart disease. The majority of infections occur in the left heart (aortic and mitral valves), but with intravenous drug use, right-sided tricuspid valve lesions are common because the pathogens are introduced into the venous system.

3. Which bacteria are most commonly associated with bacterial endocarditis?
Endocarditis can be classified as acute or subacute, depending on the time course. Acute infections occur within days to weeks, and patients are extremely sick during this time. **Acute infections** are most often due to streptococci or staphylococci. **Subacute infections** present with milder symptoms and are characterized by a consistently low-grade illness for 3–4 weeks; they are frequently caused by *Streptococcus viridans* and group D streptococci such as *Streptococcus bovis*. — think colon cancer perforation
Note: Bacterial endocarditis that occurs soon after prosthetic valvular surgery is commonly due to *Staphylococcus epidermidis* and is believed to result from intraoperative contamination.

CASE 4

A 20-year-old man presents for the evaluation of a new genital lesion. He returned from spring break last week and noticed a painless ulcer on his scrotum. He is quite concerned and admits to several instances of unprotected intercourse. Physical exam reveals a well-demarcated, 2-cm painless lesion with a raised border on the anterior aspect of the scrotum, as shown below. The remainder of the exam is unremarkable.

Lyme = Syph = Spyrochete

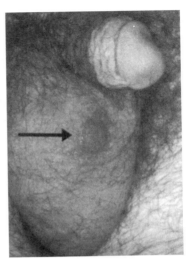

Scrotal lesion. (From Brochert A: Platinum Vignettes: Microbiology. Philadelphia, Hanley & Belfus, 2003, p 29, with permission.)

1. What is the most likely diagnosis?

Syphilis, which is caused by the organism *Treponema pallidum* and is acquired through broken epithelium or mucosal contact.   Chancre - painless ulcer

2. Based on the presentation, what stage of syphilitic infection does the patient probably have?

Syphilis progresses through three different stages: primary, secondary, and tertiary syphilis. This patient displays the painless chancre on the genitals, which is the classic sign of primary syphilis and appears 3–6 weeks after contact. This lesion is highly infectious and continuously sheds motile spirochetes. The primary stage lasts 4–6 weeks and then resolves, often fooling patients into thinking that they are cured.

3. What stage of syphilis would you suspect in a patient with a diffuse maculopapular rash?

This presentation is classic for secondary syphilis. The secondary stage of syphilis begins approximately 6 weeks after the primary chancre has healed. This phase is characterized by a generalized maculopapular rash with or without the fleshy, painless genital warts called condyloma lata. The second stage of syphilis resolves in 6 weeks, and the disease enters the latent phase. If not treated, approximately one-third of patients with secondary syphilis progress to tertiary syphilis.

4. Suppose the patient does not seek treatment and presents 10 years later with a regurgitant murmur heard best over the right second intercostal space and a pathologic ataxic gait. What is the likely diagnosis?

Tertiary syphilis, the end stage of the disease. This stage can develop anywhere from 5 to 35 years after the initial infection. Tertiary syphilis is a systemic disease with three major components: granulomatous change (gummas), cardiovascular syphilis, and neurosyphilis. Inflammatory destruction is the pathophysiologic mechanism inherent to all three components. Cardiovascular syphilis may result in aortic valve insufficiency and aortic aneurysm, whereas neurosyphilis can cause tabes dorsalis, a condition that involves degeneration of the dorsal column of the spinal cord and subsequent ataxia.

5. What tests definitively diagnose syphilis?

Direct visualization by dark-field microscopy can be done during the active phases of stage one and two by obtaining a sample from the lesion and observing the motile spirochetes. Serologic tests were developed to answer the need for a syphilis screen. The Venereal Disease Research Laboratory (VDRL) and rapid plasmin reagin (RPR) tests were developed to detect antibodies against certain components released after cell death. Both are nonspecific treponemal tests and, if positive, require a more specific measure, the fluorescent treponemal antibody, absorbed test (FTA-ABS). The key point is that the VDRL and the RPR are effective screening methods for at-risk patients.

6. How should you treat the patient?

Luckily, syphilis is one of the easiest diseases to treat. Administer penicillin G or, if the patient is penicillin-allergic, tetracycline or doxycycline. Only primary and secondary syphilis can be cured with medication. Antibiotics typically do nothing for tertiary syphilis.

7. Later that night, the patient calls you at home with serious concerns about an allergic reaction to penicillin. He states that several hours after being treated he developed a new rash, along with fever, headache, and muscle aches. What probably happened?

The patient has probably suffered from a common reaction to the penicillin treatment of syphilis, known as the Jarisch-Herxheimer reaction. This side effect of treatment is due to the immune system's reaction to the lysis of treponemes. When exposed to the tremendous load of foreign antigens, the body releases interleukin-1 and tumor necrosis factor alpha, causing fever and possibly shock. This entity should not be confused with an allergy to penicillin; it requires only treatment of symptoms and close monitoring.   IL1   TNFα

CASE 5

A frantic mother brings her 8-year-old son for an emergent visit. She is concerned about an enlarging rash located on the child's back. She adds that he has been complaining of a flu-like illness since the family's return from a hiking trip in New England, during which her son was bitten by a tick. On exam you appreciate a large, well-demarcated, 20-cm erythematous rash with central clearing and some regional adenopathy.

1. What is the most likely diagnosis?

Lyme disease, caused by the spirochete *Borrelia burgdorferi*. This organism is transmitted from the bite of an *Ixodes* tick, endemic to the woodlands of New England.

2. What stage of Lyme disease should you suspect in this child?

The patient has manifestations consistent with stage 1 or "early localized" Lyme disease. Lyme disease is similar to syphilis in that both illnesses are caused by the dissemination of an infectious spirochete and progress through three stages: an early localized stage, an early-disseminated stage and a late stage (stage 1, 2, and 3, respectively). This patient is in stage 1, which consists of the expanding erythematous lesion known as erythema chronicum migrans. A flu-like syndrome and regional adenopathy often accompany the rash of stage 1 Lyme disease.

3. How would your diagnosis change if the patient presented with a similar history but had complaints of various painful swollen joints and a diffuse macular rash all over his body?

The patient is most likely suffering from stage 2 or early disseminated Lyme disease. This stage is characterized by the spread of *Borrelia burgdorferi* to four components of the body: joints, heart, nervous tissue, and skin. Migratory musculoskeletal pains develop, usually affecting the large joints such as the knee. Affected joints become swollen, and tender. Cardiac complications vary from conduction block to myocarditis, whereas neural issues range from viral meningitis to nerve palsies, most classically Bell's palsy. The skin lesions of stage 2 Lyme disease are similar to stage 1 rashes but are smaller and more widely distributed over the body surface.

4. If the patient does not seek treatment, what is the likelihood that he will progress to stage 3 Lyme disease?

The late stage of Lyme disease (stage 3) occurs in only 10% of untreated patients and is characterized by the development of chronic arthritis, which involves multiple large joints, and progressive central nervous system disease.

5. **What is the treatment for Lyme disease? Name a preventative measure.**

Lyme disease is effectively treated with penicillin or doxycycline. Recently, an effective vaccination has been developed.

CASE 6

While you are in Pakistan on a medical mission, a patient presents with an 8-week history of fever, night sweats, and a productive cough at times tinged with blood (hemoptysis). He has lost 20 pounds during this time and has been generally fatigued and weak. A chest x-ray reveals a pulmonary infiltrate, and a purified protein derivative (PPD) skin test is positive. The patient reports that the same test was negative 1 year ago. A sputum stain for acid-fast bacilli is positive.

1. **What is the presumptive diagnosis?**

Tuberculosis, due to *Mycobacterium tuberculosis*.

Note: This is a presumptive rather than definitive diagnosis because several other occasionally pathogenic mycobacteria, such as *Mycobacterium avium-intracellulare* (MAC), can produce a similar clinical presentation and acid-fast stain result.

2. **How is the disease primarily transmitted?**

Aerosolization of contaminated respiratory secretions (e.g., coughing).

3. **Why is the acid-fast stain required to visualize this bacterium?**

M. tuberculosis does not stain well with Gram stain but does react to the acid-fast stain. For this reason it is called an acid-fast bacterium.

4. **Does the patient most likely have primary tuberculosis, latent tuberculosis, or recrudescent (secondary) tuberculosis?**

Because his previous PPD test was negative, he most likely has primary tuberculosis, which results from initial infection with the organism. More specifically, he probably has a "progressive" primary infection, in which symptoms manifest. This distinction is made because most patients who become infected with the mycobacteria do not develop symptoms. Latent tuberculosis develops after symptoms (if there were any) of primary tuberculosis have resolved and is due to tubercle bacilli residing in macrophages. Recrudescent tuberculosis develops after some form of immunologic compromise that allows the latent tubercle bacilli to begin proliferating again.

Note: About 10% of patients infected with tuberculosis in the United States eventually have a recrudescence. Miliary tuberculosis occurs when the bacilli are transmitted and cause foci of infection throughout the body.

5. **What are the first-line drugs for treating tuberculosis? Why are they always used in combination?**

First-line drugs include isoniazid (also used for prophylaxis), rifampin, ethambutol, streptomycin, and pyrazinamide. They are used in combination because of the high incidence of resistance. In the U.S., in fact, about 10–15 % of isolates have resistance to one of these drugs even before treatment is started.

6. **If the patient is treated with isoniazid as part of his regimen, why should he also receive supplemental pyridoxine?** Vit B6

One of the main side effects of isoniazid is a peripheral neuropathy, which results when the drug stimulates excretion of pyridoxine and creates a relative pyridoxine deficiency. One of the features of pyridoxine deficiency is peripheral neuropathy.

Note: The most common side effect, for which isoniazid is famous, is liver damage. It can even cause a full-blown hepatitis with nausea, vomiting, jaundice, and right upper quadrant pain.

P450 induter
PCR B GQ

7. If the patient is treated with rifampin as part of his regimen, why may he need larger doses of opioid analgesics for pain control in other illnesses and injuries?
Rifampin induces hepatic p450 enzymes, including those that metabolize opioids.

8. Three weeks after starting a therapeutic regimen with rifampin and isoniazid the patient complains of orange urine. What is the probable cause?
Orange urine is a well-known and common side effect of rifampin. Rifampin also often turns sweat, tears, and contact lenses an orange color.

9. Why is the standard treatment regimen so prolonged?
Several characteristics of the tubercle bacilli make it difficult to control quickly. One problem is its intracellular location, where drugs do not penetrate well. In addition, the bacillus is often found in large cavities with avascular centers, which drugs also have difficulty in penetrating. Finally, the tubercle bacillus has a very slow generation time.

10. Is cell-mediated immunity or humoral immunity more important for fighting tuberculosis? Why?
Because the tubercle bacillus resides intracellularly in macrophages, cell-mediated immunity, which targets intracellular pathogens, is more important.

11. How does the PPD skin test (Manteoux test) work?
PPD (purified protein derivative) is made from the bacterial cell wall of *M. tuberculosis*. When injected into the immune system of a person who has been exposed to the tubercle bacilli, PPD elicits a type IV hypersensitivity response, which manifests as an indurated area at the site of injection within about 48 hours.

12. Why is reactivation tuberculosis more likely to occur in the apical lungs rather than the lower lobes?
Because mycobacteria are obligate aerobes, the higher oxygen tension in the apex of the lung facilitates their growth. However, primary infections are more likely to occur in the lower segments where the bacteria are initially deposited.

13. What type of necrosis is associated with granulomatous cell death in tuberculosis?
Caseous necrosis, which has a cheesy white appearance.
Note: Other types of necrosis include liquefactive (e.g., stoke), coagulative (e.g., myocardial infarction), fatty (e.g., pancreatitis), and gangrenous necrosis (e.g., bacterial infection).

14. How can TB cause the urinalysis to show microscopic pyuria and hematuria (with red blood cell casts) in the face of a sterile culture?
Hematogenous spread of tuberculosis to the kidneys, causing pyelonephritis. Tuberculosis is notoriously difficult to culture and is not cultured routinely, unless specifically requested.

15. How can TB cause the patient to become acutely ill, with marked hypotension, hyponatremia, hyperkalemia, and an abdominal CT scan that shows bilateral adrenal involvement?
Tubercular invasion of the adrenal glands, causing hemorrhagic destruction of the adrenal glands and mineralocorticoid deficiency. This condition is known as the Waterhouse-Friderichsen syndrome.
also c̄ Neisseria

16. Why may Pott's disease be suspected in a patient with TB who has a new onset of back pain but denies any trauma that might explain the pain?
Hematogenous spread of tuberculosis to the spine, causing vertebral osteomyelitis, is sometimes called Pott's diseases.

17. VIRAL, FUNGAL, AND PARASITIC DISEASES

Bahair Ghazi, Dave Brown, and Thomas Brown

BASIC CONCEPTS

Virology

1. What structural components are used to categorize viruses?
Viruses can be classified according to the following structural components:
- Nucleic acid (RNA vs. DNA, single-stranded vs. double-stranded, single or segmented pieces)
- Capsid symmetry (icosahedral vs. helical)
- Size
- Presence or absence of an envelope

2. Since there are a great number of RNA viruses, which two components are most helpful in creating subdivisions?
The two major distinguishing features of any RNA virus are its capsid symmetry (icosahedral or helical) and its nucleic acid polarity. The nucleic acid polarity is either positive (+) or negative (−). Viruses with + sense have RNA strands that can function directly as messenger RNA (mRNA).

3. How are the DNA virus families classified?
DNA viruses are classified according to the presence or absence of an envelope and the structure of the DNA (linear vs. circular). Only the Parvovirus family is single-stranded; all other viruses have double-stranded DNA.

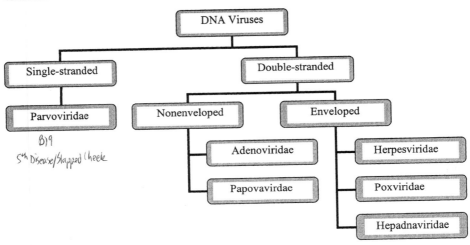

Classification of DNA virus families.

273

4. Name the DNA virus families and their medically important members.

FAMILY	MEMBERS	DISEASE
Parvoviridae (single-stranded)	Parvovirus B19	Fifth's disease and aplastic crisis in sickle cell anemia
Herpesviridae (enveloped)	Herpes simplex virus (HSV) 1 and HSV 2	Oral and genital lesions
	Varicella zoster virus (VZV)	Chicken pox (varicella) and herpes zoster (shingles)
	Epstein-Barr Virus (EBV)	Infectious mononucleosis
	Cytomegalovirus (CMV)	CMV retinitis, congenital infections, mono
	Human herpes virus (HHV) 6 and HHV 7	Roseola infantum (exanthema subitum)
	HHV 8	Kaposi's sarcoma
Poxviridae (enveloped)	Variola	Smallpox
	Molluscum contagiosum virus	Small, wart-like tumors
Hepadnaviridae (enveloped)	Hepatitis B	Hepatitis
Adenoviridae (nonenveloped)	Adenovirus	Conjunctivitis, pneumonia, pharyngitis
Papovaviridae (nonenveloped)	Human papillomavirus (HPV)	Serotypes 16 and 18 cause cervical dysplasia
	JCV	Multifocal leukoencephalopathy in immuno-suppressed patients

Note: If you can remember that these few viruses account for all of the medically relevant DNA viruses, then by deduction any other virus must be an RNA virus!

5. Using the clinical descriptions below, name the most likely virus.

DESCRIPTION	MOST LIKELY VIRUS
Rash with "slapped-cheek" appearance	Parvovirus B19
Descending maculopapular rash, Koplik's spots	Measles (rubeola)
Typically causes gastroenteritis but may cause paralysis via destruction of anterior horn cells	Poliovirus (fecal oral)
Cervical cancer in sexually active smoker	HPV (serotypes 16,18)
Parotitis, orchitis, and possible sterility in males	Mumps virus
Cataracts leading to blindness in newborns	Rubella virus
Painful vesicular lesions in dermatomal pattern; virus remains dormant in dorsal root ganglion	Varicella virus
Acute retinitis in patient with AIDS	CMV retinitis
Genital warts	HPV (serotypes 6,11)
Painful genital vesicular lesions	HSV-2 (occasionally HSV-1)
Hepatitis in pregnant women with high mortality rate	Hepatitis E
Teenager with fatigue, splenomegaly, and atypical lymphocytosis; positive heterophile antibody test	Epstein-Barr virus (EBV)
Gastroenteritis on cruise ship	Norwalk virus

(Cont'd.)

DESCRIPTION	MOST LIKELY VIRUS
Common cause of gastroenteritis in children	Rotavirus
Common cold viruses	Coronaviruses, rhinoviruses
Most common cause of bronchiolitis in children	Respiratory syncytial virus (RSV)
Undergoes segmental rearrangement of genome; can cause pneumonia or predispose to pneumonia	Influenza
Severe encephalitis following an animal bite	Rabies virus
Neonatal encephalitis	HSV or CMV

Mycology

6. What are the two morphologies of pathogenic fungi?
   Filamentous (molds) and unicellular (yeast). An example of a filamentous mold is *Aspergillus* species, which cause pneumonia with "fungus balls." *Cryptococcus neoformans* is a unicellular (yeast) fungus that is also encapsulated; it is known for causing cryptococcal meningitis.

7. What is meant by the term *dimorphic fungi*? Name two pathogens that are dimorphic.
   Dimorphic fungi can exist in either the filamentous (mold) or the unicellular (yeast) form, depending on environmental signals. *Histoplasma capsulatum* and *Candida albicans* are dimorphic fungi that can cause pathogenic infections. *H. capsulatum* causes systemic mycoses common in the Ohio and Mississippi River Valleys; *Candida* species cause various infections, the more serious occurring in immunocompromised patients.

8. What arm of the adaptive immune system is generally involved in eradicating fungi?
   Most fungi are intracellular; therefore, cell-mediated immunity, which targets intracellular organisms, is primarily responsible.
   Note: Many of the systemic fungal infections typically only occur in patients with severely compromised immune systems, especially with defects in cell-mediated immunity.

9. How do the antifungal "azole" agents work?
   All azole agents inhibit the synthesis of ergosterol, a key component of fungal cell membranes. Examples include ketoconazole, itraconazole, and miconazole.
   Note: Ketoconazole inhibits hepatic enzymes as well as adrenal and gonadal steroid synthesis. This latter effect may explain the frequent reversible gynecomastia that develops in men who take this drug.

10. How do amphotericin and nystatin work?
   Both agents bind to ergosterol in the fungal membrane, creating pores that allow entry or escape of tightly regulated substances.
   Note: Amphotericin is highly nephrotoxic.

11. Name the most likely fungal organism.

DESCRIPTION	MOST LIKELY FUNGAL ORGANISM
Diffuse interstitial markings on chest x-ray in HIV-positive patient who presents with shortness of breath. Positive silver stain.	*Pneumocystis carinii*
Thrush in cancer patient receiving high dose chemotherapy	*Candida albicans*
HIV patient with signs and symptoms of meningitis, with positive Indian ink stain on lumbar puncture	*Cryptococcus neoformans*

(Cont'd.)

DESCRIPTION	MOST LIKELY FUNGAL ORGANISM
Lung granulomas in individual in Ohio River Valley	*Histoplasma capsulatum*
Tinea cruris, corporis, pedis	*Trychophyton, Epidermophyton, Microsporum* species (not all organisms cause all three diseases)
Lung granulomas in San Joaquin Valley	*Coccidiomycosis* species
Fungus ball in cavitary lung lesion	*Aspergillus* species
Systemic mycoses involving lungs, bone, and skin	*Blastomyces* species
Lymphangitis after getting stuck with a thorn	*Sporothrix schenkii*
Severe rhinocerebral infection in diabetic ketoacidosis	Mucormycosis (due to one of several different fungi)

Parasitology

12. What are protozoa? List the medically important ones and their associated diseases.

Protozoa are single-celled eukaryotic organisms.

PROTOZOAN	ASSOCIATED DISEASE
Entamoeba histolytica	Amebic dysentery (may cause liver abscess)
Giardia lamblia	Giardiasis (diarrhea after drinking contaminated water)
Cryptosporidium species	Diarrhea in immunocompromised person
Trichomonas vaginalis	Trichomoniasis
Plasmodium falciparum, P. vivax, P. ovale, P. malariae	Malaria
Toxoplasma gondii	Toxoplasmosis
Leishmania species	Leismaniasis
Trypanosoma brucei	African sleeping sickness (African trypanosomiasis)
Trypanosoma cruzi	Chagas disease (American trypanosomiasis)

13. What is the main difference between primaquine and the other antimalarial agents?

Primaquine is the only agent that can eradicate the dormant hepatic forms that both *Plasmodium vivax* and *P. ovale* are capable of maintaining. The major drawback to primaquine is that in patients with G6PD deficiency it can cause hemolytic anemia.

14. From the description specify the most likely protozoal organism.

DESCRIPTION	MOST LIKELY PROTOZOAL ORGANISM
Abdominal ultrasound reveals liver cysts or abscesses in patient with dysentery anchovy paste	*Entamoeba histolytica*
Watery, foul-smelling diarrhea after recent camping trip	*Giardia lamblia*
Recurrent fever, chills, and sweats in patient returning from Africa; peripheral blood smear shows abnormal RBCs of all ages infected with "merozoites"	*Plasmodium falciparum*

15. What is the difference among cestodes, nematodes, and trematodes?

All three are helminths (worms). Cestodes are flatworms (tapeworms), whereas nematodes are roundworms. Trematodes are flukes, which are simply small helminths.

16. From the description specify the helminth and treatment of infection.

DESCRIPTION	MOST LIKELY HELMINTHIC ORGANISM	TREATMENT
Trematode infections		
Hematuria after swimming in the Nile	*Schistosoma hematobium*	Praziquantel
Gastrointestinal involvement from inflammatory reaction to eggs; snail as intermediate host.	*Schistosoma mansoni* *Schistosoma japonicum*	Praziquantel
Biliary stricture in patient in southeast Asia	*Clonorchis sinensis*	Praziquantel
Transmitted by eating raw crab meat, resulting in GI and pulmonary involvement	*Paragonimus westermani*	Praziquantel
Cestode infections		
Infection from eating pork, causing cysts to encrust in brain (seizures, headache, vomiting)	*Taenia solium* (cysticercosis)	Surgery! (and various antiparasitic drugs)
Transmitted by undercooked beef (mostly asymptomatic)	*Taenia saginatum*	Niclosamide
Extremely long intestinal tapeworm that causes vitamin B12 deficiency and anemia	*Diphyllobothrium latum*	Niclosamide
Ingestion of eggs in dog feces, causing cysts in liver, lungs, and brain; rupture of cysts causes allergic reaction.	*Echinococcus granulosis*	Niclosamide
Nematode infections		
Anal itching with white worms visible in perianal region	*Enterobius vermicularis* (pinworm)	Mebendazole
Intestinal infection, but worms pass from intestine to lungs	*Ascaris lumbricoides*	Mebendazole
Transmitted by direct skin penetration; attaches to intestinal mucosa, causing chronic blood loss and anemia	*Necator americanus*	Mebendazole

CASE 1

A 45-year-old woman presents with complaints of a "flu-like" illness. The patient is currently employed as a nurse and has recently had to take several days off for sick leave. She states that approximately 1 month ago she started feeling fatigued and feverish. Soon after she developed a vague right upper quadrant abdominal pain that she describes as "achy." Her symptoms have not improved in the past month and in fact have worsened. Last week she noticed that her urine was darker than usual. She is quite concerned about being infected with HIV due to a needle stick exposure a few months earlier. On exam you appreciate a jaundiced, ill-appearing woman with right upper quadrant tenderness to palpation. You order liver enzymes and serology assays for viral hepatitis. The liver enzymes aspartate aminotransferase (AST) and alanine aminotransferase (ALT)are markedly elevated, and the hepatitis serology assays are positive for HbcAB IgM and HBsAg.

1. What is the most likely diagnosis?

Acute hepatitis B infection. Hepatitis B can be acute or chronic (infection persists beyond 6 month). Acute hepatitis B often presents weeks to months after infection with constitutional symptoms, right upper quadrant abdominal pain, and jaundice. Because hepatitis B is transmitted parenterally, she may have been infected by the needle stick.

2. Why are AST and ALT values elevated?

Hepatitis is an inflammatory disease of the liver. The viral particles infect hepatocytes, and in an effort to clear the infection the host immune system destroys infected cells, resulting in hepatocyte necrosis and massive leakage of hepatic enzymes. The AST and ALT are markers of hepatocyte death, *not* liver function.

3. For what three different antigens do hepatitis B profiles test?

All antigens (or antibodies to these antigens) for which the hepatitis B profiles test are structural components of the virus: surface antigen (HbsAg), core antigen (HbcAg), and "e" antigen (HbeAg).

Note: The surface antigen is the first to appear and the last to disappear in most infections with HBV. The "e" antigen is involved in viral replication and is a marker of viral infectivity.

ABBREVIATION	MEANING	SIGNIFICANCE
HBsAg	Hepatitis B surface antigen	Indicates active infection
HBsAb	Hepatis B surface antibody	Indicates successful eradication of infection or immunized status
HBcAb IgM	Hepatitis B core antibody IgM	First antibody produced in acute hepatitis B infection; may still be present shortly after resolution but disappears after several months
Total HbcAb	Total antibody to hepatitis B core antigen	Positive after resolved infection, but HBcIgM becomes negative
HBeAg	Hepatitis B "e" antigen	Indicates high level of viral infectivity

4. Which antibody shows up first in acute HBV infection?

HBcAb IgM. The presence of this antibody and HbsAg indicates acute infection. The presence of this antibody and absence of HbsAg indicates a recent, resolved acute infection.

5. What is the "core window" in hepatitis B infections?

The core window is the time frame in which hepatitis surface antigen (HbsAg) has disappeared, but the antibody to this antigen (HBsAb) has not yet appeared.

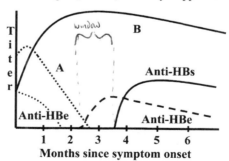

Temporal course of humoral response to hepatitis B infection. A = HbsAg, B = anti-HBcAb. (From Brochert A: Platinum Vignettes: Microbiology. Philadelphia, Hanley & Belfus, 2003, p 51, with permission.)

6. Can HBsAb (IgG) indicate active infection?

No. The presence of HBsAb indicates resolution of infection and immunity.

7. Which of the serologic tests is positive 6 months after hepatitis B vaccination?

Only the surface antigen is used to vaccinate; six months later it would not be present (nor would any other antigens). The only antibody present is HBsAb.

8. Based on serology, how can we differentiate people who have been vaccinated and people who have cleared an infection?

Only patients who have cleared an infection have antibody to the core antigen (HBcAb) in addition to surface antigen (HBsAb). People who have been vaccinated have built antibody to the surface antigen only and have not been exposed to the core antigen, since it is not part of the vaccine. They have only HBsAb.

9. What other viruses cause hepatitis? What is their usual course of infection?

Hepatitis A, C, D, and E are RNA viruses. Hepatitis B is the only DNA virus that commonly causes hepatitis. Hepatitis A and E are acute infections transmitted by the fecal-oral route. Hepatitis B, C, and D usually cause chronic infections and are transmitted parenterally (sexual contact, intravenous drug use). The "chronic" viruses are so labeled because they persist beyond 6 months; it is important to realize that any of the hepatitis viruses can cause an acute infection with the classic presenting signs. Hepatitis D is a uniquely defective virus. It requires that the host be infected with hepatitis B before it can cause any disease.

10. How is viral hepatitis treated? How does treatment relate to the temporal course of the specific viral disease?

Hepatitis A is treated with passive immunization through the administration of pooled IgG and supportive care. A vaccine is available to certain people and those traveling to high-risk areas. Active hepatitis B is treated with alpha-interferon and lamivudine. The hepatitis B vaccine is now routinely administered to children and high-risk people such as yourself (healthcare workers). Hepatitis C is treated with combination therapy consisting of alpha-interferon and ribavirin. The best treatment for hepatitis D is in the prevention of hepatitis B infection. At this time hepatitis E is treated with supportive care.

VIRUS	MECHANISM OF INFECTION	TEMPORAL COURSE	TREATMENT
Hep. A	Fecal-oral	Acute	Pooled IV Ig, vaccine for travelers
Hep. E	Fecal-oral	Acute	Symptomatic relief
Hep. B	Parenteral (IV drug use, sex, mother-child)	Acute or chronic	Vaccine for high-risk people, alpha interferon and lamivudine
Hep. C	Parenteral (IV drug use, sex, mother-child)	Chronic	Alpha interferon and ribavirin
Hep. D	Parenteral (IV drug use, sex, mother-child)	Chronic	Prevention of hepatitis B infection through vaccination

CASE 2

A 45-year-old man complains of fever, stiff neck, and a mild but consistent headache. On questioning he indicates that he developed an upper respiratory tract infection 1 week ago. He also mentions that he has vomited several times and cannot tolerate bright lights. Physical exam reveals nuchal rigidity and positive Kernig and Brudzinski signs. A CT scan identifies no contraindications to lumbar puncture. Immediately after a spinal tap is performed, the patient is started on empirical antibiotics. Cerebrospinal fluid (CSF) analysis reveals lymphocytosis, with normal glucose and slightly elevated protein. A Gram stain of the CSF reveals many white blood cells (WBCs) with a predominance of lymphocytes but no organisms.

1. What is the diagnosis?

The most likely diagnosis based on clinical presentation and CSF analysis is acute aseptic meningitis.

2. What causes aseptic meningitis?

Aseptic meningitis is an inflammation of the meninges caused by nonbacterial pathogens. Over 80% of aseptic meningitis diagnoses are due to viral infections (commonly enteroviruses), but other causes may include mycobacteria, fungi, *Rickettsia* species, spirochetes, malignancies, and medications.

3. How do the CSF findings differ between viral, bacterial, and fungal meningitis?

	WBCS	GLUCOSE	PROTEIN
Viral (aseptic)	Predominantly lymphocytes	Normal	Normal to slightly elevated
Fungal	Predominantly lymphocytes	Low	Normal to elevated
Bacterial	Predominantly neutrophils	Low	High

4. Why is the distinction between aseptic meningitis and bacterial meningitis important?

Prognosis and treatment vary tremendously depending on whether the cause of the meningitis is viral or bacterial. Acute bacterial meningitis can be a life-threatening disease and often responds well to antibiotics. In contrast, aseptic meningitis is usually self-limited. After 48 hours of negative CSF cultures, the present patient will be taken off the antibiotics and monitored for any change in course.

Note: In contrast to viral meningitis, viral encephalitis (in which both the meninges and the brain itself become inflamed) can frequently result in a devastating outcome.

18. BIOSTATISTICS

Thomas Brown and Dave Brown

BASIC CONCEPTS

1. What does the sensitivity of a diagnostic test measure?

The sensitivity is a measure of how effective a diagnostic test can detect (sense) the disease in a patient with the disease (true positive). If you consider a population of people with a given disease, the more sensitive the test is, the higher the percentage of people with the disease will have a positive test.

Note: Sensitivity can be calculated by dividing the number of true positives by the total number of persons tested with the disease (e.g., a/(a+c) in the 2 × 2 table).

Presence of disease

		+	−
Test result	+	True positives (a)	False positives (b)
	−	False negatives (c)	True negatives (d)

2. What does the specificity of a diagnostic test measure?

The specificity of a test is a measure of how effectively a diagnostic test can detect health or the absence of disease in a patient without the disease (true negative). It is an indication of how specific a positive test result is for the disease that it is designed to detect. The greater the number of different diseases or conditions that can cause a positive test result, other than the disease that the test is designed to detect, the less specific the test is.

Note: Specificity can be calculated by dividing the number of true negatives by the total number of people tested who do not have the disease (true negatives plus false positives), or d/(b+d) in the 2 × 2 table.

3. Cover the right-hand column and define each of the terms in the left-hand column.

TERM	DEFINITION
True positive	A positive test result in someone who has the disease
False positive	A positive test result in someone who does not have the disease
True negative	A negative result in someone who does not have the disease
False negative	A negative result in someone who has the disease.

4. How does the sensitivity of a test relate to its specificity?

In general, the more sensitive the cutoff for a positive result becomes, the less specific it is. Conversely, the more specific the cutoff for a test becomes, the less specific it is (see figure, next page).

Note: For screening tests for serious diseases that can be treated effectively if detected, a greater sensitivity (often at the expense of specificity) is desired.

5. What is meant by the reliability of a test?

Reliability measure the degree of agreement in the result of a test when it is performed by different examiners. For example, when a finding on a chest x-ray is read by numerous different radiologists in the same way, the chest x-ray is a reliable test for that finding. However, if there is massive disagreement among radiologists about whether or not that finding is present, the chest x-ray is unreliable for that finding.

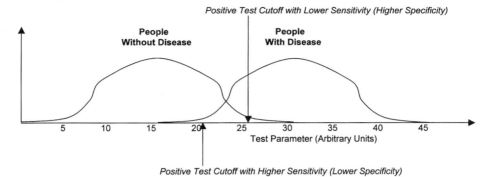

Relationship between sensitivity and specificity.

6. What is meant by the validity of a test?

Validity measures how well the test result corresponds to what it is claimed to measure. For example, in a patient with calcified arteries, the usual blood pressure cuff may give erroneous pressure readings because of the arterial stiffness, making that test of blood pressure invalid.

7. In statistical analyses of differences between groups, a p value is often given to reflect how significant the difference is. What is the meaning of the p value?

At its most basic level, the p value reflects the probability that the difference observed between groups could occur by chance alone. For example, if the p value is 0.05, there is a 5% probability that the observed difference could have been due entirely to random chance and not to whatever intervention was used in the experiment. Nevertheless, most scientists consider a difference "significant" if there was less than a 5% ($p < 0.05$) chance that the difference could have occurred by random chance. Obviously, the smaller the p value, the smaller the probability that any difference was due to chance and the more convincing it is that the intervention is responsible for the difference.

8. What determinants can be used to evaluate the existence of a causal relationship between two variables?

1. Consistency (e.g., the more studies that support the hypothesis, the better)
2. Strength of correlation (e.g., the higher the relative risk, the better)
3. Biologic plausibility (e.g., colon cancer is unlikely to be caused by ultraviolet exposure)
4. Temporality (cause must precede disease outcome)
5. Supportive experimental studies (e.g., animal studies)
6. Dose-response relationship (e.g., higher exposure leads to more frequent disease)

9. What is the difference between prevalence and incidence?

Prevalence is the percentage or number of the population that has the disease. For example, 25% of Americans are obese; thus the prevalence of obesity is 25%. Incidence refers to how many or what percentage of people develop a disease within a given time frame (usually annually). Thus, if 300,000 people are newly diagnosed with diabetes each year, the annual incidence of diabetes is 300,000.

10. How do the incidence and duration of a disease affect its prevalence?

The higher the incidence and the longer the duration of the disease, the greater the prevalence. This is because many chronic diseases (e.g., arthritis) are unlikely to result in rapid death. Indeed, most patients may die with chronic diseases rather than from them. Diseases that have a short duration (e.g., meningitis), either because they result in rapid death or because they resolve quickly, have a low prevalence in the population.

11. What does the standard deviation of a population represent?
The standard deviation has both a mathematical and a conceptual meaning. Mathematically, if one takes all the members of a population within one standard deviation of the mean (both above and below), these members will constitute 68% of the total population. If two standard deviations from the mean are taken, these members will constitute 95% of the total population. Conceptually, the standard deviation is a measure of how "spread out" the population is. The larger the standard deviation, the further along the scale one has to go in both directions to include 64% or 95% of the population.

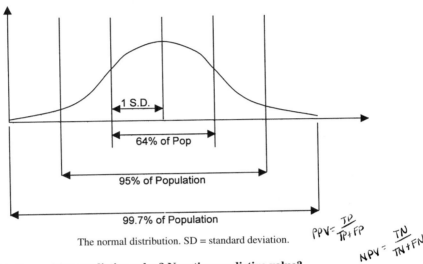

The normal distribution. SD = standard deviation.

$$PPV = \frac{TP}{TP + FP}$$

$$NPV = \frac{TN}{TN + FN}$$

12. What is the positive predictive value? Negative predictive value?
The positive predictive value is the probability that, given a positive test result, the disease in question is actually present. The negative predictive value is the probability that, given a negative result, the disease in question is absent.

13. What is the positive likelihood ratio?
The positive likelihood ratio reflects the degree to which a positive test result increases the probability that the disease in question is present. The higher the ratio, the more likely it is that disease is present. This ratio is calculated as the sensitivity divided by 1– specificity. For example, if the sensitivity is 85% and the specificity is 90%, the positive likelihood ratio is $0.85/(1-0.9) = 8.5$. Consequently, the more sensitive and specific the test is, the higher the positive likelihood ratio. The positive likelihood ratio is now widely used in evidence-based medicine because of the ease with which it can be used to calculate the positive predictive value of a test.

14. How is the positive likelihood ratio used to calculate the positive predictive value?
1. Convert the prevalence of a disease to a ratio (e.g., 20% to 1:4).
2. Multiply the first part of the ratio (1) by the positive likelihood ratio (8.5):

$$8.5 \times 1:4 = 8.5:4$$

3. Convert the ratio back to a percentage: $8.5/(8.5 + 4) = 0.68$ or 68%.

15. The following list is a sample distribution pattern representing the ages of 11 patients seen by a physician on a given day: 1, 2, 3, 3, 3, 4, 5, 5, 7, 8, 80. What are the mean, median, and mode for the ages of these patients?
The mean is simply the average of the sample. In this example, the mean would be 11 ($121/11 = 11$). The **median** is the number above and below which lies half the subjects. In this

example, the number 4 has equal numbers of subjects on either side. The mode is the number with the highest frequency, in this case the number 3.

16. Is the mean or the median more representative of central tendency in this sample?
The median is less affected by outliers (e.g., 80) than the mean and is therefore a better representation of central tendency than the mean, particularly for small sample sizes containing multiple outliers. However, keep in mind that because the mean encompasses all individuals in a study, it has much more statistical power than either the median or mode.

17. Is this sample "skewed" at all? If so, in which direction?
This sample population is positively skewed to the right because of the outlier value 80.

CASE 1

Blood pressure is monitored regularly in a group of 500 adult men. The mean blood pressure for the group is reported as 130 ± 10 mmHg, and the coefficient of variation is noted to be small. The blood pressure measurements within the group are described as having a normal distribution.

1. What does "130 ± 10 mmHg" mean with respect to the distribution of blood pressure in this sample?
The "130 mmHg" refers to the mean blood pressure of the sample, whereas the "10 mmHg" refers to the standard deviation. A standard deviation of 10 mmHg implies that 68% of the population had blood pressure between 120 mmHg and 140 mmHg. For 95% of the population of this study, the blood pressure is within two standard deviations of the mean, or within 110 mmHg and 150 mmHg.

2. What does it mean when the blood pressure in this population is said to be "normally distributed"?
If the magnitude of the analyzed variable (in this case, blood pressure) is plotted against the frequency of each magnitude, the curve takes on a "bell-shaped" form that is well described by a specific mathematical equation. This equation can be used to calculate the standard deviation accurately.

3. What does a small coefficient of variation for the sample in the above study imply?
The coefficient of variation (CV) is used to express the standard deviation as a percentage of the sample mean. The CV can be highly informative. Standard deviation typically decreases with increasing sample size, such that a good study may have a small coefficient of variation. For example, the above study expresses blood pressure as x = 130 ± 10 mmHg. In this study, the CV = $10/130 \times 100 = 7.6$ %.
Note: Smaller sample sizes are associated with larger coefficients of variation. For example, if blood pressures were measured in 10 men as opposed to 500, one may get a value such as 130 ± 60 mm Hg. In this case, CV equals $(60/130 \times 100)$ 46%.

4. What percentage of the men in this study had a blood pressure (a) between 120 and 140 mmHg? (b) between 110 and 150 mmHg? (c) above 150 mmHg? (d) below 110 mmHg?
(a) 64%; (b) 95%; (c) 2.5%; (d) 2.5%.

CASE 2

A 27-year-old man complains of fatigue and general malaise for the past several months. Although his past medical history is unremarkable, his history is significant for the use of intravenous drugs and unprotected sex with prostitutes. With the patient's consent, you

decide to screen him for HIV infection, using a test with a reported sensitivity of 95% and specificity of 75%.

1. Why does it make sense to use a screening test with a high sensitivity, even at the cost of specificity, for this patient?

Screening tests in general—and particularly for life-threatening diseases such as HIV infection—should have a high sensitivity so that they can "pick up" the disease if it is present. Because screening tests in general must be inexpensive, this high sensitivity may come at the cost of suboptimal specificity. However, because it is much more important not to miss disease (i.e., few false-negative results) than it is to inconvenience (or even traumatize) someone with a false-positive result, this discrepancy is considered acceptable.

2. If the patient tests positive, is it reasonable to tell him that you are 95% confident that he truly has the disease?

Not at all. Sensitivity and specificity values simply represent how good a test is and perhaps whether the test is ideal for screening large populations for a given disease. No conclusions whatsoever can be applied to a given patient based on the result of a test. In other words, if the man tests positive for HIV infection, we have no way of determining whether this is a true positive or a false positive unless we can calculate the positive predictive value for this test. Positive predictive value depends on additional information, as discussed in the next case.

3. What if the test is negative? Can you tell the patient that you are 75% confident that he does not have HIV?

Again, such a statement cannot be made unless you know the negative predictive value of the test, which was not provided.

4. Both a 90-year-old grandmother and the young man in this vignette both are positive for HIV using this test. Are they equally likely to have the disease?

No—and this question addresses the important concept of using screening tests appropriately. The goal of clinicians is selective testing only of people at higher risk for developing a given disease. The positive predictive value of a test depends on the prevalence of the disease in the tested population as well as on the specificity and sensitivity of the test.

Note: As an analogy, consider the havoc that would be created if physicians screened all females under the age of 20 for breast cancer by performing annual mammograms. Such testing would yield numerous false positives, necessitating unnecessary referrals and expensive work-ups by specialists, not to mention the unneeded anxiety caused to patients. Using this same test to screen only woman over 40 makes a bit more sense, because the number of true positives will increase and the number of false positives will decrease due to the increased prevalence of breast cancer with aging.

CASE 3

In a town of 1000 people, the prevalence of coronary heart disease (CHD) across all age groups is 20% (as shown by angiography, the gold standard). You have created a wonderfully inexpensive screening test that you believe is both highly sensitive and specific for detecting CHD.

		Coronary heart disease	
		+	−
New test	+	180 (a)	80 (b)
	−	20 (c)	720 (d)

1. Given the 2 × 2 table above, what is the sensitivity of this new test?

Sensitivity can be calculated by dividing the number of true positives by the total number of persons tested with the disease, or a/(a+c) in the 2 × 2 table. There were 180 true positives of the

200 patients tested who had disease, yielding a sensitivity of 180/200 or 90%. This means that this test detects (senses) the disease in 90% of people who have the disease.

2. What is the specificity of this new test?

Specificity can be calculated by dividing the number of true negatives by the total number of people tested who do not have the disease (true negatives plus false positives), or d/(b+d) in the 2×2 table. Since there were 720 true negatives and 80 false positives, the specificity of this test is 720/800 or 90%.

3. What should you tell the patient if his test comes back positive and he asks, "Hey, Doc, does this mean I have coronary heat disease?"

An accurate answer requires calculation of the positive predictive value (PPV), which is the probability that a person with a positive test result actually has the disease. PPV is calculated as the number of true positives divided by the total number of positives (true and false). This calculation requires knowledge of sensitivity and specificity of the test as well as the prevalence of the disease to generate the number of true positives (tp) and false positives (fp).

For the above example, given the fact that the disease prevalence is 20% and the sensitivity and specificity of the screening test are both 90%, the PPV of a positive test result equals 69% (see calculation below). You should tell the patient that he is only 69% likely to have CHD based on his positive test result.

$$
\begin{aligned}
\text{PPV} &= \text{tp}/(\text{tp} + \text{fp}) \\
&= 180/180 + 80 \\
&= 69\% \\
\text{True positives} &= (\text{test sensitivity}) \times (\text{people with disease}) \\
&= 0.90 \times 200 \\
&= 180 \\
\text{False positives} &= (1 - \text{test specificity}) \times (\text{people without disease}) \\
&= 0.10 \times 800 \\
&= 80
\end{aligned}
$$

4. How is the negative predictive value calculated?

The negative predictive value (NPV) is the probability that the disease is absent if the test is negative. It is calculated as true negatives divided by both true negatives and false negatives: tn/(tn + fn).

5. Using the same example, calculate the NPV.

$$
\begin{aligned}
\text{NPV} &= \text{tn}/(\text{tn} + \text{fn}) \\
&= 720/(720 + 20) \\
&= 0.97 \text{ or } 97\% \\
\text{True negatives} &= (\text{test specificity}) \times (\text{people without disease}) \\
&= 0.90 \times 800 \\
&= 720 \\
\text{False negatives} &= (1 - \text{test sensitivity}) \times (\text{people with disease}) \\
&= 0.10 \times 200 \\
&= 20
\end{aligned}
$$

Therefore, 97% of the people in this sample who had a negative test result would not have the disease.

CASE 4

In 1979 a study was initiated on employees at a nuclear power plant to determine whether an association exists between radiation exposure and cancer rates. Five hundred employees with high-level radiation exposure and 500 employees with very limited exposure were

followed for 20 years, and the incidence of cancer was compared in the two groups throughout this time. The results are depicted in the 2 x 2 table shown below.

Cancer

		+	−
Exposure	+	50	450
	−	5	495

1. What type of study design is this?

This is a (prospective) cohort study because participants are classified on the basis of exposure, not disease (as with a case-control study). Furthermore, it was an ongoing study in which the complications associated with radiation exposure were analyzed as they occurred.

2. What is the difference between a prospective cohort study and a retrospective cohort study?

In a prospective cohort study participants with a given exposure are followed over time to see whether there is an increased or decreased frequency of disease development. In a retrospective cohort study, a group of people who were exposed some time in the past are evaluated to see whether they have a higher frequency of the disease. In both cases, the study population is *grouped according to exposure.*

3. What is the major limitation of cohort studies?

Although the groups may be distinct from each other according to the factor under study, many other factors may be different between the groups and have the potential to influence outcome. For example, a cohort study found that people who eat more beta-carotene had a lower incidence of lung cancer. However, this finding did not take into account that people who ate more beta-carotene may eat substantially more fruits and vegetables in general, which itself may be protective from cancer. In fact, when a randomized trial was done, beta-carotene supplementation actually *increased* the risk of lung cancer.

Note: When other variables that are not under study (or are not controlled for) influence the outcome of a study, they are called *confounding* variables.

4. Given the 2 × 2 table above, what is the relative risk for cancer in the exposed group?

In a 2 × 2 table, relative risk (RR) is determined by comparing incidence rates in exposed individuals (I_E) to incidence rates in nonexposed individuals (IN_E), as shown below. Thus, the relative risk for the employees exposed to radiation is 10 times greater than the risk for the nonexposed employees.

$$RR = \frac{I_E}{IN_E} = \frac{a/a+b}{c/c+d} = \frac{50/500}{5/500} = 10$$

5. What is meant by attributable risk and attributable risk percent? Calculate both for the above example.

Attributable risk (AR), also called the absolute risk, is the incidence of disease in the exposed group caused solely by exposure. It can be calculated by the difference in incidence rates between exposed and nonexposed groups, as shown below for the above example.

$$AR = I_E - IN_E$$
$$= 50/500 - 5/500$$
$$= 45/500$$
$$= 0.09$$

This attributable risk of 0.09 implies that 9% of people exposed to radiation developed cancer as a result of that exposure (i.e., which could be attributed to that exposure).

The attributable risk percent (AR%) is a measure of the percentage of people who were exposed and developed the disease, and the development of disease was due to the exposure. It can be calculated by dividing the attributable risk by the incidence of disease in the exposed group:

$$AR\% = AR/I_E \times 100$$
$$= 0.09/0.10 \times 100$$
$$= 90\%$$

The AR% of 90% implies that 90% of people who were exposed to radiation and developed cancer developed their cancer as a result of the radiation.

6. What experimental design overcomes the shortcomings of the cohort study?

The best experimental design, which is the one least susceptible to confounding and bias, is the randomized, blinded, controlled trial. In this trial design participants are randomly allocated to treatment or control groups, thereby reducing considerably any confounding factors.

Note: A double-blind, placebo-controlled trial is one in which neither the investigator nor the study subjects know who is receiving the treatment.

CASE 5

Information pertaining to social habits (e.g., tobacco exposure) was gathered from two groups of people in an attempt to discern any association between tobacco exposure and lung cancer. Group A consisted of 1000 people with lung cancer. Group B consisted of 1000 similarly aged people without lung cancer. Participants were queried about their cumulative exposure to cigarette smoke, either firsthand or secondhand. Group A included 900 smokers, whereas group B included only 200 smokers.

1. What type of study design is this?

This is a case-control study because the study was composed of two groups, those already having the disease ("cases") and those free of disease ("controls"). The difference in the historical frequency of a "potential risk factor" is compared between the groups. Case-control studies are retrospective studies, because one goes back in time in comparing exposure between the two groups. If exposure levels vary between the two groups, an association between exposure and disease may be present. However, it is important to realize that a valid statistical association between two variables (e.g., exposure and disease) does not prove a causal relationship.

2. What information is provided by an odds ratio?

An odds ratio measures the relative frequency of exposure to the variable under study in the group (e.g., smoking) with the disease (e.g., lung cancer) in comparison with the control group in a case-control study.

3. What is the odds ratio for smoking in this sample?

Because 900/1000 or 0.9 of group A were smokers and 200/1000 or 0.2 were smokers in group B, the odds ratio for smoking in patients with lung cancer (group A) is 0.9/0.2 = 4.5. That is, people with lung cancer in this study were 4.5 times more likely to smoke than people without lung cancer.

4. What is meant by the term *bias*? Which study design best eliminates bias?

Bias is *systematic* error that affects one study group more than the other. It differs from *random* error, which typically affects both groups equally and should not adversely affect the study. Randomized clinical trials control most effectively for bias whereas a case-control study controls least effectively for bias. Other types of study designs (e.g., cohort, cross-sectional) vary somewhere between these two extremes in their ability to eliminate bias.

5. What are the major limitations of a case-control study design? Which types of bias are likely to be found?

As explained, case-control studies simply uncover an association between two variables but do not establish a causal relationship. In addition, data retrieval in these studies can be compromised by so-called interviewer bias and recall bias.

Interviewer bias refers to the tendency of interviewers to assume that a person with disease has been exposed to risk factors, whereas the healthy person has not. For example, the interviewer might ask a person with lung cancer the question, "How many packs per day did you smoke?," whereas a healthy person might be asked the question, "You never smoked, did you?"

Recall bias refers to the tendency of a person with disease to exaggerate their exposures and the tendency of a healthy person to minimize their exposures. For example, a woman with a child who has been born with a birth defect might recall many more chest x-rays during her pregnancy than a woman with healthy children.

6. How does a retrospective case-control study differ in design from a retrospective cohort study?

These studies differ largely with respect to how subjects are classified and selected. In a case-control study, subjects are classified based on the presence or absence of disease. By contrast, in a retrospective cohort study, subjects are classified based on the presence or absence of exposure. Only then is disease status determined.

INDEX

Page numbers in **boldface type** indicate complete chapters.